Photosynthetic Protein-Based Photovoltaics

T0199232

Photosynthetic Protein-Based Photovoltaics

Edited by
Swee Ching Tan

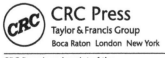

CRC Press
Taylor & Francis Group
Boca Raton London New York

CRC Press is an imprint of the
Taylor & Francis Group, an **informa** business

CRC Press
Taylor & Francis Group
6000 Broken Sound Parkway NW, Suite 300
Boca Raton, FL 33487-2742

First issued in paperback 2022

© 2019 by Taylor & Francis Group, LLC
CRC Press is an imprint of Taylor & Francis Group, an Informa business

No claim to original U.S. Government works

ISBN 13: 978-1-03-240178-2 (pbk)
ISBN 13: 978-1-4987-2489-0 (hbk)

DOI: 10.1201/9781315120249

Publisher's Note
The publisher has gone to great lengths to ensure the quality of this reprint but points out that some imperfections in the original copies may be apparent.

Visit the Taylor & Francis Web site at
http://www.taylorandfrancis.com

and the CRC Press Web site at
http://www.crcpress.com

Dedication

This book is specially dedicated to my lovely wife, Hazel, who has always been my pillar to give me unwavering support. To my two cute daughters, Valerie and Estella, your smiles are the most powerful magic potion to brighten up my day and to freshen up my mind to conquer this book-writing journey.

To my parents and parents-in-law, no words are strong enough to express how thankful Hazel and I are that you help take care of our children.

To my sister, thanks for doing free babysitting at times.

Contents

Preface

Nature is regarded as an implicit school of engineering because its biological systems have emerged as a result of rigorous evolutionary experimentations with incredible design solutions. The heart of it is photosynthesis, a solar-powered process that sustains life on Earth. With rising concerns about the need for cost-effective and sustainable photovoltaic technologies, photosynthesis stands as an ideal model to mimic and adopt in the emerging and future solar technologies. The prime objective of this book is to help to lay a bridge between the insights gained from the natural photosynthetic processes/machineries and physics/engineering of photovoltaic devices, so that researchers and engineers from diverse disciplines such as biochemistry, solid-state physics, electrochemistry, and photovoltaics shall draw inspiration and contribute to the growing interdisciplinary research on sustainable energy harvesting.

The book is designed in such a way that it can provide students and professionals of science and engineering disciplines with a comprehensive and accurate account of the basic principles and the recent progress in the field of biophotovoltaics. It essentially focuses only on the "non-living" biohybrid systems integrated with proteins and pigments isolated from plants and bacteria rather than on systems involving live cells. The book offers an eclectic mix of concepts and approaches from various disciplines of science and engineering, with sufficient illustrations and a light narrative tone for ease of understanding.

With a motivational account on how photosynthesis can impact future energy technologies, Chapter 1 briefs some of the limitations in the conventional solar cells and highlights the need to learn from nature to improve the emerging solar energy conversion devices. Integrating proteins from plants or bacteria in a device setup requires a basic understanding of some of the existing photovoltaics devices, their structures, and functions. Hence a review of the basic device architectures, components, and working mechanisms of two main fields of photovoltaics, namely dye-sensitized solar cells (DSSC) and organic bulk heterojunction (BHJ) solar cells, is outlined in the subsequent chapters (Chapters 2 and 3). The working of these devices, in general, relies on the concepts of materials chemistry and photonics, with DSSCs interfacing with electrochemistry in addition and BHJs involving solid-state physics. These concepts inevitably apply to biophotovoltaics as well, though there are more complexities in the construction and working of the device when there is a biological component in it. With a concise note on the structure and function of the different photosynthetic proteins, Chapter 4 throws light on that hub of all photosynthetic organisms, which is the nanoscale reaction center (RC) where the charge separation begins. The RC is the most efficient molecular system that drives the solar energy into electrical (and in turn chemical) energy conversion. The physics of charge separation process, dynamics, and kinetics of electron transfer in the RCs are presented in Chapter 4. With these chapters, the reader might get a good instinct on how these proteins can be used in photovoltaics. Chapter 5 presents an account of the progress made in the last decade in integrating the proteins in electrochemical cells, with a focus on different immobilization routes and the ensuing charge transfer modes.

Chapter 6 chronicles the most recent and emerging approaches in designing bio-photovoltaics and discusses the device physics in these systems in conjunction with insights from photonics and electronics. Highlighting the limitations in the present approaches, the book sheds light on new device architectures and possible future directions, which are outlined in Chapters 6 and 7.

About the Editor

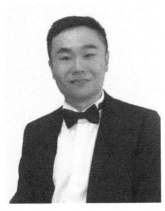

Swee Ching Tan received his bachelor's degree in Physics from the National University of Singapore (NUS). He then worked for Hewlett Packard Enterprise Singapore and Ireland as a laser process and equipment engineer to develop new technologies for silicon micromachining. At Hewlett Packard, he made two major contributions that helped the company to achieve major cost-cutting goals and to increase the throughput within his department. He was honored with the Award for Outstanding Achievement for these contributions to the company. He subsequently gained PhD admission to the University of Cambridge's Electrical Engineering Department with scholarships from Cambridge Commonwealth Trust and the Wingate Foundation. His PhD work, under the supervision of Professor Sir Mark Welland, involved using photosynthetic proteins as light-absorbing materials for solar cells. After completing his PhD, Dr. Tan moved to the Department of Materials Science and Engineering at the Massachusetts Institute of Technology to become a postdoctoral associate working on nanoelectronics. He is currently an assistant professor in the Department of Materials Science and Engineering with NUS Faculty of Engineering.

Dr. Tan's research interests span a wide range of areas in the fields of energy and environmental sciences. The area of biohybrid photovoltaics is a core expertise of his research lab with a number of new device architectures developed in recent years. Dr. Tan's research group has achieved breakthrough energy-harvesting performances using natural and engineered photoproteins. His research group is also working on developing organic ionic conductors and work-function engineering for applications in energy harvesting and photosensing electronic devices. Bridging the spheres of energy and environment sciences, the research group is also focusing on developing low-energy and low-cost air filtration and thermal comfort technologies. By engineering super-hygroscopic materials and hierarchically structured solar absorbers, the research team led by Dr. Tan aims to develop clean water technologies that could generate potable water not only from seawater but also out of humid air.

Contributors

Tianyu Bai
Department of Chemistry
Southern University of Science and
Technology
Shenzhen, P. R. China

Feng He
Department of Chemistry
Southern University of Science and
Technology
Shenzhen, P. R. China

Michael R. Jones
School of Biochemistry
University of Bristol
Bristol, United Kingdom

Ajay K. Kushwaha
Discipline of Metallurgy Engineering
and Materials Science
Indian Institute of Technology Indore
Indore, India

Di Sheng Lee
Department of Biological Engineering
Massachusetts Institute of Technology
Cambridge, Massachusetts

Daize Mo
Department of Chemistry
Southern University of Science and
Technology
Shenzhen, P. R. China

Krishnaiah Mokurala
International Centre for Materials
Science
Jawaharlal Nehru Centre for Advanced
Scientific Research
Bangalore, India

Nagaraju Mokurala
Discipline of Metallurgy Engineering
and Materials Science
Indian Institute of Technology Indore
Indore, India

Yoke Keng Ngeow
Department of Biological Sciences
National University of Singapore
Singapore

Sai Kishore Ravi
Department of Materials Science and
Engineering
National University of Singapore
Singapore

Anuraj Singh Rawat
Department of Materials Science and
Engineering
National University of Singapore
Singapore

Siddhartha Suman
Discipline of Metallurgy Engineering
    and Materials Science
Indian Institute of Technology Indore
Indore, India

Swee Ching Tan
Department of Materials Science and
    Engineering
National University of Singapore
Singapore

Leilei Tian
Department of Materials Science and
    Engineering
Southern University of Science and
    Technology
Shenzhen, P. R. China

Vishnu Saran Udayagiri
Department of Materials Science and
    Engineering
National University of Singapore
Singapore

1 Learning from Nature to Improve Solar Energy Conversion Devices

Di Sheng Lee, Yoke Keng Ngeow, and Swee Ching Tan

CONTENTS

1.1 INTRODUCTION

Global energy consumption models envisage that human civilization would require 46 TW of energy in 2100, which is a few times greater than current global energy consumption.[1] Coupled with an increasing world population, the emerging economies of India and China will pose great challenges to global energy demand. Now, fossil fuels account for most of the global energy demand, and the consumption is even more for developed countries. What's more, oil production is estimated to decline around 2007–2038,[2] but recent studies suggest that oil production level has already reached its apex.[3] Even if oil reserves run out, coal and gas remain to be exploited.[4] Therefore, the exigent issue is not the fossil fuel constraint but the repercussions of burning fossil fuel, which releases a staggering amount of CO_2 into the atmosphere. The CO_2 level would rise to that of primordial times if every drop of fossil fuel remaining on our planet is burned.[5] In the last 400,000 years, atmospheric CO_2 levels were stable at ~250 ppm but have risen sharply to 400 ppm.[6,7] The current staggering atmospheric CO_2 level is the culprit behind global warming; if global warming is left unchecked, it will spell doom not only for human civilization but also for all lives on Earth. For example, at atmospheric CO_2 levels of 450 ppm, irreversible coral reef damage is likely to happen.[8] A level of 550 ppm would cause the melting of the West Antarctic ice sheet, the rising of sea level for 4–6 m,[8] and the extinction of a 35% of flora and fauna.[9] At levels of 650 ppm, thermohaline circulation would be disrupted, and local climate would change considerably.[9] Some global climate change models[10] suggest that the potential effects could be more serious than previously anticipated;[9,11,12] as such, it is imperative to keep the CO_2 level below 450 ppm. Since CO_2 emission is unlikely to be cut down soon, and the fact that CO_2 is stable in the atmosphere for a long period of time, it is improbable that the CO_2 level could be kept below 450 ppm. Hoffert and coworkers calculated that in order to keep atmospheric CO_2 levels below 450 ppm, we would need to use 11 TW of CO_2-emission-free fuel by 2025.[1] In other words, we are running out of time as we urgently need a CO_2 emission-free technology capable of producing energy equivalent to the global annual energy consumption rate in 2000 (13 TW) within 10 years. However, we are still heavily dependent on fossil fuels for many years to come; thus, it is important to minimize carbon dioxide release into the atmosphere and to develop carbon dioxide sequestration technologies as soon as possible.[13] Hand in hand with this is definitely the development of highly efficient clean energy technologies.

Unlike wind, geothermal, and hydroelectric energy, solar energy is one of the most copious (178,000 TW year^{-1}) and accessible sources of clean energy.[15] Solar energy can be economically viable even in regions where sunlight is scarce. The bottleneck, however, is the development of affordable photovoltaic systems with high efficiency. In fact, an area of 634 × 634 (equivalent to 4.4% of the Sahara desert) is enough for today's commercial solar cells to supply global annual energy consumption.[16] Yet, the costs of constructing and installing such extended solar systems are still much higher compared to those of fossil fuels. Hence, we have two challenges ahead. The first is to develop more efficient solar energy systems. Existing solar capture technologies are improving on a daily basis.[17,18] In the foreseeable future, solar systems will be more affordable as biomimetic materials inspired by natural photosynthesis would improve the current solar systems.[19,20] The second is to implement a carbon tax as well as include the costs related to decommissioning nuclear power plants and radioactive waste in order to increase the competition in the energy market. The sun provides solar energy at a rate of 172,500 TW to our planet annually. Since incident sunlight is reflected and absorbed by the atmosphere, only ~65,000 TW of it reaches the hydrosphere and 15,600 TW of it falls on land (Figure 1.1).[21] To better appreciate the power of the sun, consider that the energy from an hour of sunlight is enough to power the total energy humanity uses in a year.[22] The sun spectrum is represented by air mass 0 (AM0), while the amount of sunlight that reaches the Earth has been reduced significantly by the atmosphere and hence is represented by air mass 1.5 (AM1.5); the air mass is the path length that light takes through the

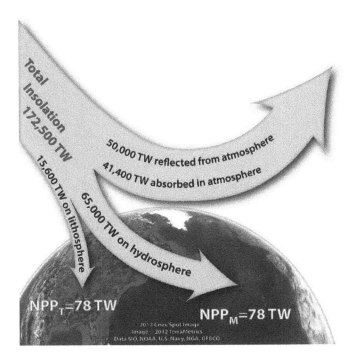

FIGURE 1.1 Rates of solar energy reaching different parts of the Earth. The sun provides solar energy at a rate of 172,500 TW to our planet annually. Since incident sunlight is reflected and absorbed by the atmosphere, only ~65,000 TW of it reaches the hydrosphere and 15,600 TW of it falls on land. (With kind permission from Springer Science+Business Media: *Photosynth. Res.*, 120, 2014, 59–70, Sherman, B.D. et al.)

atmosphere (Figure 1.2). To fully make use of sunlight, solar-energy converters have to be sufficiently cheap, robust, and efficient; however, current solar technologies are a far cry from being the primary energy source for humanity.

Mother Nature's photosynthesis might be the solution to our energy crisis as this elegant process has undergone billions of years of evolution to increase its efficiency to capture the sun's energy.[24,25] Biological cells evolved highly efficient and sophisticated molecular machineries that can adapt to different environmental conditions. Balzini et al. wrote, "An intelligent approach toward the design of artificial systems for solar energy conversion is to take the natural solar energy conversion sequence (i.e., the light reactions of photosynthesis) as a model and see whether the natural devices can be replaced by artificial ones."[26] As such, photochemists have long foreseen the potentials hidden within the natural solar systems, and recent progress in obtaining atomically resolved structures have shed light on the photosynthetic molecular machinery in terms of structure and function that so elegantly converts sunlight into useful chemical energy. These seminal discoveries were made on the purple bacteria, which is an anaerobic photosynthetic bacteria. Comparable to the role of

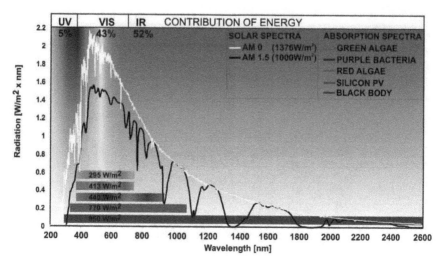

FIGURE 1.2 Solar energy distribution and capture. The sun spectrum is represented by AM0 (white line), while the amount of sunlight that reaches the Earth has been reduced significantly by the atmosphere and is represented by AM1.5 (black line). The air mass is the path length that light takes through the atmosphere (Figure 1.2). On the surface of the Earth, 5% of the sunlight is in the ultraviolet (300–400 nm) region, while 43% and 52% of the sunlight are in the visible (400–700 nm) infrared region, respectively. The absorption spectra of some of the most common light-harvesting systems are shown: green plants, purple bacteria, red algae, and typical silicon photovoltaic (PV) panels. Photosyntheic organisms and silicon PV panels have different absorption properties. (Kruse, O. et al., *Photoch. Photobio. Sci.*, 4, 957–970, 2005. Reproduced by permission from The Royal Society of Chemistry.)

the hydrogen atom in understanding basic physics and chemistry in earlier times of the scientific era, the photosynthetic machinery of purple bacteria with its multicomponent organization holds the key to unlock the secrets behind the functions and mechanisms of molecular machineries in photosynthetic organisms. Although purple bacteria have similar solar energy conversion as those of green plants, purple bacteria's ones are simpler and better understood. As such, the photosynthetic machinery of purple bacteria is chosen as a model of biomimicry as a green plant's two-photosystem photosynthetic machinery is quite complicated. In purple bacteria, the photosynthetic process occurs across a cell membrane and is facilitated by some membrane proteins. It makes use of both visible and near-infrared photons. Antenna systems are employed to collect sunlight and maximize the absorption of wavelengths obtainable from the surroundings. Within the antenna, electronic excitation transfers from one chromophore to another and eventually to a reaction center, where charge separation occurs across the bilayer and where the excitation energy is converted to chemical energy. A bacteriochlorophyll "special pair" near the outside of the cell membrane and a series of steps involving several donor-acceptor cofactors are involved. It is possible to build a more energy-efficient artificial reaction center that employs fewer redox centers.[27] Even though most wavelengths of the visible region can be efficiently trapped by photosynthetic organisms (Figure 1.2), the energy required to split water and reduce carbon dioxide is similar to that of red photons. Therefore, in the light-harvesting pigments, higher energy photons are converted to red photons of ~1.8 eV, and the rest of the energy is degraded to heat. In other words, in photosynthetic organisms, energy is lost not only to maintain their metabolism and survival but also in degrading high-energy photons to the energy of red photons.

Purple bacteria's biological functionalities are governed by the law of physics. The photosynthetic apparatus of purple bacteria provides sufficient energy for its survival even under low sunlight irradiation. How is this feat achieved? The answer may lie in the fact that nature arranges its photosynthetic apparatus in an architecture of reaction centers, pigments, and protein complexes but not many copies of reaction centers. This multicomponent organization is the key feat of engineering since it allows energy in the photosynthetic apparatus to flow in many different ways. Photosynthesis research has attracted scientists from diverse backgrounds such as physics, molecular genetics, structural biology, and chemistry to name a few. Back then, the idea of many pigment molecules embedded in a symmetrical and hierarchical architecture posed a big challenge to physicists to describe excitation transfer through quantum physics.[28] The term "exciton" was introduced to photosynthesis research, which was originally invented in solid-state physics.[29] Unlike excitation of crystals in solid-state physics, excitations in photosynthetic systems are relatively random and disordered. Fluorescence resonance energy transfer (FRET) applies to such pigment molecules in a solution; therefore, photosynthetic proteins are somewhere between crystals and fluids.[30] While electron transfer in chemical systems is influenced by many factors, only three factors matter in biological systems: distance, free energy, and reorganization energy.[27] The BChl system in the photosynthetic apparatus is arranged in a hierarchical fashion: higher-energy BChls are arranged further away from the reaction centers. BChl molecules are strongly coupled, enabling exciton states to be formed from coherent delocalization of excitation over a substantial part of the ring. Some of the key experimental techniques involved in characterizing the photosynthetic apparatus include hole-burning spectroscopy, time-resolved femtosecond spectroscopy,[31] nonlinear absorption spectroscopy,[32] high-resolution fluorescence spectroscopy[33] as well as single-molecule spectroscopy.[34] Theoretical methods include, but are not limited to, bioinformatics and structure prediction,[35,36] molecular dynamics,[37] quantum chemistry,[38] the theory of exciton systems,[30] stochastic quantum mechanics,[39] and advanced condensed matter theory.[40] Evolution has engendered the pigments of light-harvesting systems to abide by a set of rules as to which wavelengths to absorb.[41] The absorbance peaks are typically tuned to the area of the spectrum where there is a peak photon flux. The reaction center pigments exhibit absorption peak at the longest wavelength available as long as the photon energy is enough to power its photochemistry.[41] On the other hand, the accessory pigments exhibit another absorption peak that aligns with the shortest wavelengths available.

In photosynthesis, electron transfers occur in the symmetrical and hierarchical architecture of antenna system, reaction center, and other cofactors. After sunlight is converted to electronic excitation energy, a cascade of electron transfer events precedes charge separation in the reaction center. The antenna system collects light and transfers the resulting electronic excitation energy to the reaction center via singlet–singlet energy transfer. In the reaction center, charge separation occurs with amazing efficiency to produce a spatially and electronically well-isolated radical pair. The resulting potential energy drives protons across the membrane to generate a charge gradient that will power the production of a high-energy biochemical fuel, adenosine triphosphate (ATP). One of the important factors attributed to this process is the overall small reorganization energy exhibited by the reaction center.[42] Non-covalent interaction arranges the donor-acceptor couples in the reaction center into well-defined transmembrane proteins. This elegant solar energy conversion approach is an archetype of the Rube Goldberg designs common in biological systems.[43] These complex yet versatile processes have prompted research on the natural photosynthetic machineries and spurred attempts to mimic them in the laboratory by designing synthetic donor-acceptor linked ensembles such as triads, tetrads, and pentads.[44–48] Major advancement has been in the last decade to use biomimicry as an approach to learn from nature's highly efficient pigment–protein complexes.[46] Integrating antennae systems with electron transfer relay systems has proven to be a viable approach to mimic photosynthesis.[48] Although the chemistry and physics behind electron transfer in natural and artificial systems have been extensively studied, synthetic systems are facing difficulties in achieving a stable and highly efficient charge separation as compared to natural photosynthesis. The ultimate ambition of artificial photosynthesis is to make use of artificial systems that can replicate the natural analog process of solar energy conversion.[49] An artificial photosystem could simplify a complicated natural photosynthetic system into its basic components and lead to a better understanding of photosynthesis and even to surpass photosynthesis itself. The first mention of artificial photosynthesis for applications in solar energy conversion dates back a century ago.[50] Today, artificial photosynthesis is burgeoning and its applications can be found in photonics, optoelectronics, sensors, and other nanotechnologies.[46,51–54] Artificial reaction centers can be assembled by using synthetic pigments as well as electron donors and acceptors that mimic natural pigments such as chlorophylls and carotenoids in a covalently bonded scaffold instead of a protein scaffold. The function of the covalent scaffold is still similar to that of the natural protein matrix, which is to control the distance and electronic coupling among the components, thus maximizing the rates of energy and electron-transfer processes. Furthermore, photosynthesis has evolved protective mechanisms to protect its photosynthetic machineries from damage caused by excess light.[55] Also, the biochemical pathways that are driving the photosynthetic process come with an inbuilt flexibility that confers adaptability of the organism to environmental changes. Hence, a successful artificial photosynthesis requires not only carefully "engineered" catalysts and charge separation units but also clever systems engineering.

1.2 LEARNING FROM PHOTOSYNTHETIC ORGANISMS

There are two main pigments in the purple bacteria for light absorption: bacteriochlorophyll a (Bchla) and carotenoids. They are bound to two types of hydrophobic integral-membrane-protein assemblies in a non-covalent fashion, forming reaction centers (RCs) and light-harvesting (LH) or antenna complexes, respectively.[56,57]

LH complexes, together with a RC, is known as the photosynthetic unit (PSU).[58] PSU functions as if it is a radiotelescope consisting of a large antenna and a transducer that turns radio signal into an electrical signal. Without the large antenna to facilitate and enhance the capture of incoming radio waves, the transducer will be useless since there will be little incoming radio waves received by the transducer.

There are two different types of LH complexes present in purple photosynthetic bacteria (*Rhodopseudomonas acidophila* and *Rhodopseudomonas palustris*): a core light-harvesting antenna (LH1) and a peripheral light-harvesting antenna (LH2).[61–63] As the name suggests, core LH1 is closely linked to the RC, forming RC-LH1 core complex. Since chlorophylls absorb some wavelengths weakly, carotenoids in proximity complement chlorophylls and transfer the resulting excitation energy to them. The Bchla molecules in LH1 and LH2 absorb at different wavelengths; this creates an energy gradient and ensures that the light harnessed in LH2 is directed "downhill" to LH1. The collected energy in LH1 is in turn channeled into a special pair of chlorophylls in the reaction center.[64] A collection of chromophores found in the transmembrane protein (Figure 1.3) is involved in a unidirectional electron-transfer event that ultimately produces a long-lived, charge-separated state across the membrane with a quantum efficiency of nearly 100%.[65] This separation of charge is necessary to generate a proton gradient across the membrane and to produce adenosine triphosphate (ATP).[45,46]

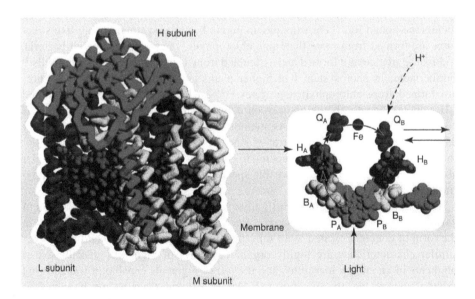

FIGURE 1.3 *Rhodobacter sphaeroides*'s reaction center. P, the primary donor bacteriochlorophyll a molecules; B, the monomeric bacteriochlorophyll a molecules; H, the bacteriopheophytin molecules; and Q, the ubiquinone molecules. The two branches are represented by the A and B subscripts. (Reproduced from *Trends Biotechnol.*, 16, Cogdell, R.J. and Lindsay, J.G., 521–527, Copyright 1998, with permission from Elsevier; Reproduced from *Curr. Biol.*, 7, Jones, M.R., R541–R543, Copyright 1997, with permission from Elsevier.)

1.2.1 REACTION CENTERS (RCs)

The RCs of the purple bacteria, which are likened to the transducer in a radio telescope, have been extensively studied in the past few decades since they can be easily isolated, and the pigments in the RCs have distinct absorption peaks.[66] The seminal work in this area started in 1984 when the structure of the RC from *Rhodopseudomonas viridis* was determined by X-ray crystallography.[67] Studies from *Rhodobacter sphaeroides* RC show that it consisted of three protein subunits—H, M, and L (Figure 1.3). Mutants containing RC are only photosynthetically active under intense solar radiation.[68] This is because the presence of the LH complexes provides additional surface area for capturing light energy. The array of electron acceptors between P and Q_A are able to minimize the back reaction by many orders of magnitude, ensuring that the electron transfer pathway is in essence irreversible (Figure 1.3). Cytochrome C re-reduces P1 on a microsecond timescale to maintain the unidirectionality of the charge-separation event, and so the quantum yield of the primary redox reactions is close to 100%.[69]

1.2.2 LIGHT-HARVESTING (LH) COMPLEXES

LH complexes are likened to a large collecting dish. Mother Nature has produced a variety of LH structures, reflecting the diversity of environments in which the organisms live. The structural organizations of LH complexes can be categorized into three types (Figure 1.4) by the position of the peripheral LH complexes relative to the membrane-bound RC.[70] For example, in purple bacteria, symmetric ring-like structures are formed from more than nine chlorophylls,[61–63] whereas in green bacteria, rod-like aggregates are formed and assembled from a large number of chlorophylls.[71] Furthermore, in photosystem I of higher plants and cyanobacteria, 2D structures are formed from chlorophyll aggregates.[72–74] Such structural diversity in natural LH complexes conceals the association between structure and function in the LH complexes. Nevertheless, scientists attempted to study and unveil LH processes by using synthetic multiporphyrin arrays[64] since porphyrins are more stable and easier to synthesize synthetically as compared to chlorophylls; moreover, they have similar absorption properties across the visible spectrum. However, huge arrays of porphyrins are difficult to synthesize.

Even though they are structurally diverse, the principles of light absorption of various LH complexes are the same.[76] Each LH complex harvests light energy in the form of coherent excited-state superpositions—excitons.[30,77] In addition, other similar characteristics are highly organized arrays of pigments, distribution of pigments in an energy hierarchy, and the use of pigments capable of transmitting exciton energy via the Förster and Dexter exciton transfer mechanisms.[78,79] The LH complexes not only contain many pigment molecules but also possess an arrangement that is optimized to maximize the number and the range of photon energies to the RCs. In other words, the LH complexes widen the range of wavelengths that can be used to power photosynthesis. By increasing the rate of charge separation per unit time in the RC, antenna systems maintain the rate of RC turnover as close as possible to the rate of its biochemical processes. Moreover,

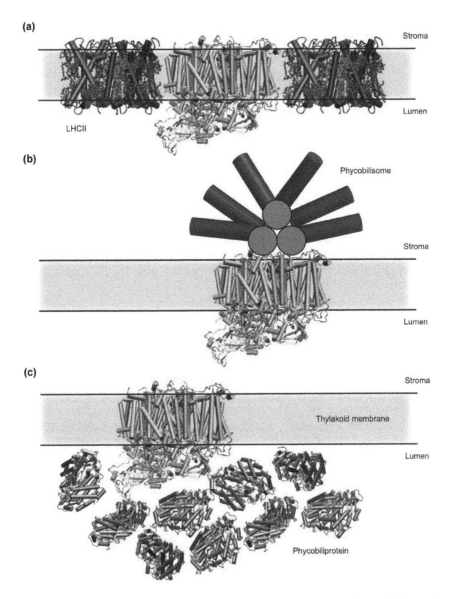

FIGURE 1.4 Various organizations of light-harvesting antenna complexes relative to the photosynthetic membrane: (a) Higher plants and green algae. (b) Cyanobacteria and red algae. (c) Cryptophytes. (Reprinted by permission from Macmillan Publishers Ltd. Scholes, G.D. et al., 3, 763–774, 2011, Copyright 2011.)

this architecture permits photosynthetic organisms to regulate the energy transfer pathways.[80] Exciton energy transfer happens when two chromophores have similar energy levels and are resonating with each other.[28] Generally, the organization of antenna complexes engenders two types of energy-transfer reactions in the PSU: (1) rapid transfer steps in antenna complex; (2) relatively slower ring–ring transfers

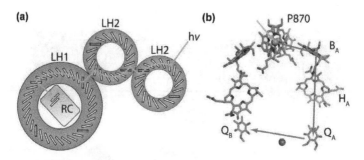

FIGURE 1.5 Electron transfer pathway in photosynthetic bacteria. (a) After a photon enters LH2, excitation energy is transferred from LH2 to another LH2, then LH1; and finally RC. (b) After charge separation occurs, electron transfers from P870 via B_A to H_A and then Q_A. The doubly reduced Q_B leaves the RC by exchanging with the reservoir of oxidized quinone in the membrane. P, the primary donor bacteriochlorophyll a molecules; B, the monomeric bacteriochlorophyll a molecules; H, the bacteriopheophytin molecules; and Q, the ubiquinone molecules. (Reproduced from *Chem. Biol.*, 17, McConnell, I. et al., 434–447, Copyright 2010, with permission from Elsevier.)

between antenna complexes. Since LH2 and LH1 complexes are in proximity of one another, it takes only about 3–4 ps to transfer energy from LH2 to LH1 (Figure 1.5). The longer distance between the B875 ring in LH1 and the primary electron donor in the RC causes the energy transfer to be 10 times slower, which takes 30–40 ps. To maximize energy transfer, the LH1 complex organizes its B875 Bchls in a large ring. The light-harvesting capacity of the LH complexes is also boosted by carotenoids as they can harvest green light and transfer the resulting energy to the Bchlas. Carotenoid pigments need to be very close to one another (~3 Å) because their short lifetime of excited states (10 ps) would be difficult to transfer energy over longer distances.[81] Different LH complexes have different energy transfer efficiencies, which vary from 30% to 100%.[82] LH complexes are physiologically flexible, and their protein expressions are controlled meticulously. For example, LH complexes increase in number under low light condition and decrease under conditions such as constant light and decreased temperature,[83] low CO_2,[84] or high light.[85–88]

1.2.3 PHOTOPROTECTION

The PSU is often described as an energy funnel in which there are pigments located at higher energy levels as they get farther away from the RC, warranting that excitation energy is directed rapidly toward the RC. However, this is a misconception since electronic excitation in a PSU is distributed comparatively evenly throughout the system.[28,89] This organization is important because underlying this is a photoprotective function that dissipates excess excitation energy back to the antenna complexes, where it could be dissipated or ideally transferred to another RC.

During periods of low irradiation, photosynthetic bacteria will rewire themselves to prevent themselves from "straving" from the shortage of light. This is done genetically to activate the replacement of LH2 complexes by LH3 complexes, which are excited at 820 nm. This higher energy level accelerates forward transfer rates and facilitates the building of an excitation funnel under a low irradiation level.[28] Natural photosynthesis (especially oxygenic photosynthesis) functions optimally under a low irradiation level and is normally saturated during midday.[55] However, under a high irradiation level, the system can be over-reduced and intermediate can have extended lifetimes, which can cause charge recombination in the RCs. For example, under a high irradiation level, the reservoir of quinone, is fully reduced, and as a result the rate of charge recombination increases. This in turn leads to the reaction between triplet state Chls and O_2 to produce highly detrimental, reactive singlet O_2 molecules. Over millions of years of evolution, photosynthetic organisms have come out with some ingenious photoprotective strategies to deal with high irradiation levels.[55] One of the clever approaches to minimize photodamage is by using a smaller LH antenna. For instance, when *Rb. Sphaeroides* is grown under a high irradiation level, LH2 decreases in amount. Instead of funneling the resulting excitation energy to RCs, the LH systems dissipate excess chlorophyll singlet excitation energy as heat.[90] For example, LH complexes can dissipate absorbed light energy through photochemical (fluorescence) and non-photochemical quenching (NPQ) processes. The mechanism behind non-photochemical quenching (NPQ) is not fully understood; nonetheless, it was found that carotenoid polyenes play an important role.[91–94] Carotenoids help to protect photosynthetic membranes from photochemical damage.[82,95,96] Since carotenoid triplet states are less energetic than singlet oxygen, they can quench the harmful triplet state Chls before they have a chance to react with O_2 to form detrimental singlet O_2 molecules. In green algae and higher plants, under a high irradiation level, the xanthophyll cycle is involved in protecting the RC of PSII against damage by dissipating excess energy as heat by means of pH or energy-dependent quenching of chlorophyll fluorescence (qE).[94,97,98]

1.3   FROM NATURAL TO BIOMIMETIC PHOTOSYNTHETIC DEVICE

Through millions of years of evolution, photosynthetic organisms have optimized solar energy harvesting and conversion through an intricate scaffold of proteins in which ordered assemblies of photofunctional chromophores and catalysts lie. Analogous to natural photosynthesis, artificial photosynthesis harvests light energy, separates charge, and transports charge to catalytic sites. Although biomimicry of natural photosynthesis is making good progress, artificial photosynthesis has yet to develop devices that are efficient and robust enough to compete with existing solar technologies. Nonetheless, better understanding of natural photosynthetic mechanisms and advances in chemical synthesis have led to the creations and designs of artificial photosynthetic systems that replicate natural processes, such as those of antenna, RC, and even proton pumps of natural photosynthesis.[99] Artificial systems made of electron donors and acceptors to mimic natural light-driven charge separation in RCs have allowed researchers to study the effect of physicochemical properties such as donor/acceptor distance and orientation, free energy of the reaction, and electronic interactions on electron transfer efficiency.[100] The next step will be to improve RC and LH complexes' functions and to combine them. We are only scratching the surface of what Mother Nature can do, and there is still plenty to learn from nature. For example, the proteins in natural RC and LH complexes are more than a scaffold. In a RC, the protein also plays a role to control the redox properties of the pigments by varying the number of hydrogen bonds between the bacteriochlorin macrocycles and the protein backbone.[101]

By using chlorophyll a together with some accessory pigments, namely carotenoids, xanthophylls, and chlorophyll b, green plants are able to make use of the entire visible part of sunlight (350–700 nm). In particular, chlorophyll a makes use of blue-violet and orange-red areas of the light visible spectrum, whereas the accessory pigments absorb the yellow green-orange region, which is at the middle of the light visible spectrum. Also, having an LH complex that organizes the chlorophyll molecules in ideal arrangement by means of using lipids and lipoproteins, without carrying out charge separation itself, permits efficient light capturing even at varying light flux; as such, under bright or diffuse light conditions, natural photosynthesis has similar efficiency. Likewise, to be as successful as natural photosynthesis, artificial systems must employ several dye molecules to harvest the entire visible light spectrum of the solar radiation.[102] However, dye molecules are often directly engaged in electron transfer, acting as if they are redox active chlorophylls within photosynthetic RCs.[103] The rich and extensive absorptions (i.e., p–p* transitions) found in chlorophyll's porphyrinoid systems could hold the key to the construction of molecular architectures with increased absorptive cross sections of the solar spectrum.[51] In replacement of lipids and lipoproteins, artificial systems could utilize surfactant micelles, lipid monolayers, vesicles, cage compounds, and even covalently linked arrays to funnel energy to a charge-separation site.[102,104,105] However, most of the covalently linked arrays are difficult to synthesize, and recent approaches make use of self-assembly instead to produce functional antenna arrays. The intricate photoprotective and regulatory mechanisms of natural photosynthesis are crucial to its success. For that reason, artificial systems should ideally possess similar mechanisms, too, to protect them from photodamage.[106] Furthermore, one-electron oxidation or reduction intermediates should be avoided in artificial systems since they are highly reactive and will produce side reactions.[102]

Natural RCs by themselves are too delicate to be used directly as solar cells. Unlike *in vivo* RCs, which are very stable, *in vitro* RCs are unstable since they exist as purified complexes that are alienated from their supporting protein scaffolds. Artificial RCs could be the solution; artificial RCS have been introduced into artificial vesicles' lipid membranes to work as light-driven proton pumps.[48] Artificial RCs possess good properties such as rapid charge separation, relatively slow charge recombination, and thus relatively long-lived charge-separated states. Therefore, by using artificial constructs consisting of artificial RCs, molecular mechanisms behind natural photosynthesis can be reconstructed and enhanced or even used to create solar biological "power packs" that can drive enzymatic reactions and machineries.[99]

Our improved understanding of natural LH complexes and improvements in synthetic and spectroscopic methods have enabled the construction of artificial LH systems.[107,108] A variety of natural LH complexes have been produced as a result of evolution. For instance, cyanobacteria have two kinds of LH complexes: phycobilisomes are used as their dominant light capturing complexes;[109] however, when cyanobacteria experience iron deficiency, an alternative, ring-like antenna made up of iron-stress-induced chlorophyll-binding protein (IsiA) is employed instead.[110,111] Artificial LH antennas have been developed by using multiporphyrin arrays,[112] porphyrin dendrimers,[64] or dendrimers based on metal complexes and organic molecules.[113] Highly branched, tree-like dendrimers enable close interaction of many chromophores in close proximity.[114] However, care must be taken when incorporating artificial LH antennas since the result may not be favorable if the LH antennas and the RCs are not properly coupled.[75]

In short, a precise control over separation, electronic coupling, angular relationships, and composition in donor and acceptor molecules is mandatory to produce efficient artificial antenna and RCs. Unlike artificial systems that use covalent interactions, natural photosynthetic systems employ non-covalent self-assembly to embed light- and redox-active components into a protein matrix. This signifies that self-assembly approaches—such as hydrogen-bonding, donor–acceptor complexation, electrostatic interactions, and p–p stacking—might provide better control to achieve ideal architectures with high directionality and selectivity.[115] Therefore, self-assembled donor–acceptor assemblies might be a substitute to existing complex, covalent molecular systems.

To advance the process of artificial photosynthesis, it is vital to develop self-assembly materials in nanoscale that can be scaled up to macroscopic dimensions to facilitate the transfer of light excitation energy from antenna to RCs.[116] Molecular charge conduits need to be implemented on the system to serve as a channel for the movement of electrons and holes from the RCs and catalytic sites.[117] The major challenge of building a self-assembly functional artificial photosynthetic system lies in the development of a component that has minimum covalent linkages that have molecular recognition properties. It is essential to fabricate molecules that interact with one another in a well-ordered manner to build integrated artificial photosynthetic systems.[117] Producing such large molecular arrays by covalent syntheses is plausible, but it is not a cost-effective method. One needs to consider the organization at molecular and supramolecular levels for developing a functional, unified, integrated photosynthetic system. Some characteristics such as donor-acceptor distances and molecular structure of the components need to be known to select a desirable candidate. Those characteristics are useful for the design of the system because the process of charge separation by solar energy in the artificial photosynthetic photosystem is susceptible to energy loss to heat due the law of thermodynamics. The self-assembly properties of a component to build the large molecular arrays may have interesting and unique properties that can only be achieved when each individual unit assembles. In short, a self-assembled antenna complex and RC is an important step toward more successful artificial photosynthesis. A good understanding of interactions such as π-stacking, hydrogen bonding, and metal-ligand bonding will be crucial to assemble complex photofunctional structures from simple building blocks.

1.4   FROM NATURAL TO BIOMIMETIC LEAF

Nature has shaped leaves to adopt cellular structures and arrangement that optimize the first step of photosynthesis, which is the capture of sunlight.[118,119] For example, epidermal cells serve as a lens to focus light,[120] cylindrical palisade parenchyma cells direct light through the leaf,[121] the spongy mesophyll,[122] and porous veins structure support the scattering of light, which further improve light path length.[118,123] Other fascinating structures found within the cells are the chloroplast that holds thylakoid membranes, which are organized in stacks, and the multiple pigments that support the transport of electrons.[119] In the effort to build a highly functional artificial photosynthetic system, it is important to pay equal attention to mimic the natural photosynthetic system in the aspects of its functions and structures (Figure 1.6). During the construction of an artificial leaf, some major criteria of the artificial functional component to be adopted from the natural photosynthetic system include the ability of the component to be excited by light and feasibility to transfer the electrons to enable charge separation. Catalysts that have a resemblance to pigments in a natural leaf are also essential to complete the process of transforming the light energy.

Regardless of the direction in which the light came from, the natural leaf has ways to optimize light absorption. Palisade parenchyma cells and spongy mesophyll cells are able to focus the light that arrives at the upper surface of the leaf and lower

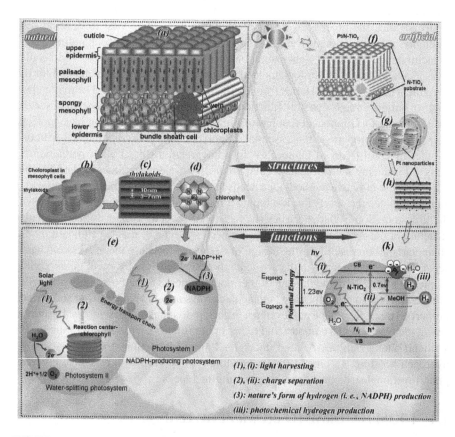

FIGURE 1.6 Comparison of the structures and functions of natural and artificial leaves. (From Zhou. H. et al.: *Adv. Mater.*, 2010, 22, 951–956. Copyright Wiley-VCH Verlag Gmbh & Co. KGaA. Reproduced with permission.)

surface of the leaf, respectively.[125] For example, the columnar cell located in the palisade layer has an elongated shape that is able to guide light through the vacuoles and intercellular air spaces,[121] whereas the less-regularly arranged spongy mesophyll cells scatter light.[122] There are many optical models developed to study how light interacts with the leaf.[126–128] Within each mesophyll cell, there are multiple chloroplasts that hold thylakoid membranes that are arranged in stacks called granum. The thylakoid membrane allows the distribution of photosynthetic pigments that are favorable to the functions of each pigment. Thylakoid membranes hence serve as a platform for photosynthetic pigments to interact with sunlight efficiently.[129] Rapid charge separation is made possible owing to the nanoscale thickness of the thylakoid membrane. The higher surface area of the thylakoid membrane that allows effective interaction between pigments and light actually provides a clue on the structure for an artificial leaf to adopt. Nanostructured materials are being fabricated to have high surface area to improve light absorption by the artificial pigments.[130–133] In order to mimic the structure of the thylakoid membrane, semiconductors can be arranged in layers in a solar cell. As the availability of light energy can vary in the environment, plants have evolved at different levels of organization to adapt to the situation.[134] To control the amount of solar radiation incident on leaves, the leaves can orientate themselves in certain patterns. At the cellular level, chloroplasts are able to rearrange to regulate light absorption. The implementation of these approaches in an artificial photosynthetic system would improve current solar energy technologies.

Inspired by the way that nature has shaped cell structure and arrangement in leaves, natural leaves were used as a biotemplate to produce N-doped TiO_2.[135] The N-doped TiO_2 mimics the structures of natural leaves in many aspects from nanoscales to macroscales, which the natural leaf utilizes to optimize light absorption. The N-doped TiO_2 was termed as artificial inorganic leaf-TiO_2 (AIL-TiO_2). The process of photosynthesis is made possible in the AIL with the association of components that are responsible for capturing light, conversion of photon energy, and catalytic processes. AIL-TiO_2 also supports the water-splitting process upon the incidence of light from the UV range to a visible range in the presence of sacrificial reagents. Such AIL that incorporated structures from natural leaves is able to show improvement in the light-harvesting process and photocatalytic activity in comparison with those doped-TiO_2 prepared using a conventional method. Using leaves as a biotemplate also offers alternatives to lower the cost of producing leaflike solar cells. Aquatic plants have adapted to their environment by having unique structures in order to carry out efficient photosynthesis.[136] Chromatophores are found in the epidermis of kelp, which aid in light harvesting. Kelp also utilizes the principle of light scattering to improve light absorption by having less ordered porous structures of the exodermis, endodermis, and pith. Hence, kelp is also a possible candidate to be used as biotemplate to produce biogenic TiO_2.[136]

In designing the artificial photosynthetic system, inspirations could be drawn not only from natural leaves but also photosynthetic organisms. By incorporating thylakoids or cyanobacteria into a 3D silica structure, such integration of a photosynthetic bioreactor in silica is an approach that is one step closer to the idea of an "artificial leaf."[138–140] The concept is not limited to thylakoids and cyanobacteria; there are various photosynthetic microorganisms to be incorporated into the "artificial leaf."

Some major issues regarding stability and efficiency of such a photosynthetic system that incorporate biological materials could be improved using genetic modification of the biological materials. The structure of the "artificial leaf" can be designed to cater to different requirements of the system. Some natural leaf surface structures of desert plants are able to reflect a great portion of the incident light to decrease the amount of solar energy received. Surfaces that are superhydrophobic are capable of reducing energy dissipitation, which in turn serves to conserve energy.[141] Given the diversity of plants on Earth, there are more strategies for improving artificial solar cells that can be inspired by Mother Earth. There are some important characteristics found in a natural photosynthetic system that are yet to be developed in an artificial photosynthetic system. An example is the capability of a natural photosynthetic system to undergo self-repair for counteracting the damage from solar radiation (Figure 1.7).[137,142] In plants, the self-repair cycles involve the synthesis of proteins that are responsible to replacing photodamaged proteins. The ability to self-repair is an adaptation acquired by plants through the course of evolution that allows them to neutralize the effects of protein degradation and to reduce the damage from solar radiation. Artificial photosynthetic devices should mimic natural self-assembly and self-repair process.[143] Moreover, in nature, a polypeptide ring that surrounds the chlorophyll serves to avoid aggregation in a natural antennae.[144] In an artificial antennae system, the material with microscale or nanoscale pores is fabricated to be selective, so that it only allows the monomers but not aggregates to pass through the pores.[145–150]

In short, a natural leaf is a model for the development of an artificial photosynthetic system because it not only incorporates processes such as photosynthesis, transpiration, and respiration that are essential for solar energy conversion, but it also provides a self-repair mechanism that responds to photodamage to maintain the proper functions. The principles of transpiration and respiration in a natural leaf have yet to be applied for the advancement in design and materials to be

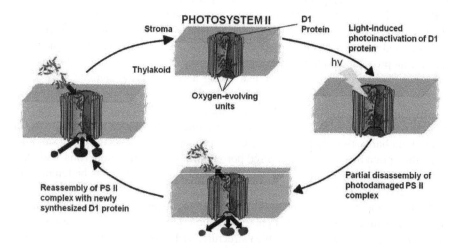

FIGURE 1.7 Self-repair mechanism in PSII. Molecular recognition of parts plays a big role in driving the self-repair cycle. (Boghossian, A.A. et al., *Energ. Environ. Sci.*, 4, 3834–3843, 2011. Reproduced by permission from The Royal Society of Chemistry.)

implemented on an artificial photosynthetic system. Hence, the ultimate goal of the development of an artificial photosynthetic system is to incorporate most, if not all, of the functions that a natural leaf possesses to utilize solar energy beautifully.

1.5   OVERVIEW

Ever since the discovery of the photoelectric effect, researchers have been trying hard to improve the conversion efficiency of sunlight into electricity through photovoltaic devices. However, there is a limiting factor in the ultimate conversion efficiency of commercial silicon solar cells, in that it can never exceed 34% according to the Shockley-Queisser efficiency limit. One possible way to overcome this barrier is to learn from Mother Nature, which has created the most efficient process to harness the power of the sun through photosynthesis. Photosynthetic organisms harvest sunlight and store the energy in chemical forms. Crucial to this process are the antenna proteins that capture sunlight and transfer it to an RC where charge separation begins. The electrons produced go through an electron transport chain to make chemical compounds that are used to fuel the organism's activities. The internal quantum yield of converting harvested light into the abovementioned electron transfer process in photosynthetic organisms is close to 100%. Owing to this attractive efficiency in photosynthetic systems, the idea of direct integration of proteins in photovoltaics has gained immense research interest in recent times,[24,151–155] In this book, a concise overview of the fundamental concepts of photosynthesis will be given with a brief account of the structure and function of some of the commonly used photosynthetic reaction centers and photosystems. The absorption properties, electron transfer processes, and kinetics within these proteins will be reviewed. Two concepts related to solar cells, namely dye-sensitized solar cells and bulk heterojunction solar cells, will be introduced to enable the readers to have a basic understanding of how solar cells work. With enough background on these concepts, the different types of protein-integrated biophotovoltaic cells, their progress, and future will be discussed.

REFERENCES

1. Hoffert, M. I.; Caldeira, K.; Jain, A. K.; Haites, E. F.; Harvey, L. D. D.; Potter, S. D.; Schlesinger, M. E. et al., **1998**, 395, (6705), 881–884.
2. Rifkin, J. *The Hydrogen Economy*. Penguin Putnam, New York: 2002.
3. Kerr, R. A. *Science* **2011**, 331, (6024), 1510–1511.
4. Goldemberg, J. *World Energy Assessment: Energy and the Challenge of Sustainability.* United Nations Publications: 2000.
5. Watson, R. T.; Albritton, D. L., *Climate Change 2001: Synthesis Report: Third Assessment Report of the Intergovernmental Panel on Climate Change.* Cambridge University Press: **2001**.
6. Petit, J. R.; Jouzel, J.; Raynaud, D.; Barkov, N. I.; Barnola, J. M.; Basile, I.; Bender, M. et al., **1999**, 399, (6735), 429–436.
7. Feldman, D. R.; Collins, W. D.; Gero, P. J.; Torn, M. S.; Mlawer, E. J.; Shippert, T. R. **2015**, 519, (7543), 339–343.
8. O'Neill, B. C.; Oppenheimer, M. *Science* **2002**, 296, (5575), 1971–1972.

9. Hughes, T. P.; Baird, A. H.; Bellwood, D. R.; Card, M.; Connolly, S. R.; Folke, C.; Grosberg, R. et al., *Science* **2003**, 301, (5635), 929–933.

10. Stainforth, D. A.; Aina, T.; Christensen, C.; Collins, M.; Faull, N.; Frame, D. J.; Kettleborough, J. A. et al., **2005**, 433, (7024), 403–406.

11. Cubasch, U.; Meehl, G.; Boer, G.; Stouffer, R.; Dix, M.; Noda, A.; Senior, C.; Raper, S.; Yap, K. In: Houghton, J. T.; Ding, Y.; Griggs, D. J.; Noguer, M.; Van der Linden, P. J.; Dai, X.; Maskell, K.; Johnson, C. A. (Eds.): *Climate Change 2001: The Scientific Basis: Contribution of Working Group I to the Third Assessment Report of the Intergovernmental Panel* **2001**, 526–582.

12. Schiermeier, Q. Cleaner skies leave global warming forecasts uncertain. *Nature*, **2005**, 435, 135.

13. Metz, B.; Davidson, O.; De Coninck, H.; Loos, M.; Meyer, L. *Carbon Dioxide Capture and Storage: Special Report of the Intergovernmental Panel on Climate Change.* Cambridge, UK: Cambridge University Press. **2005**.

14. Sherman, B. D.; Vaughn, M. D.; Bergkamp, J. J.; Gust, D.; Moore, A. L.; Moore, T. A. *Photosynthesis Research* **2014**, 120, (1), 59–70.

15. Miyamoto, K. *Renewable Biological Systems for Alternative Sustainable Energy Production. Food & Agriculture Org.*: **1997**; Vol. 128.

16. Harder, N. P.; Peter, W. *Semiconductor Science and Technology* **2003**, 18, (5), S151.

17. Shaheen, S. E.; Ginley, D. S.; Jabbour, G. E. *MRS Bulletin* **2005**, 30, (1), 10–19.

18. Hagberg, D. P.; Yum, J.-H.; Lee, H.; De Angelis, F.; Marinado, T.; Karlsson, K. M.; Humphry-Baker, R. et al., *J Am Chem Soc* **2008**, 130, (19), 6259–6266.

19. Lewis, N. S.; Nocera, D. G. *Proceedings of the National Academy of Sciences* **2006**, 103, (43), 15729–15735.

20. Lewis, N. S.; Crabtree, G. **2005**.

21. Sorensen, B., *Renewable Energy: Physics, Engineering, Environmental Impacts, Economics & Planning.* Elsevier, Burlington, MA: **2011**.

22. Tsao, J.; Lewis, N.; Crabtree, G. *U.S. Department of Energy* **2006**.

23. Kruse, O.; Rupprecht, J.; Mussgnug, J. H.; Dismukes, G. C.; Hankamer, B. *Photochemical & Photobiological Sciences* **2005**, 4, (12), 957–970.

24. Ravi, S. K.; Tan, S. C. *Energy & Environmental Science* **2015**, 8, (9), 2551–2573.

25. Ravi, S. K.; Swainsbury, D. J.; Singh, V. K.; Ngeow, Y. K.; Jones, M. R.; Tan, S. C. *Advanced Materials* **2018**, 30, (5).

26. Balzani, V.; Campagna, S.; Denti, G.; Juris, A.; Serroni, S.; Venturi, M. *Accounts of Chemical Research* **1998**, 31, (1), 26–34.

27. Moser, C. C.; Dutton, P. L. *Biochimica et Biophysica Acta (BBA): Bioenergetics* **1992**, 1101, (2), 171–176.

28. Ritz, T.; Damjanović, A.; Schulten, K. *ChemPhysChem* **2002**, 3, (3), 243–248.

29. Scholes, G. D.; Rumbles, G. **2006**, 5, (9), 683–696.

30. Van Amerongen, H.; Valkunas, L.; Van Grondelle, R. *Photosynthetic Excitons.* World Scientific: 2000.

31. Amesz, J.; Hoff, A. J. *Biophysical Techniques in Photosynthesis.* Springer Science & Business Media, Dordrecht, the Netherlands: **2006**; Vol. 3.

32. Leupold, D.; Voigt, B.; Beenken, W.; Stiel, H. *FEBS Letters* **2000**, 480, (2–3), 73–78.

33. Zhang, J.-P.; Fujii, R.; Qian, P.; Inaba, T.; Mizoguchi, T.; Koyama, Y.; Onaka, K.; Watanabe, Y.; Nagae, H. *The Journal of Physical Chemistry B* **2000**, 104, (15), 3683–3691.

34. van Oijen, A. M.; Ketelaars, M.; Köhler, J.; Aartsma, T. J.; Schmidt, J. *Science* **1999**, 285, (5426), 400–402.

35. Hu, X.; Schulten, K. *Biophysical Journal* **1998**, 75, (2), 683–694.

36. Koepke, J.; Hu, X.; Muenke, C.; Schulten, K.; Michel, H. *Structure* **1996**, 4, (5), 581–597.

37. Xu, D.; Schulten, K. *Chemical Physics* **1994**, 182, (2), 91–117.

38. Damjanović, A.; Ritz, T.; Schulten, K. *Physical Review E* **1999**, 59, (3), 3293–3311.
39. Sundström, V.; Pullerits, T.; van Grondelle, R. *The Journal of Physical Chemistry B* **1999**, 103, (13), 2327–2346.
40. Damjanović, A.; Kosztin, I.; Kleinekathöfer, U.; Schulten, K. *Physical Review E* **2002**, 65, (3), 031919.
41. Kiang, N. Y.; Siefert, J.; Blankenship, R. E. *Astrobiology* **2007**, 7, (1), 222–251.
42. Guldi, D. M. *Chemical Society Reviews* **2002**, 31, (1), 22–36.
43. Gould, S. J., *Ever since Darwin: Reflections in Natural History.* WW Norton & Company: New York, 1992.
44. Connolly, J.; Bolton, J.; Fox, M.; Chanon, M. *By MA Fox, M. Chanon, Elsevier* **1988**, 303.
45. Wasielewski, M. R. *Chemical Reviews* **1992**, 92, (3), 435–461.
46. Gust, D.; Moore, T. A.; Moore, A. L. *Accounts of Chemical Research* **1993**, 26, (4), 198–205.
47. Kurreck, H.; Huber, M. *Angewandte Chemie International Edition in English* **1995**, 34, (8), 849–866.
48. Gust, D.; Moore, T. A.; Moore, A. L. *Accounts of Chemical Research* **2001**, 34, (1), 40–48.
49. Balzani, V. *Electron Transfer in Chemistry.* Wiley, New York: 2001.
50. Ciamician, G. *Science* **1912**, 36, (926), 385–394.
51. Kadish, K.; Guilard, R.; Smith, K. M. *The Porphyrin Handbook: Applications of Phthalocyanines.* Academic Press, San Diego, CA, 2012.
52. Balzani, V.; Moggi, L.; Scandola, F. Towards a supramolecular photochemistry: Assembly of molecular components to obtain photochemical molecular devices. In *Supramolecular Photochemistry*, Balzani, V. (Ed.) Springer, Dordrecht, the Netherlands: 1987; pp 1–28.
53. Meyer, T. J. *Accounts of Chemical Research* **1989**, 22, (5), 163–170.
54. Lee, D. S.; Qian, H.; Tay, C. Y.; Leong, D. T. *Chemical Society Reviews* **2016**, 45, (15), 4199–4225.
55. Demmig-Adams, B.; Adams, W.; Mattoo, A. *Photoprotection, Photoinhibition, Gene Regulation, and Environment.* Springer Science & Business Media, Dordrecht, the Netherlands: 2006; Vol. 21.
56. Zuber, H.; Cogdell, R. J., Structure and organization of purple bacterial antenna complexes. In *Anoxygenic Photosynthetic Bacteria*, Blankenship, R. E.; Madigan, M. T.; Bauer, C. E., Eds. Springer: Dordrecht, Netherlands, 1995; pp. 315–348.
57. Roy, C.; Lancaster, D.; Ermler, U.; Michel, H. The structures of photosynthetic reaction centers from purple bacteria as revealed by x-ray crystallography. In *Anoxygenic Photosynthetic Bacteria*, Blankenship, R. E.; Madigan, M. T.; Bauer, C. E., Eds. Springer: Dordrecht, the Netherlands, 1995; pp. 503–526.
58. Aagaard, J.; Sistrom, W. R. *Photochemistry and Photobiology* **1972**, 15, (2), 209–225.
59. Cogdell, R. J.; Lindsay, J. G. *Trends in Biotechnology* **1998**, 16, (12), 521–527.
60. Jones, M. R. *Current Biology* **1997**, 7, (9), R541–R543.
61. McDermott, G.; Prince, S. M.; Freer, A. A.; Hawthornthwaite-Lawless, A. M.; Papiz, M. Z.; Cogdell, R. J.; Isaacs, N. W. **1995**, 374, (6522), 517–521.
62. Papiz, M. Z.; Prince, S. M.; Howard, T.; Cogdell, R. J.; Isaacs, N. W. *Journal of Molecular Biology* **2003**, 326, (5), 1523–1538.
63. Roszak, A. W.; Howard, T. D.; Southall, J.; Gardiner, A. T.; Law, C. J.; Isaacs, N. W.; Cogdell, R. J. *Science* **2003**, 302, (5652), 1969–1972.
64. Imahori, H. *The Journal of Physical Chemistry B* **2004**, 108, (20), 6130–6143.
65. Deisenhofer, J.; Epp, O.; Miki, K.; Huber, R.; Michel, H. *Nature* **1985**, 318, 618–624.
66. Zinth, W.; Wachtveitl, J. *ChemPhysChem* **2005**, 6, (5), 871–880.
67. Deisenhofer, J.; Epp, O.; Miki, K.; Huber, R.; Michel, H. *Journal of Molecular Biology* **1984**, 180, (2), 385–398.

68. Jones, M. R.; Visschers, R. W.; Van Grondelle, R.; Hunter, C. N. *Biochemistry* **1992**, 31, (18), 4458–4465.

69. Wraight, C. A.; Clayton, R. K. *Biochimica et Biophysica Acta (BBA): Bioenergetics* **1974**, 333, (2), 246–260.

70. Scholes, G. D.; Fleming, G. R.; Olaya-Castro, A.; van Grondelle, R. **2011**, 3, (10), 763–774.

71. Olson, J. M. *Photochemistry and Photobiology* **1998**, 67, (1), 61–75.

72. Zouni, A.; Witt, H.-T.; Kern, J.; Fromme, P.; Krauss, N.; Saenger, W.; Orth, P. **2001**, 409, (6821), 739–743.

73. Jordana, P.; Fromme, P.; Witt, H. T.; Klukas, O.; Saenger, W.; KrauB, N. *Nature* **2001**, 411, 909–917.

74. Ben-Shem, A.; Frolow, F.; Nelson, N. **2003**, 426, (6967), 630–635.

75. McConnell, I.; Li, G.; Brudvig, G. W. *Chemistry & Biology* **2010**, 17, (5), 434–447.

76. Cogdell, R. J.; Gardiner, A. T.; Hashimoto, H.; Brotosudarmo, T. H. P. *Photochemical & Photobiological Sciences* **2008**, 7, (10), 1150–1158.

77. Hu, X.; Damjanović, A.; Ritz, T.; Schulten, K. *Proceedings of the National Academy of Sciences* **1998**, 95, (11), 5935–5941.

78. Van Grondelle, R. *Biochimica et Biophysica Acta (BBA)-Reviews on Bioenergetics* **1985**, 811, (2), 147–195.

79. van Grondelle, R.; Dekker, J. P.; Gillbro, T.; Sundstrom, V. *Biochimica et Biophysica Acta (BBA)-Bioenergetics* **1994**, 1187, (1), 1–65.

80. Bailey, S.; Grossman, A. *Photochemistry and Photobiology* **2008**, 84, (6), 1410–1420.

81. Larkum, T. *Trends in Plant Science* 1, (8), 252.

82. Frank, H. A.; Cogdell, R. J. *Photochemistry and Photobiology* **1996**, 63, (3), 257–264.

83. Maxwell, D. P.; Falk, S.; Trick, C. G.; Huner, N. P. A. *Plant Physiology* **1994**, 105, (2), 535–543.

84. Teramoto, H.; Nakamori, A.; Minagawa, J.; Ono, T.-a. *Plant Physiology* **2002**, 130, (1), 325–333.

85. Escoubas, J. M.; Lomas, M.; LaRoche, J.; Falkowski, P. G. *Proceedings of the National Academy of Sciences* **1995**, 92, (22), 10237–10241.

86. Yang, D.-H.; Webster, J.; Adam, Z.; Lindahl, M.; Andersson, B. *Plant Physiology* **1998**, 118, (3), 827–834.

87. Durnford, D. G.; Price, J. A.; McKim, S. M.; Sarchfield, M. L. *Physiologia Plantarum* **2003**, 118, (2), 193–205.

88. Melis, A.; Neidhardt, J.; Benemann, J. R. *Journal of Applied Phycology* **1998**, 10, (6), 515–525.

89. Ritz, T.; Park, S.; Schulten, K. *The Journal of Physical Chemistry B* **2001**, 105, (34), 8259–8267.

90. Chow, W. S.; Lee, H.-Y.; He, J.; Hendrickson, L.; Hong, Y.-N.; Matsubara, S. *Photosynthesis Research* **2005**, 84, (1), 35–41.

91. Yamamoto, H. Y. *Pure and Applied Chemistry* **1979**, 51, (3), 639–648.

92. Adams, W. W.; Demmig-Adams, B. *Planta* **1992**, 186, (3), 390–398.

93. Horton, P.; Ruban, A. V.; Walters, R. G. *Annual Review of Plant Physiology and Plant Molecular Biology* **1996**, 47, (1), 655–684.

94. Müller, P.; Li, X.-P.; Niyogi, K. K. *Plant Physiology* **2001**, 125, (4), 1558–1566.

95. Cohen-Bazire, G.; Stanier, R. Y. **1958**, 181, (4604), 250–252.

96. Siefermann-Harms, D. *Physiologia Plantarum* **1987**, 69, (3), 561–568.

97. Demmig-Adams, B.; Adams, W. W. *Trends in Plant Science* **1996**, 1, (1), 21–26.

98. Frank, H. A.; Brudvig, G. W. *Biochemistry* **2004**, 43, (27), 8607–8615.

99. Moore, T. A.; Moore, A. L.; Gust, D. *Philosophical Transactions of the Royal Society B: Biological Sciences* **2002**, 357, (1426), 1481–1498.

100. Page, C. C.; Moser, C. C.; Chen, X.; Dutton, P. L. **1999**, 402, (6757), 47–52.

101. Lin, X.; Murchison, H. A.; Nagarajan, V.; Parson, W. W.; Allen, J. P.; Williams, J. C. *Proceedings of the National Academy of Sciences* **1994**, 91, (22), 10265–10269.
102. Kalyanasundaram, K.; Graetzel, M. *Current Opinion in Biotechnology* **2010**, 21, (3), 298–310.
103. Hammarström, L.; Styring, S. *Philosophical Transactions of the Royal Society of London B: Biological Sciences* **2008**, 363, (1494), 1283–1291.
104. Kirstein, S.; Daehne, S. *International Journal of Photoenergy* **2006**, 2006, 21.
105. Allwood, J. L.; Burrell, A. K.; Officer, D. L.; Scott, S. M.; Wild, K. Y.; Gordon, K. C. *Chemical Communications* **2000**, (9), 747–748.
106. Gust, D.; Moore, T. A.; Moore, A. L. *Accounts of Chemical Research* **2009**, 42, (12), 1890–1898.
107. Gust, D. *Nature* **1997**, 386, (6620), 21–22.
108. Frischmann, P. D.; Mahata, K.; Wurthner, F. *Chemical Society Reviews* **2013**, 42, (4), 1847–1870.
109. Grossman, A. R.; Bhaya, D.; He, Q. *Journal of Biological Chemistry* **2001**, 276, (15), 11449–11452.
110. Bibby, T. S.; Nield, J.; Barber, J. **2001**, 412, (6848), 743–745.
111. Boekema, E. J.; Hifney, A.; Yakushevska, A. E.; Piotrowski, M.; Keegstra, W.; Berry, S.; Michel, K. P.; Pistorius, E. K.; Kruip, J. **2001**, 412, (6848), 745–748.
112. Nakamura, Y.; Aratani, N.; Osuka, A. *Chemical Society Reviews* **2007**, 36, (6), 831–845.
113. Serroni, S.; Campagna, S.; Puntoriero, F.; Loiseau, F.; Ricevuto, V.; Passalacqua, R.; Galletta, M. *Comptes Rendus Chimie* **2003**, 6, (8–10), 883–893.
114. Balzani, V.; Credi, A.; Venturi, M. *ChemSusChem* **2008**, 1, (1–2), 26–58.
115. Guldi, D. M.; Luo, C.; Swartz, A.; Scheloske, M.; Hirsch, A. *Chemical Communications* **2001**, (12), 1066–1067.
116. Wasielewski, M. R. *The Journal of Organic Chemistry* **2006**, 71, (14), 5051–5066.
117. Wasielewski, M. R. *Acc. Chem. Res.* **2009**, 42, (12), 1910–1921.
118. Niinemets, Ü.; Sack, L. Structural determinants of leaf light-harvesting capacity and photosynthetic potentials. In *Progress in Botany*, Esser, K.; Lüttge, U.; Beyschlag, W.; Murata, J., Eds. Springer: Berlin, Germany, 2006; pp. 385–419.
119. Shimoni, E.; Rav-Hon, O.; Ohad, I.; Brumfeld, V.; Reich, Z. *The Plant Cell* **2005**, 17, (9), 2580–2586.
120. Smith, W. K.; Vogelmann, T. C.; DeLucia, E. H.; Bell, D. T.; Shepherd, K. A. C. *BioScience* **1997**, 47, (11), 785–793.
121. Vogelmann, T. C.; Martin, G. *Plant, Cell & Environment* **1993**, 16, (1), 65–72.
122. DeLucia, E. H.; Nelson, K.; Vogelmann, T. C.; Smith, W. K. *Plant, Cell & Environment* **1996**, 19, (2), 159–170.
123. Nikolopoulos, D.; Liakopoulos, G.; Drossopoulos, I.; Karabourniotis, G. *Plant Physiology* **2002**, 129, (1), 235–243.
124. Zhou, H.; Li, X.; Fan, T.; Osterloh, F. E.; Ding, J.; Sabio, E. M.; Zhang, D.; Guo, Q. *Advanced Materials* **2010**, 22, (9), 951–956.
125. Poulson, M. E.; Vogelmann, T. C. *Plant, Cell & Environment* **1990**, 13, (8), 803–811.
126. Maier, S. W.; Lüdeker, W.; Günther, K. P. *Remote Sensing of Environment* **1999**, 68, (3), 273–280.
127. Kumar, R.; Silva, L. *Applied Optics* **1973**, 12, (12), 2950–2954.
128. Govaerts, Y. M.; Jacquemoud, S.; Verstraete, M. M.; Ustin, S. L. *Applied Optics* **1996**, 35, (33), 6585–6598.
129. Ort, D. R.; Yocum, C. F. Electron transfer and energy transduction in photosynthesis: An overview. In *Oxygenic Photosynthesis: The Light Reactions*, Ort, D. R.; Yocum, C. F.; Heichel, I. F., Eds. Springer: Dordrecht, the Netherlands, 1996; pp. 1–9.
130. Maeda, K.; Eguchi, M.; Youngblood, W. J.; Mallouk, T. E. *Chemistry of Materials* **2008**, 20, (21), 6770–6778.

131. Peng, T.; Ke, D.; Cai, P.; Dai, K.; Ma, L.; Zan, L. *Journal of Power Sources* **2008**, 180, (1), 498–505.
132. Lakshminarasimhan, N.; Bae, E.; Choi, W. *The Journal of Physical Chemistry C* **2007**, 111, (42), 15244–15250.
133. Li, Q.; Chen, L.; Lu, G. *The Journal of Physical Chemistry C* **2007**, 111, (30), 11494–11499.
134. Ruban, A. V. *Communicative & Integrative Biology* **2009**, 2, (1), 50–55.
135. Li, X.; Fan, T.; Zhou, H.; Chow, S.-K.; Zhang, W.; Zhang, D.; Guo, Q.; Ogawa, H. *Advanced Functional Materials* **2009**, 19, (1), 45–56.
136. Zeng, M.; Li, Y.; Mao, M.; Bai, J.; Ren, L.; Zhao, X. *ACS Catalysis* **2015**, 5, (6), 3278–3286.
137. Boghossian, A. A.; Ham, M.-H.; Choi, J. H.; Strano, M. S. *Energy & Environmental Science* **2011**, 4, (10), 3834–3843.
138. Meunier, C. F.; Rooke, J. C.; Leonard, A.; Xie, H.; Su, B.-L. *Chemical Communications* **2010**, 46, (22), 3843–3859.
139. Meunier, C. F.; Rooke, J. C.; Leonard, A.; Van Cutsem, P.; Su, B.-L. *Journal of Materials Chemistry* **2010**, 20, (5), 929–936.
140. Meunier, C. F.; Dandoy, P.; Su, B.-L. *Journal of Colloid and Interface Science* **2010**, 342, (2), 211–224.
141. Koch, K.; Bhushan, B.; Barthlott, W. *Progress in Materials Science* **2009**, 54, (2), 137–178.
142. Melis, A. *Trends in Plant Science* 4, (4), 130–135.
143. Ham, M.-H.; Choi, J. H.; Boghossian, A. A.; Jeng, E. S.; Graff, R. A.; Heller, D. A.; Chang, A. C. et al., **2010**, 2, (11), 929–936.
144. Zhou, H.; Fan, T.; Zhang, D. *ChemCatChem* **2011**, 3, (3), 513–528.
145. Calzaferri, G. *Topics in Catalysis* **2010**, 53, (3), 130–140.
146. Calzaferri, G.; Lutkouskaya, K. *Photochemical & Photobiological Sciences* **2008**, 7, (8), 879–910.
147. Brühwiler, D.; Dieu, L.-Q.; Calzaferri, G. *CHIMIA International Journal for Chemistry* **2007**, 61, (12), 820–822.
148. Maas, H.; Calzaferri, G. *Angewandte Chemie International Edition* **2002**, 41, (13), 2284–2288.
149. Minkowski, C.; Pansu, R.; Takano, M.; Calzaferri, G. *Advanced Functional Materials* **2006**, 16, (2), 273–285.
150. Yatskou, M. M.; Meyer, M.; Huber, S.; Pfenniger, M.; Calzaferri, G. *ChemPhysChem* **2003**, 4, (6), 567–587.
151. Ravi, S. K.; Udayagiri, V. S.; Suresh, L.; Tan, S. C. *Advanced Functional Materials* **2018**, 28, 1705305.
152. Ravi, S. K.; Yu, Z.; Swainsbury, D. J. K.; Ouyang, J.; Jones, M. R.; Tan, S. C. *Advanced Energy Materials* **2017**, 7, 1601821.
153. Singh, V. K.; Ravi, S. K.; Ho, J. W.; Wong, J. K. C.; Jones, M. R.; Tan, S. C. *Advanced Functional Materials* **2018**, 28, 1703689.
154. Pamu, R.; Sandireddy, V. P.; Kalyanaraman, R.; Khomami, B.; Mukherjee, D. *The Journal of Physical Chemistry Letters* **2018**, 9, 970–977.
155. Robinson, M. T.; Armbruster, M. E.; Gargye, A.; Cliffel, D. E.; Jennings, G. K. *ACS Applied Energy Materials* **2018**, 1, (2), 301–305.

2 Developments in Electrodes and Electrolytes of Dye-Sensitized Solar Cells

Ajay K. Kushwaha, Nagaraju Mokurala,
Krishnaiah Mokurala, and Siddhartha Suman

CONTENTS

2.1   INTRODUCTION

Global warming is the most challenging problem of the present era that arises due to extensive and uncontrolled use of fossil fuels/conventional energy sources. Switching toward renewable energy sources could be a suitable option to overcome the global warming problem. In some content, energy research is very much inclined toward nonconventional, renewable, and environmentally friendly energy sources. Moreover, conventional energy sources are limited; thus, development of non-conventional energy resources is an important task. Among various nonconventional energy sources, solar light has sufficient energy supply that is required for humans on Earth. If the solar energy that strikes on Earth in an hour can be harvested by any means, it will be more than enough to use for an entire year by humans.[1] However, the major challenge is to convert this energy into a usable form and create efficient storage that allows its usage when solar light is not available.

Harvesting of solar energy is possible in various ways, and solar cells have shown excellent potential to convert solar energy (light) into electrical energy. However, limited/lower efficiency of solar cells is the major concern, along with materials cost, processing, durability, and cost per unit power generation—all of which are existing challenges. To resolve these challenges, various types of materials and solar cell devices have been demonstrated and fabricated by different researchers.[2] In similar content, dye-sensitized solar cells (DSSCs) came into the picture due to interesting features such as easy processing and low-cost materials usability. Although DSSCs are prominent in various fronts, cell stability, durability, and low efficiency are existing tasks to be addressed. Several attempts have been made by various researchers across the globe to find solutions for these challenges of DSSCs. In the last decade significant progress has been observed in efficiency enhancement of DSSCs, as shown in Figure 2.1. The porphyrin dyes were used to increase the cell efficiency by using TiO_2 as anode and even using ruthenium as a dye to enhance cell efficiency.[3] Mesoscopic photoanode-based DSSCs were reported by Takeru Bessho et al. in 2010; they integrated porphyrin chromophore to bridge the dye, which resulted in a new conjugate leading to efficiency of 11%.[4] The light-harvesting nature of plants was studied by Li et al. in 2013,[5] and the idea was to use artificial chlorophylls to develop the DSSCs, which have shown 12.3% efficiency. Recently, a low-cost carbon material with triiodide was incorporated by Bora et al.[6] in 2017 to develop a low-cost device that has shown 13% efficiency.[7] Much more work has been done in the past several years, and it has been noted that DSSCs have achieved a fair amount of efficiency; further efforts are being made to develop more efficient DSSC devices.

The research and development in dye-sensitized solar cells (DSSCs) are trending high, and such enhancement in efficiency is achieved by optimization of photoanode design, sensitizers/dyes, and electrolytes. The development of stable photoanode materials with economical production cost is an important concern for energy conversion. Most of the presented photoanode have shown facile fabrication with low-cost precursors that leads to fabrication of relatively inexpensive solar cells. In the present chapter, recent advancements in the areas of photoanode, cathode, and electrolytes are presented. The progress on sensitizer development for DSSCs is also discussed. The dye-sensitized solar cell has the ability to develop efficient cells by addressing the various issues of electrodes and electrolyte design.

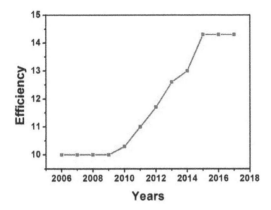

FIGURE 2.1 Enhancement in efficiency of DSSCs (with TiO_2 photoanode) within last 10 years' time frame. (From Li, S.-L. et al., *Chem. Commun.*, 2, 2792, 2006; Bessho, T. et al., *Angew. Chemie: Int. Ed.*, 49, 6646–6649, 2010; Li, L.-L. and Diau, E.W.-G., *Chem. Soc. Rev.*, 42, 291–304, 2013; Bora, A. et al. *Electrochim. Acta*, 259, 233–244, 2017; Campbell, W.M. et al. *J. Phys. Chem. C*, 111, 11760–11762, 2007; Han, L. et al. *Energy Environ. Sci.*, 5, 6057, 2012; Son, D.Y. et al., *J. Phys. Chem. C*, 118, 16567–16573, 2014; Yella, A. et al., *Angew. Chemie: Int. Ed.*, 53, 2973–2977, 2014; Yao, Z. et al. *J. Am. Chem. Soc.*, 137, 3799–3802, 2015; Huang, C.Y.C.L. et al., *Thin Solid Films*, 4, 153–158, 2016.)

In comparison with silicon-based solar cells, the power conversion efficiency (PCE) of DSSCs is moderate; however, fabrication cost is lower—and that makes it a preferred and prospective future device for harvesting of solar energy.

2.2 COMPONENTS AND WORKING PRINCIPLE OF DYE-SENSITIZED SOLAR CELLS (DSSCs)

The invention of a dye-sensitized solar cell (DSSC) is attributed to Brian O'Regan and Michael Gratzel, who in 1991 successfully developed an efficient DSSC device.[14] The solar cell was based on the design of a photoelectrochemical cell, in which a thin layer of solar light active material was sandwiched between two transparent conducting films, as shown in Figure 2.2. The light active material is commonly known as *"dye"* or *"sensitizer."* Doped tin oxides with TiO_2 films or nanostructures are commonly used as conducting transparent electrodes. The sensitizer or dye is loaded on a metal-oxide platform. This platform helps in transportation of photo-generated charge carriers and is known as a photoanode. The DSSC consists of one more electrode called a cathode. Moreover, an electrolyte material is filled in between these two electrodes to complete the energy conversion process. These components of the DSSC are briefly discussed as follows.

2.2.1 PHOTOANODE

A photoanode is mostly fabricated by transparent conducting of oxides and a layer of metal-oxide film or nanostructures. It works as a platform for loading of dye or

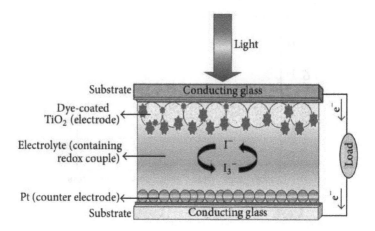

FIGURE 2.2 Schematic diagram of dye-sensitized solar cells (DSSCs) with titanium dioxide (TiO_2) nanoparticles as photoanode and platinum as counter electrodes. (Reproduced from Kushwaha, R. et al. *J. Energy*, 2013, 1–12, 2013 of Hindavi.)

sensitizer. The photoanode is transparent in nature for visible light, so that photons can transmit towards dye to harvests solar energy. It deals with injection, collection, and transportation of photogenerated charges to produce electrical energy. In a typical device, the size of the photoanode is normally decided by the kind of material chosen. TiO_2 is commonly applied and an intensively investigated material due to its high chemical stability and wide bandgap. Several techniques have been developed for direct growth of TiO_2 thin film on conducting electrodes. In Section 2.4 of this chapter, further discussion about different growth process for metal oxides films, nanostructures, and composite materials is presented.

2.2.2 COUNTER ELECTRODE

The counter electrode, also known as auxiliary electrode, is one of the essential components to complete the circuit in the electrochemical cell. The counter electrode should be inert in nature—for example, Pt, Au, graphite, glassy carbon kind of materials. The reason for the electrode to be inert is it should not participate in the reaction. In the DSSC, the current flows from working electrode to counter electrode; therefore, the surface area of the counter electrode must be higher than the working electrode. The area of the counter electrode should not become a limiting factor in the kinetics of the process. It can also be explained as the interface where the oxidized species present in the electrolyte solution are reduced.[16] The counter electrode plays a vital role to support the redox mechanism, where counter electrode performs the reduction mechanism in the electrolyte thereby oxidizing the photovoltaic electrode. Usually, platinum-coated FTO glass substrate is used as a counter electrode because it offers better electron transfer in reverse order with less resistance. Graphite, carbon black[17] and carbon nanotubes,[17] and graphene[18] on FTO have also been demonstrated as counter electrodes as discussed in Section 2.5.

2.2.3 Sensitizer

Absorption/harvesting of the solar light is the main feature of the sensitizer or dye that governs the performance of the DSSCs. It converts the light energy into electrical energy by means of electron-hole generation. The sensitizer's properties and loading amount have a significant role in light-harvesting and power efficiencies. The sensitizer should have a nature to harvest a wider spectrum of solar energy, and it should also adopt the surface of the photoanode to inject electrons.

2.2.4 Electrolyte

The electrolyte consists of ions for the interaction with electrodes, where redox reaction takes place to have the electrons flow toward the counter electrode for successful completion of the process. The overall performance of the DSSC is affected by leakage, evaporation, stability of the electrolyte, and reaction with sensitizer and electrode materials.[19–21] Therefore, the electrolyte has direct impact on DSSC efficiency, and a careful consideration of the electrolyte is required to design a more efficient solar cell.[20] The liquid electrolytes have received more attention due to their high ionic conductivity; however, solid or semisolid electrolytes are also gaining popularity due to their ease of processing in devices and better stability.[21] A more detailed discussion on electrolytes is given in Section 2.6.

2.2.5 Working Principle of Dye-Sensitized Solar Cell

In the DSSC, the light-harvesting process starts when the photon interacts with photosensitizer. The sensitizer absorbs the photon and reaches an electronically excited state (X^*), as shown in Figure 2.3. At an excited state, the photosensitizer delivers an electron to the conduction band of the photoanode. The process is called injection of electron. This electron moves through the mesoporous structure of the photoanode to reach the collector electrode (transparent conducting electrode). Since the sensitizer is in contact with the electrolyte that has a mediator in the form of an iodide, it brings back the sensitizer to a normal state. There is no change in chemical composition of the reactants; thus, an overall energy conversion take place. The step-by-step working principle is described as follows.[22]

Step 1: Initially, the sensitizer/dye is in a ground state (S). When the photon of appropriate energy is illuminated on the cell, dye molecules acquire the energy and excite to a higher energy level, as depicted in Equation (2.1).

$$S + hv = S^*$$ (2.1)

Step 2: The excited molecules (S^*) inject the electron to the conduction band of the photoanode. Due to a difference in energy level of photoanode material and sensitizer/dye, free motion of electrons takes place. Now, the excited molecule converts into an oxidized molecule (S^+) as shown in Equation (2.2).

$$S^* \rightarrow S^+ + e^-$$ (2.2)

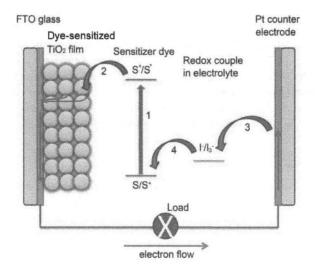

FIGURE 2.3 Working principle of DSSC, sensitizer absorbs the illuminated photons (sunlight) and produces electron-hole pairs followed by separation and collection of electrons. (Wu, Y. and Zhu, W., *Chem. Soc. Rev.*, 42, 2039–2058, 2013. Reproduced by permission of The Royal Society of Chemistry.)

The electron transfer takes place in a microsecond to millisecond time range. During this time, there are several chances to have a recombination of photogenerated charge carriers. It has an adverse effect on photovoltaic performance. Therefore, control over an undesired recombination should be seriously considered during device design and fabrication. Sensitizer molecular enhancement is commonly adopted to reduce the recombination. This is done by orienting the molecular structure in such a way that the photogenerated charge should get more time for separation leading to lower recombination.[23]

Step 3: The oxidized molecule (S^+) that is generated due to the emission of electrons is returned to its original state by reacting iodide molecules, as depicted in Equation (2.3)

$$2S^+ + 3I^- \rightarrow 2S + I_3^- \tag{2.3}$$

Step 4: Due to the interaction of the electrolyte with the counter electrode, iodide ions are regenerated by reducing the triiodide on the cathode part of the cell, as depicted in Equation (2.4).

$$I_3 + e^- \rightarrow 3I^- \tag{2.4}$$

Regeneration of charges is a very important factor in getting better efficiency. The electrolyte of the DSSC consists of ions to get transfer from one place to another; therefore, the mediator must get ready to regenerate charges. This should not absorb sunlight to avoid losses comprising photon to current. The drawback of using a liquid electrolyte is the leakage taking place in the device and the corrosive nature of the material;

therefore, researchers have been exploring ways to replace the liquid electrolyte with an alternative redox system.[24]

The interaction between the LUMO orbitals of the sensitizer/dye and the accepting states of the metal-oxide electrode are generally overlapping in nature. The distance between both the parts shows a strong injecting phenomenon. Thus, the excitation of the photosensitizer will result in migration of the electron to the electrode surface.[23] Now, the electrons are getting transported to the collector part of the anode, a phenomenon known as diffusion process.

2.3   CHARACTERIZATION AND PERFORMANCE MEASUREMENT OF DYE-SENSITIZED SOLAR CELL

The efficiency of a dye-sensitized solar cell is calculated in a similar manner to other solar cells. The *I-V* curve provides information related to power generated by the cell including various other parameters. The performance of a DSSC was evaluated based on photovoltage, photocurrent, fill factor, solar-to- electrical energy conversion, and photocurrent converting factor. The current-voltage (*I-V*) plot in dark and light represents the performance of the solar cell, as depicted in Figure 2.4. The open-circuit potential is measured, when there is no load, and it implies flow of zero current and the voltage across the cell is at maximum value (V_{oc}). The other important parameter is short-circuit current (I_{sc})—when both the contact of the DSSC is connected, the connection allows a large amount of current to flow and have a zero potential across it. When the current reaches to its maximum value, it is said to be a short- circuit current. The points located in between the open-circuit voltage and short-circuit current develop maximum power, known as the maximum power point.

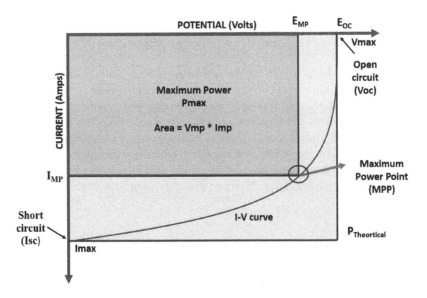

FIGURE 2.4   *I-V* plot for performance evaluation of dye-sensitized solar cell.

At this point, the solar cell produces maximum power. The point where the power reaches maximum is located as I_{mp} and V_{mp} in the graph.

Photocurrent conversion efficiency is the measurement of overall quantum phenomena of charges that are getting generated due to a single source of light equivalent to one sun. The charge generation only occurs when the light of suitable wavelength is illuminated on a solar cell device leads to the movement of a photoelectron toward the external load. The light harvesting at a wavelength can be expressed in terms of quantum yield of injected electron; this arises from the sensitizer into the conduction band. The photocurrent conversion efficiency is largely dependent upon the amount of dye getting adsorbed or loaded onto the metal oxide platform. The photocurrent conversion efficiency of the DSSC can be calculated using the following formula.[25]

$$\eta = \frac{V_{oc} \times I_{sc} \times FF}{P_{in}}$$

where:

V_{oc} is the value of open-circuit voltage
I_{sc} is the value of short-circuit current
FF is the fill factor
P_{in} is the input power

The current value (I_{sc}) is measured when the DSSC is short-circuited and illuminated with solar light.[26] The short-circuit current can be evaluated as follows.

$$I_{sc} = qG\left(L_n + L_p\right)$$

where:

q is the value of charge in electron volts
G is generation rate
L_n and L_p are the electron and hole diffusion lengths, respectively

To achieve higher photocurrent, the dye must have a large sunlight-harvesting capability and very strong interaction between sensitizer and the surface.

The open-circuit potential is the potential difference between the terminals of the cell under the illumination of light in an open-circuit condition. The value of photovoltage of the DSSC should be maximum as it corresponds to the energy gap between the conduction band of the sensitizer to the electrolyte. However, in practical cases the value of the photovoltage is less than the theoretical value due to the recombination of electrons with electrolyte and dye. The open-circuit potential can be given as follows.[26]

$$V_{oc} = \frac{nkT}{q} \ln\left(\frac{I_L}{I_o} + 1\right)$$

where:

n is the ideal factor
K is the value of Boltzmann constant
T is the value of temperature in kelvin

q is the value of charge

I_L is the light-generated current

I_o is the dark saturation current

Fill factor indicates toward the amount of maximum power output delivered in response to the input power to the cell. This is determined by the curve drawn between the current density and the voltage applied and the area between the curves.[26]

$$\text{Fill Factor}\left(\text{FF}\right) = \frac{I_{mp} \times V_{mp}}{I_{sc} \times V_{oc}}$$

where:

I_{mp} is the current at maximum point

V_{mp} is the corresponding voltage at maximum power point

V_{oc} is the value of open circuit voltage

I_{sc} is the value of short circuit current

2.4 DEVELOPMENTS IN PHOTOANODES

The photoanode is the most important component of the DSSC and strongly influences the performance of the cell. Mostly metal oxides have been applied as photoanode in DSSCs; however, a variety of other materials have also been proposed and demonstrated. Here, various metal-oxides and hybrid materials-based electrodes are discussed to get an idea of their role in the DSSC. Moreover, introduction of various kinds of nanostructures in the photoanode is also reviewed, and their impact on solar cell performance is presented.

2.4.1 METAL-OXIDES (TiO_2, ZnO, SnO_2 and Nb_2O_5) BASED PHOTOANODE

The role of the photoanode in the DSSC is to support/load the dye molecules and provide an efficient path for electron transfer/injection. The TiO_2 is the most commonly used material for the photoanode along with other metal oxides such as ZnO and SnO_2. The wide bandgap, excellent chemical stability, low cost, and non-toxicity of TiO_2 are the major criteria to select it as photoanode material. A mesoporous TiO_2 (titania) layer-based photoanode has shown reasonably good performance, and its efficiency was further improved by placing a dense (compact) layer of titania between the mesoporous layer and the TCO substrate. Introduction of a scattering layer of large titania particles over the mesoporous layer is also demonstrated. It improves the light-harvesting capability of the photoanode.[27–29] Thus, the overall photoanode had a compact titania layer (25–50 nm thick) followed by a 12–14 µm mesoporous titania layer and scattering layer of 4–5 µm.[28] The function of the dense layer is to prevent the direct contact between the electrolyte interface and FTO, which effectively prohibits charge recombination at the FTO and mesoporous layer (TiO_2) interface.[28] The task of the mesoporous TiO_2 layer (to provide sufficiently high surface area) is to adsorb dye molecules and to transport electrons that are injected by the sensitizer.[27] The mesoporous TiO_2 films with particles size around 20–25 nm and pore diameter around 12 nm have shown optimum performance

TABLE 2.1

TiO$_2$ Nanoparticles-Based Photoanode for DSSC, Synthesized Using Various Methods and Their Power Conversion Efficiencies

Synthesis Method	Photocurrent (mA.cm^{-2})	Open-Circuit Voltage (V)	Fill Factor (%)	Efficiency (%)	References
Hydrothermal	9.64	0.815	68	5.45	33
Two-step hydrothermal	14.80	0.756	63	7.06	34
Electrospray	9.19	0.77	71	6.81	35
Freezer drying	14.83	0.73	65	6.97	36
Sol-gel	10.09	0.69	52	9.70	37
Electric discharge	—	—	—	5.37	38

of the DSSCs.[27,30,31] TiO$_2$ nanoparticles-based photoanodes have achieved 14.3% power conversion efficiency.[32] The fabrication process of TiO$_2$ nanoparticles/photoanodes also plays a significant role in governing the performance of the DSSC. Table 2.1 compares the performance of the DSSC, in which TiO$_2$ nanoparticles photoanodes are synthesized using different methods.

Although TiO$_2$ nanoparticles-based photoanodes have shown excellent potential for the DSSC, the electron ejection and transportation are not very efficient due to the mesoporous nature and presence of large grain boundaries. The amount of dye loading is relatively higher in nanoparticles photoanodes as compare to thin film based photoanode. However, there is a possibility to accommodate more dye molecules in the photoanode by surface-engineering and nanostructuring the photoanode. Therefore, various morphologies of TiO$_2$ nanostructures were investigated by different researchers.[39–42] A few examples are nanorods,[43] nanofibers,[44] nanotubes,[42] nanowires[45] of TiO$_2$, as compared in Figure 2.5. These nanostructures were synthesized using a variety of methods including hydrothermal, solvothermal, DC reactive magnetron sputtering, and microwave assisted, etc. Table 2.2 depicts that single crystalline nanorods have shown better performance because they offer direct electrical transport to electrodes.[46]

1-D nanostructures such as oriented nanorods/nanotubes/nanowires provide a better directional way to enhance the charge separation and electron transport.[47–51] Higher surface areas have better potential to simplify the dye absorption movement, increase the optical absorption due to light scattering effects, and decrease the recombination loss.[52] Also, 3-D hierarchical nanostructures of TiO$_2$ materials are proposed for the photoanode of the DSSC. These 3-D hierarchical structures enhance the light-harvesting, dye-loading capability of the photoanode[53] and also provide a higher specific pore volume.[54] The combination of nanowires/nanoparticles has rendered the PCE of the DSSC around 6.01%.[55] The experimental and theoretical investigations have proven the suitability of TiO$_2$ material in the photoanode of the DSSC. It is anonymously accepted that improvement in electrical conductivity of the photoanode can further boost DSSC performance; therefore, several other semiconducting metal oxides are also investigated to use as photoanode materials.

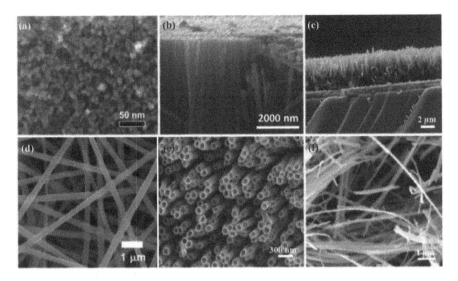

FIGURE 2.5 SEM images of TiO$_2$ nanostructures that display a variety of morphologies such as (a) nanoparticles (Reproduced from Dalod, A.R.M. et al., Beilstein J. Nanotechnol., 8, 304–312, 2017.), (b) nanorods (Reproduced from *Thin Solid Films*, 577, Meng, L. et al., 103–108, Copyright 2015, with permission from Elsevier.), (c) cross-sectional view of nanorods (Reproduced with permission from Yang, M. et al., *J. Phys. Chem. C*, 115, 14534–14541, 2011. Copyright 2011 American Chemical Society.), (d) nanofibers (Reproduced with permission from Chuangchote, S. et al., *Appl. Phys. Lett.*, 93, 5–8, 2008. Copyright 2010 by the American Institute of Physics.), (e) nanotubes (Reproduced with permission from Sharmoukh, W. and Allam, N.K., *ACS Appl. Mater. Interfaces*, 4, 4413–4418, 2012. Copyright 2012 American Chemical Society.), and (f) nanowires. (Reproduced from *Phys. Lett.*, 365, Zhang, Y.X. et al., 300–304, Copyright 2002, with permission from Elsevier.)

TABLE 2.2
Different Morphologies of TiO$_2$ Photoanode and PCE Efficiency of DSSC

Morphology of TiO$_2$	Synthesis Methods	Photocurrent (mA.cm^{-2})	Open Circuit Voltage (V)	Fill Factor (%)	Efficiency (%)	References
Nanorods	Hydrothermal	17.75	0.75	70	9.2	39
Nano-fibers	Electro spun	22.4	0.64	72	10.30	47
Nanotubes	Anodization	22.60	0.79	55	9.8	48
Nanowires	Sol-gel	13.10	0.71	57	5.40	49
	Hydrothermal	13.97	0.82	64	7.34	45
	One step solvothermal	17.38	0.687	74	8.90	50
	Two-step hydrothermal	13.60	0.78	68	7.20	51
	Dip coating	16.22	0.792	77.5	9.95	13

Zinc oxide is another popular and widely studied material for the photoanode of the DSSC due to its similar properties as TiO_2. The facile synthesis of ZnO nanostructures with controlled growth makes it very promising. ZnO also has a wide bandgap that is suitable for developing transparent photoanode. The large exciton energy, more abundance, high electron mobility, and low crystallization temperature are added advantages in ZnO.[59] Further, a higher flat-band potential of ZnO can effectively contribute to enhance the open-circuit voltage of the cell.[60] The DSSC has shown a 3.92% and 7.07% power conversion efficiency when ZnO nanoparticles and nanosheets were used as photoanode material.[60,61] There are different routes for synthesis of ZnO nanostructures as reported by various researchers, and this has significant impact on DSSC performance. The ZnO photoanode with different morphologies of nanostructure and their efficiencies are shown in Table 2.3. Figure 2.6 shows few examples of the ZnO morphologies (nanoparticles, nanowires, nanosheets, nanorods, nanofibers, etc.) that have been adopted in photoanode to fabricate DSSC. ZnO nanorods-nanosheets hierarchical architecture,[62] photoanode was demonstrated to develop the flexible DSSC. The ZnO nanostructures-based photoanode has shown moderate efficiency of the DSSC. The comparison in J–V characteristics of DSSCs can be seen in Figure 2.7, when two different morphologies

TABLE 2.3
The DSSC Performance of Metal-Oxides Photoanode Based DSSC Using Different Morphology

Morphology of Metal-Exide Photoanodes	Photocurrent (mA.cm^{-2})	Open Circuit Voltage (V)	Fill Factor (%)	Efficiency (%)	References
ZnO-nanosheets	19.53	0.58	0.63	7.07	61
ZnO-nanoparticles	16.09	0.57	0.59	5.40	67
ZnO-nanoflowers	5.50	0.65	0.53	1.90	83
ZnO-nanotubes	11.51	0.69	0.22	1.60	84
ZnO-nanofibres	8.45	0.49	0.40	1.66	85
ZnO-nanodisk	6.92	0.69	52.50	2.49	86
ZnO-nanocones	15.00	0.64	0.45	4.36	87
SnO$_2$-nanoparticles	12.7	0.677	0.50	4.30	70
SnO$_2$-nanoflake	5.17	0.32	39	0.62	71
SnO$_2$-nanoflowers	4.36	0.43	36	1.11	88
SnO$_2$-nanotubes	7.99	0.49	0.27	1.06	72
SnO$_2$-Thin film	2.07	0.23	30.37	0.14	71
SnO$_2$-nanofibers	14.9	0.702	50	5.44	70
SnO$_2$-nanowires	5.7	0.522	49.5	2.22	89
SnO$_2$-nanobelt	16.91	0.690	51	5.76	59
Nb$_2$O$_5$-nanorod	11.2	0.74	66	6.03	75
Nb$_2$O$_5$-fibers	6.68	0.77	59	3.05	90
Nb$_2$O$_5$-nanopores	10	0.7	58	4.1	81
Nb$_2$O$_5$-nano-channel	17.6	0.639	39	4.48	79
Nb$_2$O$_5$-nanoforest	6.6	0.71	49	2.41	82

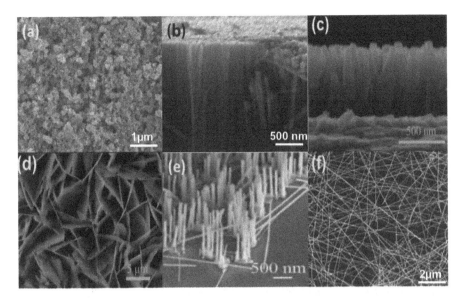

FIGURE 2.6 SEM images of ZnO nanostructures having different morphologies: (a) nanoparticles (Reproduced from Ref. 60 with permission of Elsevier), (b) nanowires (Reproduced from *Ceram. Int.*, Zi, M. et al., 1–6, Copyright 2014, with permission from Elsevier.), (c) cross-sectional image of nanowires (Reproduced from *Ceram. Int.*, Zi, M. et al., 1–6, Copyright 2014, with permission from Elsevier.), (d) nanosheets (Lin, C.-Y. et al., *Energy Environ. Sci.*, 4, 3448, 2011. Reproduced from The Royal Society of Chemistry.), (e) nanorods (Reproduced with permission from Wang, X. et al., *Nano Lett.*, 4, 423–426, 2004. Copyright 2004 American Chemical Society.), and (f) nanofibers. (Reproduced from *Ceram. Int.*, Zi, M. et al., 1–6, Copyright 2014, with permission from Elsevier.)

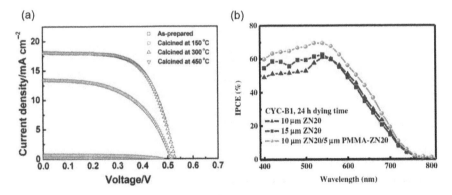

FIGURE 2.7 J–V characteristic of the DSSCs based on (a) ZnO nanosheets-based photoanode, when heat treated at different temperatures. (Lin, C.-Y. et al., *Energy Environ. Sci.*, 4, 3448, 2011. Reproduced by permission of The Royal Society of Chemistry.) (b) photoanode fabricated using different size of ZnO nanoparticles. (Reproduced *J. Power Sources*, 246, Lee, C.P. et al., 1–9, Copyright 2014, with permission from Elsevier.)

named as nanosheets and nanoparticles are adopted in the photoanode. Although ZnO has shown excellent potential as photoanode materials, the instability in acidic dye/media, high charge recombination, and huge surface defects are the existing challenges.

SnO_2 is another alternative material that has been demonstrated to apply in the photoanode. It has a faster rate of electron capture by the redox electrolyte and higher electron mobility.[68] It has better stability in comparison to TiO_2 and ZnO.[68] However, the slow electron diffusion, high electron recombination, lower surface area, and lower conduction band edge compared to another metal oxide are limiting factors for SnO_2. These challenges can be solved by optimizing the size and morphology of the SnO_2 nanostructure. SnO_2 nanoparticles based photoanode has some limitation that is, faster recombination of electrons with electrolyte. However, it was reported that by controlling the shape and structure of SnO_2, the performance of the DSSC can be improved.[69] Also, 1-D nanostructures of SnO_2 are considered as photoanode material to overcome the recombination of electrons. The various morphologies (Figure 2.8)—that is, nanotubes and porous nanofibers of SnO_2—have been reported and their comparative performances are presented in Table 2.3. Although the conductivity and stability are better in the case of SnO_2 photoanode, the performance of the SnO_2 photoanode-based DSSC is lower in comparison to TiO_2-based and ZnO-based photoanodes.

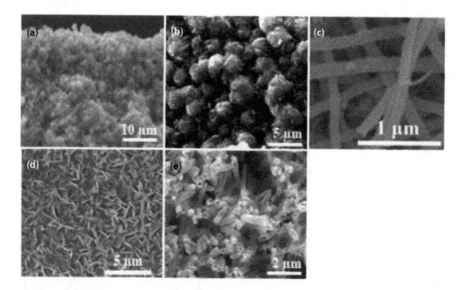

FIGURE 2.8 SEM images of SnO_2 photoanodes having different morphologies: (a) nanoparticles (Wang, Y.-F. et al., *RSC Adv.*, 3, 13804, 2013. Reproduced by permission of The Royal Society of Chemistry.), (b) nanoflowers (Reproduced with permission from Elumalai, N.K. et al., *J. Phys. Chem. C*, 116, 22112–22120, 2012. Copyright 2012 American Chemical Society.), (c) nanowires (Reproduced with permission from Elumalai, N.K. et al., *J. Phys. Chem. C*, 116, 22112–22120, 2012. Copyright 2012 American Chemical Society.), (d) nanoflakes (Reproduced from *Optik (Stuttg).*, 147, Bu, I.Y.-Y., 39–42, Copyright 2017, with permission from Elsevier.), and (e) nanotubes. (Gao, C. et al., *Nanoscale*, 4, 3475, 2012. Reproduced by permission of The Royal Society of Chemistry.)

Nb_2O_5 is also frequently investigated. It exhibits higher electron injection efficiency and offers high open-circuit potential due to the high conduction band edge.[73] Nb_2O_5 has shown a unique feature that was demonstrated in anode materials as well as cathode materials. It is also applied as a blocking layer in the DSSC to reduce the loss of the electrons by recombination with the electrolyte.[74] The highest efficiency achieved to date using Nb_2O_5 nanorods photoanode is around 6%.[75] Nanostructures of Nb_2O_5 have been synthesized by various methods, and different morphologies of Nb_2O_5 photoanode such as nanoparticles, nanorods, nanofibers, nanochannels, and nanoporous are reported, as shown in Figure 2.9. The impact of the morphology of the photoanode materials (Nb_2O_5) on DSSC performance are compared from literature, as shown in Table 2.3.

Literature on metal oxides-based photoanode conclude that the mesoporous nature of metal oxide nanoparticles plays a vital role in DSSCs' performance. The mesoporous nature improves the dye adsorption and also the transport of photogenerated charge carriers.[28] The most commonly used metal oxides are TiO_2, ZnO, SnO_2, and Zn_2SnO_4, etc. Among these oxides, TiO_2 photoanode-based DSSCs have demonstrated the highest efficiency of 14.3% by proper selection of electrolyte, dye, and Pt/graphene composite counter electrode.[32] However, lower

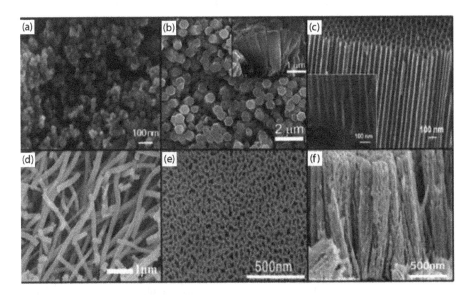

FIGURE 2.9 SEM image of Nb_2O_5 photoanode having different morphologies. (a) particle film (Rani, R. A. et al., *J. Mater. Chem. A*, 2, 15683–15703, 2014. Reproduced by permission of The Royal Society of Chemistry.), (b) nanorods (He, J. et al., *J. Mater. Chem. C*, 2, 8185–8190, 2014. Reproduced by permission of The Royal Society of Chemistry.), (c) nanochannels (Reproduced with permission from Ou, J.Z. et al., *ACS Nano*, 6, 4045–4053, 2012 Copyright 2012 American Chemical Society.), (d) nanofiber (Qi, S. et al., *J. Mater. Chem. A*, 2, 8190, 2014. Reproduced by permission of The Royal Society of Chemistry.), (e) nanopores (Wei, W. et al., *Chem. Commun.*, 48, 4244, 2012. Reproduced by permission of The Royal Society of Chemistry.), and (f) nanoforests. (Reproduced with permission from Ghosh, R. et al., *ACS Appl. Mater. Interfaces*, 3, 3929–3935, 2011. Copyright 2011 American Chemical Society.)

electrical properties (low electrical conductivity and mobility) of TiO_2 and lack of wide-range light absorption dye (UV to NIR region) limit the device performance.[76] Future research involving improvement of the electrical properties of TiO_2 (for example, doping with metal Nb), improvement in dye-loading capacity, and development of wider light absorption dyes is ongoing work in the DSSC field. On the other hand, ZnO is not stable in the most efficient dyes containing acidic groups, which are required for attaching the dye on the surface. In that sense, the tin oxide (SnO_2) is an attractive photoanode material, but it shows poor photovoltaic performance due to faster recombination dynamics and lower isoelectric point, leading to poor dye loading on its surface.[68] Therefore, understanding of charge recombination mechanisms in the ZnO-based and SnO_2-based DSSCs is essential for further improving the devices.

2.4.2   HYBRID MATERIAL FOR PHOTOANODE

Recently, a graphene-TiO_2 composite was reported as the photoanode has shown excellent potential for the DSSC as compared to the pure graphene and pure TiO_2.[25] Incorporation of graphene into TiO_2 increases the electron transport rate because of its fast charge carriers and high electrical conductivity. The composite also has better thermal stability, optical transparency, and electrocatalytic activity. Moreover, graphene is a low-cost material with transparency for visible light that is the primary need of DSSC electrodes. The graphene-TiO_2 composite electrode was developed by a dip-coating method, in which TiO_2 was coated on FTO substrate followed by preparation of graphene on TiO_2 nanosheets. The composite film was developed by a blade-coating method and resulted in a power conversion efficiency of 5.77%.[91] Graphene reduces recombination of the electron and enhances the transport of the photogenerated charges. In another study, reduced graphene and TiO_2 nanocomposite-based photoanode was developed that has shown an 8.51% efficient solar cell.[92] In 2009, a TiO_2-MWCNT nanocomposite was reported as the photoanode for the DSSC with a 7.4% efficiency.[93] The authors of that report proposed that nanocomposite photoanode rendered an efficient charge transfer from TiO_2 to multi-walled carbon nanotubes and had a better electron transport rate. Figure 2.10 shows the photocurrent density-voltage curve of TiO_2-MWCNT nanocomposite photoanode and ZnO–TiO_2 nanocomposite photo anode. In 2011, Zn_2SnO_4–SnO_2 hetero-junction nanocomposite (ZTO–SnO_2) was reported as the photoanode for the DSSC with a 1.29% power conversion efficiency.[94] The ZnO/SnO_2 core-shell nano-needle arrays were reported for the photoanode (Figure 2.11), and the photoanode was synthesized by a two-step process that had a result around 4.71%.[95] The core/shell structure nano-needle surface defects for suppressing the recombination led to an increase in the open- circuit voltage. The Zinc–tin oxide (ZnO–SnO_2) nanostructures were also developed and applied to fabricate the photoanode with 4.72% PCE.[59] Table 2.4 compares the hybrid material-based photoanodes and their efficiency. Although hybrid material has better potential for photoanodes, the reported power conversion efficiencies are lower compared to metal oxide. Therefore, further steps are required to explore the real potential of hybrid electrodes.

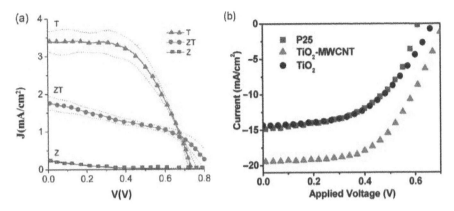

FIGURE 2.10   J-V characteristics of DSSC with (a) ZnO–TiO$_2$ nanocomposite (green), TiO$_2$ (red), ZnO (blue) photoanodes. (Reproduced with permission from Manthina, V. et al., *J. Phys. Chem. C*, 116, 23864–23870, 2012. Copyright 2012 American Chemical Society.) (b) TiO$_2$-MWCNT composite (red), TiO$_2$ (black), P25 (blue) photoanodes. (Reproduced with permission from Muduli, S. et al., *ACS Appl. Mater. Interfaces*, 1, 2030–2035, 2009. Copyright 2009 American Chemical Society.)

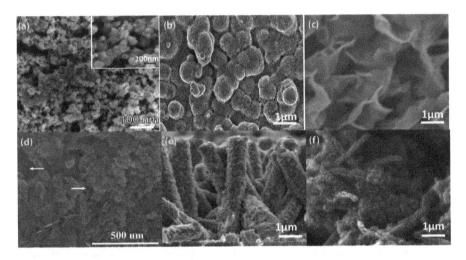

FIGURE 2.11   Hybrid photoanodes, (a) ZTO–SnO$_2$ (Reproduced from *J. Alloys Compd.*, 509, Li, B. et al., 2186–2191, Copyright 2011, with permission from Elsevier.), (b) Zn$_2$SnO$_4$ modified SnO$_2$ hierarchical microspheres (Reproduced from *Mater. Lett.*, 76, Liu, M. et al., 215–218, Copyright 2012, with permission from Elsevier.), (c) CaCO$_3$ coated SnO$_2$ on conductive glass (FTO) (Reproduced from *J. Photochem. Photobiol. A Chem.*, 295, Bhande, S.S. et al., 64–69, Copyright 2014, with permission from Elsevier.), (d) TiO$_2$ nanosheets/graphene composite (Fan, J. et al., *J. Mater. Chem.*, 22, 17027, 2012. Reproduced by permission of The Royal Society of Chemistry.), (e) ZnO–TiO$_2$ nanocomposite (Reproduced with permission from Manthina, V. et al., *J. Phys. Chem. C*, 116, 23864–23870, 2012. Copyright 2012 American Chemical Society.), and (f) Growth of TiO$_2$ on MWCNTs. (Reproduced with permission from Muduli, S. et al., *ACS Appl. Mater. Interfaces*, 1, 2030–2035, 2009. Copyright 2009 American Chemical Society.)

TABLE 2.4
Hybrid Material-Based Photoanodes and Their Performance in DSSC

Composite Photoanodes	Photocurrent (mA.cm^{-2})	Open Circuit Voltage (mV)	Fill Factor (%)	Efficiency (%)	References
TiO$_2$ nanosheets/graphene composite	16.8	606	56	5.77	91
TiO$_2$ on MWCNTs	21.9	701	49	7.37	93
ZTO–SnO$_2$	2.85	706	65	1.29	94
ZrO$_2$ coated TiO$_2$	3.98	578	55	2.27	99
SnO$_2$ NPs-MgO	16.60	650	64	6.91	100
SnO$_2$ NPs-CaCO$_3$	11.4	681	69	5.4	101
SnO$_2$ NPs-SrTiO$_3$	9.5	580	62	3.4	102
SnO$_2$ NPs-ZnO	6.49	597	62	2.4	103
SnO$_2$ NPs-NiO	3.91	598	52	1.21	103
SnO$_2$ NPs-CuO	0.87	475	70	0.29	103
SnO$_2$ nanosheets-CaCO$_3$	16.07	720	45	5.17	97
SnO$_2$ nanosheets-ZrO$_2$	12.96	690	47	3.96	97
Meso SnO$_2$–Al$_2$O$_3$	10.1	705	51	3.6	104
NWs based SnO$_2$-Zn$_2$SnO$_4$	7.22	570	74	3.05	105

2.5 DEVELOPMENTS IN COUNTER ELECTRODE

A counter electrode (CE) is one of the vital components in dye-sensitized solar cells (DSSCs).[106] The primary task of the CE is to act as a electrochemical catalyst for reducing the I$_3^-$/I$^-$ that helps in regeneration of the dye after electron injection.[106–108] Another function of the CE is to collect the electrons from the external circuit.[106–108] The CE characteristics such as transparency, conductivity, surface area, porous nature, catalytic activity, and stability affect the DSSCs' performance.[106–113] The ideal CE should have 80% optical transparency at 550 nm, lower sheet resistance (R$_S$, <20 Ω-sq.), smaller charge transfer resistance (R$_{CT}$, 2–3 Ω-cm^2), high chemical corrosion resistance, electrochemical and mechanical stability, and strong adhesion with TCO.[106–113]

The most commonly used counter electrode is platinum (Pt) because of its superior electrochemical catalytic activity and conductivity.[106] Owing to its limited availability and higher cost, the usage of platinum in DSSCs attributes for an increase in the overall cost of the cells.[106,108] Hence, it is imperative to develop low-cost CE materials that should have high electrochemical catalytic activity for the reduction of I$_3^-$/I$^-$ in the electrolyte, high conductivity, and good stability similar to that of Pt electrode.[106] There has been a considerable effort to replace platinum with carbon-based materials (for example, carbon black, carbon nanotubes, and graphene), conducting polymers, and inorganic compounds (i.e., metal oxides, metal sulfides, metal nitrides, and metal carbides).[106–113] The purity of the starting materials and the processing technique play important roles in electrical conductivity and electrocatalytic activity of CE materials, which have an impact on the performance of DSSCs.[111]

2.5.1 Carbon Materials and Their Hybrid Counter Electrodes

Numerous carbon materials (graphene, reduced graphene oxide [RGO], carbon nanotubes [CNTs], activated carbon, graphite, mesoporous carbon [MC], and carbon black, etc.) have been substituted instead of a platinum electrode in DSSCs due to their superior electrical conductivity, large surface area, and low cost.[111,113] The recent development of different carbon-based CEs using iodine-based and cobalt electrolyte and ruthenium-based dye are given in Table 2.5. The DSSCs fabricated with platinum composite (Au/GNP [graphene nanoplatelet]) have demonstrated the highest photo-conversion efficiency of 14.3%.[32] SEM images of CNT counter electrodes fabricated

TABLE 2.5
Progress in Counter Electrodes Materials for DSSCs

CEs Materials	J_{sc} (mA/cm^2)	V_{oc} (mV)	FF	η (%)
Pt				
$Pt_{0.02}Co$	18.53	0.735	0.75	10.23
$CoPt_{0.1}$	17.92	0.735	0.728	9.59
NiCu/Pt	18.37	0.758	0.696	9.66
NiPt	16.15	0.763	0.737	9.08
Pt_3Ni	17.46	0.730	0.718	9.15
Cu/Fe/Pt	15.94	0.726	0.70	8.21
Pt/NiO	18.38	0.825	0.625	9.48
$W_{18}O_{49}$	17.37	0.73	0.68	8.58
$WO_{2.72}$	14.90	0.77	0.70	8.03
NbO_2	13.90	0.81	0.70	7.88
Fe_3O_4	16.23	0.693	0.63	7.65
SnO_2	16.18	0.506	0.36	2.96
Pt/SnO_2	16.24	0.731	0.74	8.83
$Ni_{0.85}Se$	24.34	0.737	0.59	10.63
$CoSe_2$	17.65	0.809	0.72	10.17
CoS	19.26	0.759	0.631	9.23
Transparent CoS/rGO	18.90	0.767	0.67	9.82
CoTe/RGO	17.41	0.770	0.69	9.18
Ni_5P_4	14.70	0.720	0.72	7.60
Mesoporous NiN	15.76	0.766	0.69	8.31
FeN/N-doped graphene	18.83	0.740	0.78	10.86
OM TiN–C	15.30	0.820	0.67	8.41
PEDOT nanofibers	17.50	0.724	0.73	9.20
PANI-SO4-F(HFIP)	17.94	0.729	0.67	8.80

Source: Wu, J. et al., *Chem. Soc. Rev.*, 2017; Theerthagiri, J. et al., *ChemElectroChem*, 2, 928–945, 2015; Yun, S. et al., *Adv. Mater.*, 26, 6210–6237, 2014; Wu, M. and Ma, T. *ChemSusChem*, 2012, 1343–1357; Tang, Q. et al., *Electrochimica Acta.*, 886–899, 2015; Saranya, K. et al., *Eur. Polym. J.*, 207–227, 2015; Thomas, S. et al., *J. Mater. Chem. A Mater. Energy Sustain.*, 2, 4474–4490, 2014; Kouhnavard, M. et al., *ChemSusChem.*, 1510–1533, 2015.

via a screen-printing CNT paste and the CVD process are shown in Figure 2.12.[114] The chemical vapor deposited carbon nanotubes (CNTs)-based CEs showed an efficiency of 10.03% as compared to other processing techniques (Figure 2.13).[114] The rate of reduction of I_3^-/I^- of the screen-printed CNT counter electrode is lower than that of Pt and CVD grown CNT-based counter electrodes due to unfavorable contact resistance between randomly oriented CNTs and the TCO.[114]

The DSSCs fabricated with hybrid carbon CEs (RGO-SWCNTs, MWCNTs-Pt, MWCNTs-NiS, MC-CNTs) showed higher performance as compared to the carbon CEs due to their improvement in electrochemical catalytic activity and electrical

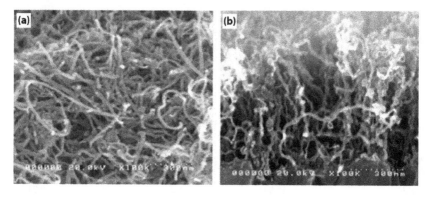

FIGURE 2.12 SEM images of (a) a screen-printing CNT paste and (b) a directly formed CNT counter electrode. (Reproduced from *Scr. Mater.*, 62, Nam, J.G. et al., 148–150, Copyright 2010, with permission from Elsevier.)

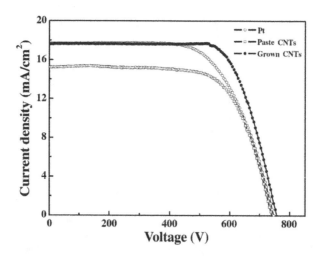

FIGURE 2.13 J–V characteristics of DSSC with counter electrodes of Pt, CNTs, paste and grown CNTs. (Reproduced from Scr. Mater., 62, Nam, J.G. et al., 148–150, Copyright 2010, with permission from Elsevier.)

conductivity.[104,106,109,111,113–115] However, the major concern for the application of multiwall CNTs and carbon CEs in DSSCs is long-term stability. Finally, the carbon-based CEs required larger thickness to obtain the desired catalytic activity, and their poor adhesion to substrates influenced the device stability.[117]

2.5.2 Conducting Polymers and Their Hybrid-Based CEs

Conducting polymers (CPs) such as polyaniline (PANI), polypyrrole (PPy), and poly(3,4-ethylenedioxythiophene) (PEDOT) have been utilized as CEs in DSSCs due to their unique properties, such as high transparency, high conductivity, and high catalytic activity for I_3^- reduction.[106,108,111,113] The optical transparency of CPs is demonstrated to construct bifacial DSSCs.[111] The transparency of the CEs was used for fabrication of semitransparent DSSCs, and it has many real-time applications such as windows, roof panels, or various decorative installations.[111] Among the CPs, PANI is one of the most commonly studied CE materials. The doping with various ions such as SO_4^{2-}, ClO_4^-, BF_4^- and Cl^- affects the morphology, porosity, increases conductivity, and electrocatalytic properties of PANI.[111] The highest efficiency of DSSCs fabricated with PANI-based CE shows around 8.88%.[118] The main problem with PANI-based CEs was the nonuniform film deposition on FTO, which led to a lower conductivity. Hence, the key challenge is to find a proper deposition process and suitable dopants (act as a pore former and also enhance surface area) that allow uniform film growth, which increases the conductivity and electrochemical catalytic activity.[111]

Polypyrrole (PPy) is another promising candidate to replace Pt from CE due to its good electrochemical catalytic activity and considerable environmental stability.[111,113] The electrochemical catalytic activity of PPy CE depends on synthesis process, dopant, and morphology.[111,113] SEM images of polypyrrole nanoparticles and films coated on FTO substrate are shown in Figure 2.14. Polypyrrole nanoparticles were well separated and have a particle diameter of 40–60 nm. The surface exhibits porous state, which is beneficial for the improvement of electrochemical catalytic activity for redox reaction. DSSCs with PPy nanoparticle-based CE showed

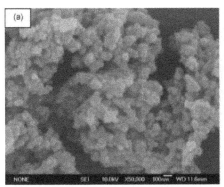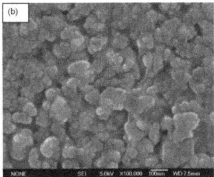

FIGURE 2.14 SEM image of (a) polypyrrole nanoparticles and (b) polypyrrole coated on FTO. (Reproduced from J. Power Sources, 181, Wu, J. et al., 172–176, Copyright 2008, with permission from Elsevier.)

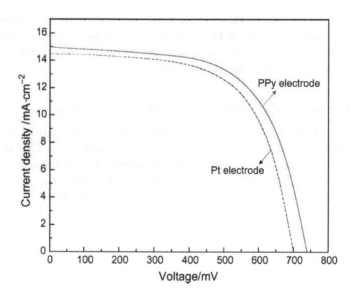

FIGURE 2.15 Photocurrent–voltage characteristics of DSSCs with PPy (red line) and Pt (black line) CEs under 100 mWcm^{-2} light irradiation. (Reproduced from *J. Power Sources*, 181, Wu, J. et al., 172–176, Copyright 2008, with permission from Elsevier.)

an efficiency of 7.66% (Figure 2.15).[119] The addition of carbon materials and metals (CNTs, RGO, Pt.) to PPy increases the electrical conductivity, facilitating the fast electron transfer, providing a large specific surface area for catalytic sites, and reducing the R_{ct} value—and all these properties improve the electrochemical catalytic activity and device performance.[120–122]

The main problem with PPy CE is its higher R_{ct}, and the conductivity of the film is also low. Many research groups are working on improving conductivity, reducing the R_{ct} of PPy film, which might improve the efficiency of the device.[111] The addition of inorganic compounds (metal oxide, metal nitrides, carbide, and sulfide) to CPs provides durability (stability) and enhances the electrical conductivity.[106–113] However, purity of starting materials and the processing technique for CPs play essential roles in device performance.[111] Until now, an unavoidable problem for CP CEs is the structural alteration in electrochemical conditions.[107,123] For example, the PEDOT:PSS film adsorbs the organic molecules in the electrolytes during the device working conditions.[123] Hence, the long-term stability of the liquid-electrolyte-based DSSCs with CP-based CEs could not attain the requirements for real solar cells.[123]

2.5.3 INORGANIC MATERIALS AND THEIR HYBRID COUNTER ELECTRODES

Several inorganic compounds such as metal oxides, metal nitrides/carbide, and metal sulfide/selenides, and their composite have been demonstrated as alternative CE materials in DSSCs.[124,125] The electrochemical catalytic activity of newly explored CE materials was screened based on the adsorption energy of iodine at the electrolyte/CE interface.[124,125] The optimum adsorption energy of iodine (E^I_{ad}) was calculated using the density functional theory and was found to be in the range of 0.33 to 1.2 eV.[124,125] The E^I_{ad} values of TiO_2, MnO_2, SnO_2, CeO_2, ZrO_2, La_2O_3, Al_2O_3, Ga_2O_3, Cr_2O_3, and Ta_2O_5 are not in the optimal range, which indicates inferior catalytic activities.[124,125] However, E^I_{ad} of these oxides can be modified by doping with $N-SnO_2$, $S-NiO$, which improves the catalytic activities.[126,127] The $WO_{2.72}$ has a hierarchical architecture composed of nanorod bundles (highly uniform 250 nm) in length (Figure 2.16a,b). The transmission electron microscopy (TEM) image (Figure 2.16b) reveals that nanorod bundles are not densely packed together. This feature is important for the CEs in DSSCs because a porous structure is desired for the electrolyte filling and subsequent catalytic reactions.[128] The morphology of the synthesized samples significantly changed after annealing.[128] DSSCs fabricated with $WO_{2.77}$ CEs have shown an efficiency of 8.03% while DSSCs with WO_3 CEs exhibited an efficiency of 4.63% (Figure 2.17), which ascribed to the oxygen content (oxygen vacancy) in oxide-based CEs (Figure 2.18).[128] The oxygen content has a vital role in the electrochemical catalytic activity of oxide-based CEs.[128]

Transition metal nitride, carbide (TiN, TiC, MoC, WC, VC, Ta_4C_3, etc.), and their hybrid CE (TiN-MC, VC-MC, WC-MC, etc.) have been attractive CE materials due to their low cost, superior electrical conductivity, intrinsic corrosion resistance toward electrolyte, and good thermal stability under different environmental conditions.[106–108,129] Figure 2.18 shows SEM images and (insets) TEM images of the synthesized Cr_2O_3, CrN, Cr_3C_2, V_2O_3, VN, VC(N), VC–MC, TiO_2, TiN, and TiC(N) and commercial VC and TiC.[129] The J–V curves for DSSCs fabricated

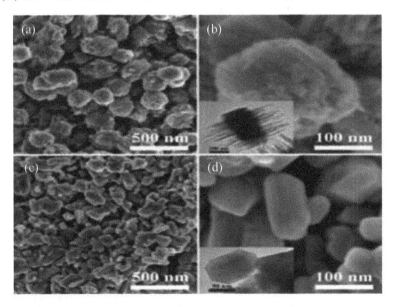

FIGURE 2.16   SEM images of the as-synthesized (a) and (b) $WO_{2.72}$ nanorod bundles (NRBs); (c) and (d) WO_3 prisms; the insets show their corresponding TEM images. (Zhou, H. et al., *Chem. Commun.*, 49, 7626, 2013. Reproduced by permission of The Royal Society of Chemistry.)

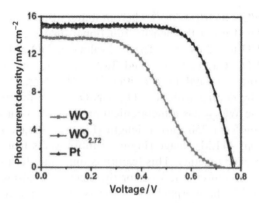

FIGURE 2.17 Photocurrent–voltage (J–V) curves of the DSSCs based on counter electrodes of Pt, WO₃. (Zhou, H. et al., *Chem. Commun.*, 49, 7626, 2013. Reproduced by permission of The Royal Society of Chemistry.)

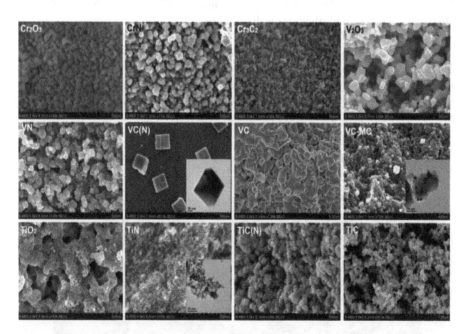

FIGURE 2.18 SEM images and (insets) TEM images of the synthesized Cr_2O_3, CrN, Cr_3C_2, V_2O_3, VN, VC(N), VC–MC, TiO_2, TiN, and TiC(N) and commercial VC and TiC. (Reproduced with permission from Wu, M. et al., *J. Am. Chem. Soc.*, 134, 3419–3428, 2012. Copyright 2012 American Chemical Society.)

using Pt, carbides, nitrides, and oxides as CEs are shown in Figure 2.19.[129] The enhancement in catalytic activity and device performance was reported for DSSCs made with N-doped carbides TiC(N), VC(N), and NbC(N)-based CEs as compared to the TiC, VC, and NbC.[107,129] The reason behind the improvement in the device performance was not clear.[129] The addition of mesoporous

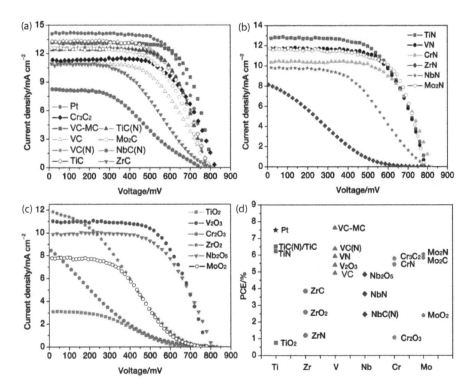

FIGURE 2.19   J–V curves for I_3^-/I^- DSCs using (a) Pt or carbide, (b) nitride, or (c) oxide CE catalysts. (d) Distribution graph showing the PCEs of these I_3^-/I^- DSCs. (Reproduced with permission from Wu, M. et al., *J. Am. Chem. Soc.*, 134, 3419–3428, 2012. Copyright 2012 American Chemical Society.)

carbon (MC) to the nitrides (TiN-MC, VC-MC, WC-MC) provided a large surface area for catalysis, which increases the catalytic activity and device performance.[129] However, the performance of DSSCs assembled TMC-based CE was lower than that of the other Pt-free CE materials; thus, poor conductivity of TMCs affects electron transportation at the interface of TMCs and substrates, which lowers the performance.[106,108,129]

Among these inorganic materials, much attention has been paid to chalcogenide semiconductors due to their good electronic properties and a wide variety of potential applications.[130–135] DSSCs fabricated with the in-situ deposition of $Co_{0.8}$ Se, and $NiSe_2$-based CEs have shown the highest efficiency of 10.63% and 10.17%, respectively, and this is the highest efficiency among all inorganic materials.[106] Among the quaternary chalcogenide semiconductor, earth-abundant quaternary chalcogenide such as Cu_2ZnSnS_4 (CZTS), Cu_2FeSnS_4 (CFTS), $Cu_2CoSn(S)_4$ (CCoTS), and Cu_2CdSnS_4 (CCdSnS) have been explored as CE materials and also showed superior performance in DSSCs.[130–135] However, the stability studied of ternary and quaternary sulfide-based CEs have yet to be reported.

The novel CE materials should have earth abundance, low cost, and low temperature solution processability; and possess superior conductivity, catalytic activity, and excellent stability (chemically, electrochemically, and environmentally in different conditions). The theortical approach is essential to validate the experimental determination in catalytic activity of CE materials. The standard stability test is necessary to design for CEs. Future development should focus on improving the efficiency and stability of counter electrodes and scaling up lab devices into a high-efficiency commercial module to compete with other PV technology.

2.6 ELECTROLYTES FOR DYE-SENSITIZED SOLAR CELLS

The electrolyte has a major role in obtaining both the efficiency and durability of the DSSCs.[136–139] The primary function of the electrolyte is dye regeneration and acting as an electrically conducting medium between the two electrodes.[136,137] The materials should possess the following properties to serve as an electrolyte in DSSCs.[136,139–141]

1. The redox potential of a redox couple should be less negative than the oxidized level of a dye molecule.
2. High conductivity ($\sim 10^{-3}$ S.cm^{-1}).
3. Fast electron transfer kinetics at counter electrodes (CEs).
4. Excellent diffusion properties are required to have a proper mass transport in the device under different irradiation conditions.
5. Desorption of the dye from the photoanode should not occur (cause).
6. Non-reactive with the sealant.
7. Negligible visible light absorption.
8. Non-corrosiveness toward CEs.
9. Good photochemical stability—and it should be stable up to $\sim 80°C$.

The electrolyte can be classified into three groups such as liquid electrolyte, quasi-solid electrolyte, and solid electrolyte.[136,141]

2.6.1 Liquid Electrolyte

Liquid electrolyte consists of a redox couple (for example I^-/I_3^-), organic solvent (acetonitrile [AN]), valeronitrile ([VN] and 1-Methyl-3-propylimidazolim iodide), and a few additives (4-tert-butyl pyridine).[136] Iodide-based redox couple has been used from the very beginning of DSSCs' research, and it has shown high conversion efficiency of up to 10%–12%.[142–144] The DSSCs fabricated with iodine-bassed electrolyte have shown good long-term stability at 60°C under the irradiance of AM 1.5G.[144] Due to the corrosive nature and light absorption in the visible region of I^-/I_3^- system,[140] great efforts have been dedicated to find alternative redox couples to replace the I^-/I_3^- system.[145–147] There are numerous alternative redox couples in electrolytes for DSSCs, such as Br^-/Br_3^-, $SCN^-/(SCN)_3^-$, $SeCN^-/(SeCN)_3^-$, TEMPO, tetraphenyldiamine, hydroquinone, thiolate/disulfide, ferrocene/ferricenium/ (Fc/Fc$^+$), copper (I/II), and a series of cobalt (II/III).[145–153,154–156,157–159]

Among these different redox couples, cobalt complexes have emerged as promising alternative mediators due to their noncorrosive nature to counter electrodes, non-volatility, and less visible light absorption.[138,160,161] Cobalt-redox couples also have more positive redox potentials than I$^-$/I$_3^-$, thus resulting in increased V_{oc} of DSSCs.[138,160,161] DSSCs fabricated using cobalt redox mediators have been achieved >14% efficiency.[32] The concentration of cobalt redox couples and its additives (lithium salt ([LiClO$_4$], 4-tert-butyl pyridine [TBP] etc.) have an impact on the stability of DSSCs.[162–166] The higher concentration of TBP increases the recombination loss during the light-soaking experiment.[162–166] Stability of DSSCs can be further improved by design of stable cobalt-redox couples and optimizing the concentration of redox couples in the electrolyte.[138,160–166] Overall, DSSCs made with cobalt-based electrolytes have shown much lower long-term stability as compared to iodide-based redox couples.[138,162–166] The leakage of liquid electrolyte, change in concentration of the electrolyte, and the detachment of the adsorbed dye on the surface of TiO$_2$ have been investigated as some of the issues restraining the long-term stability of the DSSCs.[166,167]

2.6.2 Quasi-Solid Electrolyte and Solid Electrolyte

Liquid electrolyte-based DSSCs possess the low stability due to the leakage and a volatile organic solvent used in electrolyte.[141,167] An efficient approach to solving the low stability issue is replacing the volatile liquid electrolyte with quasi-solid electrolyte (QS) or solid-state hole conductor (p-type semiconductors).[168,169] The quasi-solid electrolyte can be prepared from liquid electrolytes by addition of nanomaterials, carbon, and a suitable gelator.[136,141] The gelators can be either polymers or nanopowders. The gelation minimizes electrolyte leakage over time and maintains a good contact between the dye and the redox mediator.[141] The highest efficiency of QS-DSSCs is higher than 10%.[169] Utilization of quasi-solid-state electrolytes improves the stability of DSSCs for a long time.[141,168,170] However, efficiencies of QS-DSSCs are relatively lower than liquid DSSCs due to lower mobility of iodide/cobalt species through the viscous medium.[136,141,170] Another issue in quasi-solid DSSCs is the poor penetration of gel electrolytes into the mesoporous photoanode.[138,141,170] Solid-state hole conductors (P-type semiconductor) can meet long-term stability requirements for DSSCs. In general, solid-state DSSCs is fabricated by using p-type semiconductors.[171,168] The inorganic p-type semiconductors such as CuI, CsSnI$_3$ and [Cu (4,40,6,60-tetramethyl-2,20-bipyridine)2] (bis(trifluoromethyl sulfonyl)imide, (Cu(II/I))) etc., has been reported in the literature.[171,168,172] The highest efficiency (11%) of solid-state DSSCs is achieved by using an amorphous Cu(II/I) conductor.[172] The DSSCs made with the solid-state electrolytes have shown good long-term stability.[168,172] The cross-sectional SEM image of a solid-state DSSC is shown in Figure 2.20. The lower performance of this device is due to poor interfacial electrolyte/electrode contacts and low conductivity and crystallization of hole-transport materials infiltrated in the mesoscopic TiO$_2$, as compared to liquid electrolyte-based DSSCs.[168,172] Future research on solid-state DSSCs is to be dedicated by solving their primary problems such as poor pore filling and inferior hole mobility in these devices.[168,172] The comparison of different electrolytes is summarized in Table 2.6.

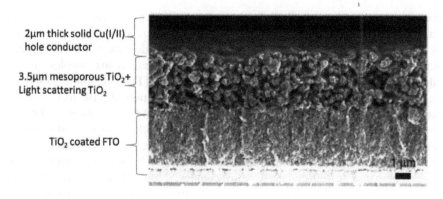

2µm thick solid Cu(I/II) hole conductor

3.5µm mesoporous TiO₂+ Light scattering TiO₂

TiO₂ coated FTO

FIGURE 2.20 Cross-sectional SEM image of a solid-state DSC without the counter electrode. (Reproduced by permission from Cao, Y. et al., *Nat. Commun.*, 8, 15390, 2007, Copyright 2007.)

TABLE 2.6
Different Electrolyte for Dye-Sensitized Solar Cell

Parameters	Iodide Liquid Electrolyte	Cobalt Liquid Electrolyte	Quasi-Solid-State Electrolyte	Solid State Electrolyte
Redox couples/	Iodide/triiodide	cobalt(II/III) redox	Gel form of Iodide or cobalt redox	Hole transporting materials (CsSnI₃)
Organic solvents	Volatile	Volatile	Reduce volatile	—
Corrosive nature	Corrosive	Less corrosive	Less corrosive	—
Efficiency (%)	11–12	14.3	10.1	11
Stability	Less	Less as compared Iodide electrolyte	Stable as compared liquid electrolyte	More stable
Limiting factors	Leakage of electrolyte and dye desorption	Leakage of electrolyte and dye desorption	Poor penetration of electrolytes into the mesoporous TiO₂	Poor interfacial electrolyte/ electrode contacts
Future scope	Non corrosive and non-volatile electrolyte (eg., DW)	Optimization of concentration of additives in electrolyte	Increase the conductivity of electrolyte	Increase the infiltration of HTM into Mesoporous TiO₂

Source: Wang, M. et al., *Nat. Chem.*, 2, 385–389, 2010; Giribabu, L. et al., *Chem. Rec.* 15, 760–788, 2015; Hamann, T.W.T. *Dalt. Trans.*, 41, 3111, 2012; Mohamad, A.A., *J. Power Sources*, 329, 57–71, 2016; Li, B. et al., *Sol. Energy Mater. Sol. Cells.*, 549–573, 2006.

2.7 ENHANCEMENT IN EFFICIENCY OF DSSC USING RELAY DYES: FOSTER RESONANCE ENERGY TRANSFER

Development of advanced and hybrid material has shown better potential to enhance the energy efficiency of dye-sensitized solar cells. The cell performance and efficiency can be significantly enhanced by improving the light absorption capability that is possible by incorporation of relay dyes. Relay dye improves the capturing of light and produces more photogenerated charges. A variety of multiple dyes are incorporated together to achieve higher energy efficiency.[173] These approaches are widely used so as to improve the efficiency as compared to conventional dyes. The limitation of earlier mono material-based dyes is with the partial use of the light energy—that is, the energy obtained from the sun is not fully utilized; thus, our process of converting light energy to electrical energy is not efficient. By using relay, a wider spectrum of light energy can be harvested and transfer of energy (FRET) to the sensitizers will take place.[174] Thus, placing multiple dyes in the electrolyte solution increases the harvesting of light. Förster resonance energy transfer (FRET) is the linking parameter between the two materials, which is used to fulfill a strong absorption coefficient of the solar spectrum.[175]

2.7.1 PRINCIPLE OF FRET

FRET can be understood by considering a molecule, which might transfer its excitation energy by a nonradiative way to another molecule, which is present at a unique distance. These molecules are bonded together through an electric field due to the dipole-dipole interaction. The process starts with a fluorophore from the donor, which gets in an excited state due to the interaction of light from outside; this causes the fluorophore to gain energy. This energy is transferred to another molecule, which is available in an acceptor due to the dipole-dipole interaction, sometimes called dipole-dipole coupling. After the transition of energy, the acceptor molecule, which is in an excited state, returns to the ground state by losing the energy due to the photon emission.[176] The efficiency of the material is calculated by quantifying the energy transfer, which is inversely proportional to the sixth power of the distance between the donor and acceptor; thus, FRET is very sensitive to the change in distance.[177] The energy transfer efficiency E is given by:[177]

$$E = \frac{R_o^6}{R_o^6 + r^6} \tag{2.5}$$

The Forster radius R_o is defined as the separation distance between the donor and acceptor, where the transfer efficiency is 50%.[177]

$$(R_0)^6 = \frac{9000 \ln(10) K^2 . \phi_D}{128 \, pi^2 N_A n^4} \left[\int_0^\infty F_D(\lambda) 3_A(\lambda) \lambda^4 d\lambda \right] \tag{2.6}$$

where:
  K is the orientation factor between donor and acceptor dipoles
  λD is the donor fluorescence quantum yield in the absence of the acceptor
  N_A is the Avogadro constant
  n is the index of refraction for the medium surrounding the donor and acceptor

$$K_{ET} = \frac{1}{(\tau_D)} \left(\frac{R_o}{r} \right)^6 \tag{2.7}$$

where:

τ_D is the lifetime of the donor excited state in the absence of the acceptor
r is the distance between donor and acceptor chromophores

FRET can be understood as presented in a schematic diagram (Figure 2.21a). The process starts with absorption of a photon of a specific energy as denoted by a straight line pointing up. The energy of the photon gets transferred to the electron present in the ground state; thus, the electron is excited from the lower energy state to the higher energy state. At an excited state, the electron goes through vibrational and internal conversion. Here, the excited electron has multiple ways of dissipating energy, which is supported by a non-radiating process (the curved arrow depicts this kind of transition). The non-radiating process is very fast; it may occur between 10^{-14} and 10^{-11} s. There is also the possibility to dissipate the energy of the excited electron by emission of a photon; the phenomena are known to be fluorescence. In case of a relay dye, the excited electron can be relaxed by transferring the energy to an acceptor molecule via a nonradiative dipole-dipole coupling between the donor and acceptor molecules of respective dyes. The intensity observed in the loss of donor fluorescence is small as compared to the gain of acceptor fluorescence; therefore, the overall intensity is increased, as shown in Figure 2.21b.[178]

Table 2.7 provides the information of two dyes incorporating together to form a unique dye for the DSSC. The unattached relay dyes start absorbing light energy

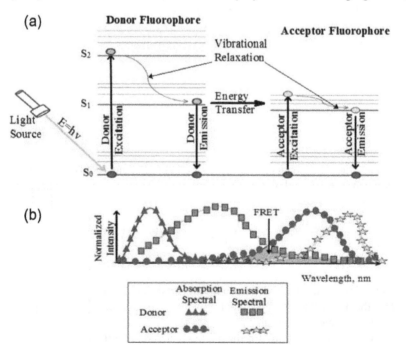

FIGURE 2.21   (a) Schematic diagram of FRET principle, (b) Absorption and emission spectra in FRET process. Schematic diagram of FRET with Intensity. (Adapted from Obeng, E.M. et al., *J. Biol. Methods*, 4, 71, 2017, with permission of Journal of Biological Methods.)

TABLE 2.7
The Various Relay Dyes and Their Respective Efficiency in DSSC

SR No.	Donor	Acceptor	ETE/V_{oc}	PCE (%)	References
1	PTCDI	TT1	0.47	3.2	180
2	DCM	TT1	0.96	4.5	181,182
3	DCM	SQ-1	0.68	1.6	177
4	N877	SQ-1	0.32	1.8	183
5	N877	SQ-1	0.14	3.6	184
6	BL302	TT1	0.70	3.8	173
7	BL315	TT1	0.67	4.1	173
8	DSSC	Phospur	0.67	3.49	185
9	DSC	GaAs	0.79	28.9	186
10	DSSC	GaAs	0.76	27	186
11	DSSC	—	1.38	1.02	187
12	DSSC	TiO/ZnO	0.76	0.69	43

photons and transfer the energy to the sensitizing dye molecule with help of the FRET principle, due to the large bandgap.[181] Multiple dyes comprise a panchromatic response of the DSSC and improve the efficiency, with the help of energy relay dyes (ERDs) incorporated into the DSSC system. High solubility increases the light-absorbing power as it increases the size by a good percent. The 95% of incident light is absorbed at the peak wavelength.[173] When phosphor is coupled with sensitizer dye, there is an improvement in efficiency, which can be observed because of the excitation energy being transferred following the FRET principle.

2.8 SUMMARY

Dye-sensitized solar cell (DSSC) has arisen as a new technology, and numerous efforts are going on to progress in the direction of an efficient material to overcome the conventional silicon-based solar cell. Progress has been made in to improve efficiency, stability, and commercialization of the cell. DSSC is one of the solar cell architectures that offers low cost and easy processing for device fabrication. Present ideas and techniques have resulted in good performance of DSSCs. The DSSCs are more sensitive than silicon and other semiconductor substrate toward the visible light, thus making them more reliable sources of power even under low light conditions. Currently, they are in the development phase, and more research is going on regarding the stability and long-lasting value of the module. While considering DSSCs, apart from efficiency, durability is also one of the major concerns for this technology. In future development of tandem cells, pn-DSSC may exceed the efficiency barrier of individual DSSC. Higher efficiency might be achieved by tailoring the geometry and other integral parts. Recently, perovskite-based material has gathered eyes due to its high stability and moderately inert state to the environment, thus making a new progress in the solar cell field.

REFERENCES

1. Würfel, P. *Physics of Solar Cells*; **2005**. published in Buch.de, Eine marke von.
2. Surek, T. **2005**, Vol. 275, pp 292.
3. Li, S.-L.; Jiang, K.-J.; Shao, K.-F.; Yang, L.-M. *Chem. Commun.* **2006**, *2* (26), 2792.
4. Bessho, T.; Zakeeruddin, S. M.; Yeh, C. Y.; Diau, E. W. G.; Grttzel, M. *Angew. Chemie: Int. Ed.* **2010**, *49* (37), 6646–6649.
5. Li, L.-L.; Diau, E. W.-G. *Chem. Soc. Rev.* **2013**, *42* (1), 291–304.
6. Bora, A.; Mohan, K.; Phukan, P.; Dolui, S. K. *Electrochim. Acta* **2017**, *259*, 233–244.
7. Peng, B.; Jungmann, G.; Jäger, C.; Haarer, D.; Schmidt, H. W.; Thelakkat, M. Systematic. *Coordin. Chem. Rev.* **2004**, 1479–1489.
8. Campbell, W. M.; Jolley, K. W.; Wagner, P.; Wagner, K.; Walsh, P. J.; Gordon, K. C.; Schmidt-Mende, L. et al., *J. Phys. Chem. C* **2007**, *111* (32), 11760–11762.
9. Han, L.; Islam, A.; Chen, H.; Malapaka, C.; Chiranjeevi, B.; Zhang, S.; Yang, X.; Yanagida, M. *Energy Environ. Sci.* **2012**, *5* (3), 6057.
10. Son, D. Y.; Im, J. H.; Kim, H. S.; Park, N. G. *J. Phys. Chem. C* **2014**, *118* (30), 16567–16573.
11. Yella, A.; Mai, C. L.; Zakeeruddin, S. M.; Chang, S. N.; Hsieh, C. H.; Yeh, C. Y.; Grätzel, M. *Angew. Chemie: Int. Ed.* **2014**, *53* (11), 2973–2977.
12. Yao, Z.; Zhang, M.; Wu, H.; Yang, L.; Li, R.; Wang, P. *J. Am. Chem. Soc.* **2015**, *137* (11), 3799–3802.
13. Huang, C. Y. C. L.; Hsu, Y. C.; Chen, J. G.; Suryanarayanan, V.; Lee, K. M. K.; Ho, K. C.; Ranga Rao, A. et al., *Thin Solid Films* **2016**, *4* (1), 153–158.
14. O'Regan, B.; Grätzel, M. A Low-Cost, *Nature* **1991**, *353*, 737–740.
15. Kushwaha, R.; Srivastava, P.; Bahadur, L. *J. Energy* **2013**, *2013*, 1–12.
16. Li, X.; Lin, H.; Zakeeruddin, S. M.; Grätzel, M.; Li, J. *Chem. Lett.* **2009**, *38* (4), 322–323.
17. Benkö, G.; Hilgendorff, M.; Yartsev, A. P.; Sundström, V. *J. Phys. Chem. B* **2001**, *105* (5), 967–974.
18. Hardin, B. E.; Hoke, E. T.; Armstrong, P. B.; Yum, J. H.; Comte, P.; Torres, T.; Fréchet, J. M. J.; Nazeeruddin, M. K.; Grätzel, M.; McGehee, M. D. *Nat. Photonics* **2009**, *3* (7), 406–411.
19. Longo, C.; Nogueira, A. F.; De Paoli, M.-A.; Cachet, H. *J. Phys. Chem. B* **2002**, *106* (23), 5925–5930.
20. Wang, P.; Dai, Q.; Zakeeruddin, S. M.; Forsyth, M.; MacFarlane, D. R.; Grattzel, M. *J. Am. Chem. Soc.* **2004**, *126* (42), 13590–13591.
21. Kay, A.; Grätzel, M. *Sol. Energy Mater. Sol. Cells* **1996**, *44* (1), 99–117.
22. Wu, Y.; Zhu, W. *Chem. Soc. Rev.* **2013**, *42* (5), 2039–2058.
23. Tang, J.; Hua, J.; Wu, W.; Li, J.; Jin, Z.; Long, Y.; Tian, H. *Energy Environ. Sci.* **2010**, *3* (11), 1736.
24. Pastore, M.; Angelis, F. De. *J. Phys. Chem. Lett.* **2012**, *3* (16), 2146–2153.
25. Low, F. W.; Lai, C. W. **2018**, *82*.
26. Energy, S. Solar Energy. *Energy Sources* **1997**, *60* (5), 245–256.
27. Ito, S.; Murakami, T. N.; Comte, P.; Liska, P.; Grätzel, C.; Nazeeruddin, M. K.; Grätzel, M. *Thin Solid Films* **2008**, *516* (14), 4613–4619.
28. Choi, H.; Nahm, C.; Kim, J.; Moon, J.; Nam, S.; Jung, D.-R.; Park, B. *Curr. Appl. Phys.* **2012**, *12* (3), 737–741.
29. Chen, Z. Y.; Hu, Y.; Liu, T. C.; Huang, C. L.; Jeng, T. S. *Thin Solid Films* **2009**, *517* (17), 4998–5000.
30. Huang, C. Y.; Hsu, Y. C.; Chen, J. G.; Suryanarayanan, V.; Lee, K. M.; Ho, K. C. *Sol. Energy Mater. Sol. Cells* **2006**, *90* (15), 2391–2397.
31. Chou, T. P.; Zhang, Q.; Russo, B.; Fryxell, G. E.; Cao, G. *J. Phys. Chem. C* **2007**, *111* (17), 6296–6302.

32. Kakiage, K.; Aoyama, Y.; Yano, T.; Oya, K.; Fujisawa, J.; Hanaya, M. *Chem. Commun.* **2015**, *51* (88), 15894–15897.

33. Zama, I.; Martelli, C.; Gorni, G. *Mater. Sci. Semicond. Process.* **2017**, *61*, 137–144.

34. Chu, L.; Qin, Z.; Yang, J.; Li, X. *Sci. Rep.* **2015**, *5* (1), 12143.

35. Zhu, T.; Li, C.; Yang, W.; Zhao, X.; Wang, X.; Tang, C.; Mi, B.; Gao, Z.; Huang, W.; Deng, W. *Aerosol Sci. Technol.* **2013**, *47* (12), 1302–1309.

36. Pai, K. R. N.; Anjusree, G. S.; Deepak, T. G.; Subash, D.; Nair, S. V.; Nair, A. S. *RSC Adv.* **2014**, *4* (69), 36821–36827.

37. Sahu, K.; Murty, V. V. S. **2015**, *2*, 567–571.

38. Chen, S.; Su, H.; Chang, H.; Jwo, C.; Ju Feng, H. *Chinese J. Chem. Phys.* **2010**, *23* (2), 231–236.

39. Kathirvel, S.; Su, C.; Shiao, Y.-J.; Lin, Y.-F.; Chen, B.-R.; Li, W.-R. *Sol. Energy* **2016**, *132*, 310–320.

40. Meng, L.; Chen, H.; Li, C.; Dos Santos, M. P. *Thin Solid Films* **2015**, *577*, 103–108.

41. Jung, W. H.; Kwak, N. S.; Hwang, T. S.; Yi, K. B. *Appl. Surf. Sci.* **2012**, *261*, 343–352.

42. Sharmoukh, W.; Allam, N. K. *ACS Appl. Mater. Interfaces* **2012**, *4* (8), 4413–4418.

43. Liu, B.; Aydil, E. S. *J. Am. Chem. Soc.* **2009**, *131* (11), 3985–3990.

44. Vu, H. H. T.; Atabaev, T. S.; Pham-Cong, D.; Hossain, M. A.; Lee, D.; Dinh, N. N.; Cho, C. R.; Kim, H. K.; Hwang, Y. H. *Electrochim. Acta* **2016**, *193*, 166–171.

45. Wu, W. Q.; Lei, B. X.; Rao, H. S.; Xu, Y. F.; Wang, Y. F.; Su, C. Y.; Kuang, D. Bin. *Sci. Rep.* **2013**, *3*, 1–7.

46. Feng, X.; Shankar, K.; Varghese, O. K.; Paulose, M.; Latempa, T. J.; Grimes, C. A. *Nano Lett.* **2008**, *8* (11), 3781–3786.

47. Chuangchote, S.; Sagawa, T.; Yoshikawa, S. *Appl. Phys. Lett.* **2008**, *93* (3), 5–8.

48. Mohammadpour, F.; Moradi, M.; Lee, K.; Cha, G.; So, S.; Kahnt, A.; Guldi, D. M.; Altomare, M.; Schmuki, P. *Chem. Commun.* **2015**, *51* (9), 1631–1634.

49. Sahu, G.; Gordon, S. W.; Tarr, M. A. *RSC Adv.* **2012**, *2* (2), 573–582.

50. Li, H.; Yu, Q.; Huang, Y.; Yu, C.; Li, R.; Wang, J.; Guo, F. et al. *ACS Appl. Mater. Interfaces* **2016**, *8* (21), 13384–13391.

51. Liu, W.; Wang, H.; Wang, X.; Zhang, M.; Guo, M. *J. Mater. Chem. C* **2016**, *4* (47), 11118–11128.

52. Momeni, M. M. *Rare Met.* **2016**, *36* (11), 865–871.

53. Ren, Z.; Guo, Y.; Liu, C.-H.; Gao, P.-X. *Front. Chem.* **2013**, *1* (November), 1–22.

54. Kim, H.-B.; Kim, H.; Lee, W. I.; Jang, D.-J. *J. Mater. Chem. A* **2015**, *3* (18), 9714–9721.

55. Suzuki, Y.; Ngamsinlapasathian, S.; Yoshida, R.; Yoshikawa, S. *Open Chem.* **2006**, *4* (3), 476–488.

56. Dalod, A. R. M.; Henriksen, L.; Grande, T.; Einarsrud, M.-A. *Beilstein J. Nanotechnol.* **2017**, *8*, 304–312.

57. Yang, M.; Ding, B.; Lee, S.; Lee, J. K. *J. Phys. Chem. C* **2011**, *115* (30), 14534–14541.

58. Zhang, Y. X.; Li, G. H.; Jin, Y. X.; Zhang, Y.; Zhang, J.; Zhang, L. D. *Chem. Phys. Lett.* **2002**, *365* (3–4), 300–304.

59. Mahmoud, S. A.; Fouad, O. A. *Sol. Energy Mater. Sol. Cells* **2015**, *136*, 38–43.

60. Lu, L.; Li, R.; Fan, K.; Peng, T. *Sol. Energy* **2010**, *84* (5), 844–853.

61. Lin, C.-Y.; Lai, Y.-H.; Chen, H.-W.; Chen, J.-G.; Kung, C.-W.; Vittal, R.; Ho, K.-C. *Energy Environ. Sci.* **2011**, *4* (9), 3448.

62. Zhu, S.; Shan, L.; Tian, X.; Zheng, X.; Sun, D.; Liu, X.; Wang, L.; Zhou, Z. Author ™ S Accepted Manuscript. *Ceram. Int.* **2014**.

63. Zi, M.; Zhu, M.; Chen, L.; Wei, H.; Yang, X.; Cao, B. *Ceram. Int.* **2014**, 1–6.

64. Wang, X.; Summers, C. J.; Wang, Z. L. *Nano Lett.* **2004**, *4* (3), 423–426.

65. Bokhari, M.; Kasi, A. K.; Kasi, J. K.; Gujela, O. P.; Afzulpurkar, N. **2015**, *11*, 56–63.

66. Mccune, M.; Zhang, W.; Deng, Y. **2012**.

67. Lee, C. P.; Chou, C. Y.; Chen, C. Y.; Yeh, M. H.; Lin, L. Y.; Vittal, R.; Wu, C. G.; Ho, K. C. *J. Power Sources* **2014**, *246*, 1–9.
68. Elumalai, N. K.; Jose, R.; Archana, P. S.; Chellappan, V.; Ramakrishna, S. *J. Phys. Chem. C* **2012**, *116* (42), 22112–22120.
69. Kay, A.; Grätzel, M. *Chem. Mater.* **2002**, *14* (7), 2930–2935.
70. Wang, Y.-F.; Li, K.-N.; Wu, W.-Q.; Xu, Y.-F.; Chen, H.-Y.; Su, C.-Y.; Kuang, D.-B. *RSC Adv.* **2013**, *3* (33), 13804.
71. Bu, I. Y.-Y. *Optik (Stuttg).* **2017**, *147*, 39–42.
72. Gao, C.; Li, X.; Lu, B.; Chen, L.; Wang, Y.; Teng, F.; Wang, J.; Zhang, Z.; Pan, X.; Xie, E. A. *Nanoscale* **2012**, *4* (11), 3475.
73. Nowak, I.; Ziolek, M. *Chem. Rev.* **1999**, *99* (12), 3603–3624.
74. Raj, C. C.; Prasanth, R. *J. Power Sources* **2016**, *317*, 120–132.
75. Zhang, H.; Wang, Y.; Yang, D.; Li, Y.; Liu, H.; Liu, P.; Wood, B. J.; Zhao, H. Directly. *Adv. Mater.* **2012**, *24* (12), 1598–1603.
76. Joshi, P.; Zhang, L.; Davoux, D.; Zhu, Z.; Galipeau, D.; Fong, H.; Qiao, Q. *Energy Environ. Sci.* **2010**, *3* (10), 1507.
77. Rani, R. A.; Zoolfakar, A. S.; O'Mullane, A. P.; Austin, M. W.; Kalantar-Zadeh, K. *J. Mater. Chem. A* **2014**, *2* (38), 15683–15703.
78. He, J.; Hu, Y.; Wang, Z.; Lu, W.; Yang, S.; Wu, G.; Wang, Y.; Wang, S.; Gu, H.; Wang, J. *J. Mater. Chem. C* **2014**, *2* (38), 8185–8190.
79. Ou, J. Z.; Rani, R. A.; Ham, M. H.; Field, M. R.; Zhang, Y.; Zheng, H.; Reece, P.; Zhuiykov, S.; Sriram, S.; Bhaskaran, M.; et al. *ACS Nano* **2012**, *6* (5), 4045–4053.
80. Qi, S.; Fei, L.; Zuo, R.; Wang, Y.; Wu, Y. *J. Mater. Chem. A* **2014**, *2* (22), 8190.
81. Wei, W.; Lee, K.; Shaw, S.; Schmuki, P. *Chem. Commun.* **2012**, *48* (35), 4244.
82. Ghosh, R.; Brennaman, M. K.; Uher, T.; Ok, M.-R.; Samulski, E. T.; McNeil, L. E.; Meyer, T. J.; Lopez, R. *ACS Appl. Mater. Interfaces* **2011**, *3* (10), 3929–3935.
83. Jiang, C. Y.; Sun, X. W.; Lo, G. Q.; Kwong, D. L.; Wang, J. X. *Appl. Phys. Lett.* **2007**, *90* (26), 263501.
84. Abd-Ellah, M.; Moghimi, N.; Zhang, L.; Heinig, N. F.; Zhao, L.; Thomas, J. P.; Leung, K. T. *J. Phys. Chem. C* **2013**, *117* (13), 6794–6799.
85. Lupan, O.; Guérin, V. M.; Ghimpu, L.; Tiginyanu, I. M.; Pauporté, T. *Chem. Phys. Lett.* **2012**, *550*, 125–129.
86. Wang, J. X.; Wu, C. M. L.; Cheung, W. S.; Luo, L. B.; He, Z. B.; Yuan, G. D.; Zhang, W. J.; Lee, C. S.; Lee, S. T. *J. Phys. Chem. C* **2010**, *114* (31), 13157–13161.
87. Chang, J.; Ahmed, R.; Wang, H.; Liu, H.; Li, R.; Wang, P.; Waclawik, E. R. *J. Phys. Chem. C* **2013**, *117* (27), 13836–13844.
88. Arote, S. A.; Tabhane, V. A.; Pathan, H. M. *Opt. Mater. (Amst).* **2018**, *75*, 601–606.
89. Gubbala, S.; Chakrapani, V.; Kumar, V.; Sunkara, M. K. *Adv. Funct. Mater.* **2008**, *18* (16), 2411–2418.
90. Kim, D.; Ghicov, A.; Albu, S. P.; Schmuki, P. *J. Am. Chem. Soc.* **2008**, 16454–16455.
91. Fan, J.; Liu, S.; Yu, J. *J. Mater. Chem.* **2012**, *22* (33), 17027.
92. Low, F. W.; Lai, C. W.; Abd Hamid, S. B. *Ceram. Int.* **2017**, *43* (1), 625–633.
93. Muduli, S.; Lee, W.; Dhas, V.; Mujawar, S.; Dubey, M.; Vijayamohanan, K.; Han, S. H.; Ogale, S. *ACS Appl. Mater. Interfaces* **2009**, *1* (9), 2030–2035.
94. Li, B.; Luo, L.; Xiao, T.; Hu, X.; Lu, L.; Wang, J.; Tang, Y. *J. Alloys Compd.* **2011**, *509* (5), 2186–2191.
95. Zhou, Y.; Xia, C.; Hu, X.; Huang, W.; Aref, A. A.; Wang, B.; Liu, Z.; Sun, Y.; Zhou, W.; Tang, Y. *Appl. Surf. Sci.* **2014**, *292*, 111–116.
96. Liu, M.; Yang, J.; Feng, S.; Zhu, H.; Zhang, J.; Li, G.; Peng, J. *Mater. Lett.* **2012**, *76*, 215–218.
97. Bhande, S. S.; Shinde, D. V.; Tehare, K. K.; Patil, S. A.; Mane, R. S.; Naushad, M.; Alothman, Z. A.; Hui, K. N.; Han, S. H. *J. Photochem. Photobiol. A Chem.* **2014**, *295*, 64–69.

98. Manthina, V.; Correa Baena, J. P.; Liu, G.; Agrios, A. G. *J. Phys. Chem. C* **2012**, *116* (45), 23864–23870.
99. Menzies, D. B.; Cervini, R.; Cheng, Y.; Simon, G. P. **2004**, 363–366.
100. Docampo, P.; Tiwana, P.; Sakai, N.; Miura, H.; Herz, L.; Murakami, T.; Snaith, H. J. *J. Phys. Chem. C* **2012**, *116* (43), 22840–22846.
101. Perera, K. A. T. A.; Anuradha, S. G.; Kumara, G. R. A.; Paranawitharana, M. L.; Rajapakse, R. M. G.; Bandara, H. M. N. *Electrochim. Acta* **2011**, *56* (11), 4135–4138.
102. Aponsu, G. M. L. P.; Wijayarathna, T. R. C. K.; Perera, I. K.; Perera, V. P. S.; Siriwardhana, A. C. P. K. *Acta: Part A Mol. Biomol. Spectrosc.* **2013**, *109*, 37–41.
103. Lee, C.; Lee, G. W.; Kang, W.; Lee, D. K.; Ko, M. J.; Kim, K.; Park, N. G. *Bull. Korean Chem. Soc.* **2010**, *31* (11), 3093–3098.
104. Ramasamy, E.; Lee, J. *J. Phys. Chem. C* **2010**, *114* (50), 22032–22037.
105. Li, Z.; Zhou, Y.; Mao, W.; Zou, Z. *J. Power Sources* **2015**, *274*, 575–581.
106. Wu, J.; Lan, Z.; Lin, J.; Huang, M.; Huang, Y.; Fan, L.; Luo, G.; Lin, Y.; Xie, Y.; Wei, Y. *Chem. Soc. Rev.* **2017**, *46* (19), 5975–6023.
107. Theerthagiri, J.; Senthil, A. R.; Madhavan, J.; Maiyalagan, T. *ChemElectroChem* **2015**, *2* (7), 928–945.
108. Yun, S.; Hagfeldt, A.; Ma, T. *Adv. Mater.* **2014**, *26* (36), 6210–6237.
109. Wu, M.; Ma, T. *ChemSusChem.* **2012**, *5*, 1343–1357.
110. Tang, Q.; Duan, J.; Duan, Y.; He, B.; Yu, L. *Electrochimica Acta.* **2015**, *178*, 886–899.
111. Saranya, K.; Rameez, M.; Subramania, A. *European Polymer Journal* **2015**, *66*, 207–227.
112. Thomas, S.; Deepak, T. G.; Anjusree, G. S.; Arun, T. A.; Nair, S. V.; Nair, A. S. *J. Mater. Chem. A Mater. Energy Sustain.* **2014**, *2* (13), 4474–4490.
113. Kouhnavard, M.; Ludin, N. A.; Ghaffari, B. V.; Sopian, K.; Ikeda, S. Challenges and prospects. *ChemSusChem.* 2015, *8* (9) 1510–1533.
114. Nam, J. G.; Park, Y. J.; Kim, B. S.; Lee, J. S. *Scr. Mater.* **2010**, *62* (3), 148–150.
115. Xiao, Y.; Wu, J.; Lin, J.; Yue, G.; Lin, J.; Huang, M.; Huang, Y.; Lan, Z.; Fan, L. *J. Mater. Chem. A* **2013**, *1* (44), 13885.
116. Chang, L.-Y.; Lee, C.-P.; Huang, K.-C.; Wang, Y.-C.; Yeh, M.-H.; Lin, J.-J.; Ho, K.-C. *J. Mater. Chem.* **2012**, *22* (7), 3185.
117. Lee, W. J.; Ramasamy, E.; Lee, D. Y.; Song, J. S. *ACS Appl. Mater. Interfaces* **2009**, *1* (6), 1145–1149.
118. Chiang, C.-H.; Chen, S.-C.; Wu, C.-G. *Org. Electron.* **2013**, *14* (9), 2369–2378.
119. Wu, J.; Li, Q.; Fan, L.; Lan, Z.; Li, P.; Lin, J.; Hao, S. *J. Power Sources* **2008**, *181* (1), 172–176.
120. Gong, F.; Xu, X.; Zhou, G.; Wang, Z.-S. *Phys. Chem. Chem. Phys.* **2013**, *15* (2), 546–552.
121. Jeon, S. S.; Kim, C.; Ko, J.; Im, S. S. *J. Phys. Chem. C* **2011**, *115* (44), 22035–22039.
122. Ahmad, S.; Yum, J.-H.; Butt, H.-J.; Nazeeruddin, M. K.; Grätzel, M. *Chemphyschem* **2010**, *11* (13), 2814–2819.
123. Yun, D.-J.; Kim, J.; Chung, J.; Park, S.; Baek, W.; Kim, Y.; Kim, S.; Kwon, Y.-N.; Chung, J.; Kyoung, Y.; et al. *J. Power Sources* **2014**, *268*, 25–36.
124. Wang, L.; Al-Mamun, M.; Liu, P.; Wang, Y.; Yang, H. G.; Wang, H. F.; Zhao, H, Mechanistic study, material screening and experimental validation. *NPG Asia Materials.* **2015**, *7*, 226.
125. Hou, Y.; Wang, D.; Yang, X. H.; Fang, W. Q.; Zhang, B.; Wang, H. F.; Lu, G. Z.; Hu, P.; Zhao, H. J.; Yang, H. G. *Nat. Commun.* **2013**, *4*.
126. Guai, G. H.; Leiw, M. Y.; Ng, C. M.; Li, C. M. *Adv. Energy Mater.* **2012**, *2* (3), 334–338.
127. Wu, M.; Lin, X.; Guo, W.; Wang, Y.; Chu, L.; Ma, T.; Wu, K. *Chem. Commun.* **2013**, *49* (11), 1058.
128. Zhou, H.; Shi, Y.; Wang, L.; Zhang, H.; Zhao, C.; Hagfeldt, A.; Ma, T. *Chem. Commun.* **2013**, *49* (69), 7626.

129. Wu, M.; Lin, X.; Wang, Y.; Wang, L.; Guo, W.; Qi, D.; Peng, X.; Hagfeldt, A.; Grätzel, M.; Ma, T. *J. Am. Chem. Soc.* **2012**, *134* (7), 3419–3428.

130. Mokurala, K.; Mallick, S. *RSC Adv.* **2017**, *7* (25), 15139–15148.

131. Mokurala, K.; Mallick, S.; Bhargava, P. *J. Power Sources* **2016**, *305*, 134–143.

132. Bathina, C.; Mokurala, K.; Ravindran, P.; Bhargava, P.; Mallick, S. *Adv. Mater. Lett.* **2016**, *7* (11), 100–150.

133. Mokurala, K.; Kamble, A.; Bathina, C.; Bhargava, P.; Mallick, S. *Mater. Today Proc.* **2016**, *3* (6), 1778–1784.

134. Fan, M.-S.; Chen, J.-H.; Li, C.-T.; Cheng, K.-W.; Ho, K.-C. *J. Mater. Chem. A* **2015**, *3* (2), 562–569.

135. He, J.; Lee, L. T. L.; Yang, S.; Li, Q.; Xiao, X.; Chen, T. *ACS Appl. Mater. Interfaces* **2014**, *6* (4), 2224–2229.

136. Jena, A.; Mohanty, S. P.; Kumar, P.; Naduvath, J.; Lekha, P.; Das, J.; Narula, H. K.; Mallick, S.; Bhargava, P.; Gondane, V. *Trans. Indian Ceram. Soc.* **2012**, *71* (May 2012), 1–16.

137. Sauvage, F. *Adv. Chem.* **2014**, *2014*, 1–23.

138. Bella, F.; Galliano, S.; Gerbaldi, C.; Viscardi, G. *Energies* **2016**, 1–22.

139. Bella, F.; Gerbaldi, C.; Barolo, C.; Grätzel, M. *Chem. Soc. Rev.* **2015**, *44* (11), 3431–3473.

140. O'Regan, B. C.; Durrant, J. R. *Acc. Chem. Res.* **2009**, *42* (11), 1799–1808.

141. Mahmood, A. *Journal of Energy Chemistry.* **2015**, *24*, 686–692.

142. Chiba, Y.; Islam, A.; Watanabe, Y.; Komiya, R.; Koide, N.; Han, L. *Jpn. J. Appl. Phys.* **2006**, *45* (No. 25), L638–L640.

143. Han, L.; Koide, N.; Chiba, Y.; Islam, A.; Komiya, R.; Fuke, N.; Fukui, A.; Yamanaka, R. *Appl. Phys. Lett.* **2005**, *86* (21), 1–3.

144. Hinsch, A.; Kroon, J. M.; Kern, R.; Uhlendorf, I.; Holzbock, J.; Meyer, A.; Ferber, J. *Appl.* **2001**, *9* (6), 425–438.

145. Yanagida, S.; Yu, Y.; Manseki, K. *Acc. Chem. Res.* **2009**, *42* (11), 1827–1838.

146. Yu, Z.; Vlachopoulos, N.; Gorlov, M.; Kloo, L. *Dalt. Trans.* **2011**, *40* (40), 10289.

147. Tsao, H. N.; Burschka, J.; Yi, C.; Kessler, F.; Nazeeruddin, M. K.; Grätzel, M. *Energy Environ. Sci.* **2011**, *4* (12), 4921.

148. Tian, H.; Sun, L. *J. Mater. Chem.* **2011**, *21* (29), 10592.

149. Wang, Z. S.; Sayama, K.; Sugihara, H. *J. Phys. Chem. B* **2005**, *109* (47), 22449–22455.

150. Teng, C.; Yang, X.; Yuan, C.; Li, C.; Chen, R.; Tian, H.; Li, S.; Hagfeldt, A.; Sun, L. *Org. Lett.* **2009**, *11* (23), 5542–5545.

151. Oskam, G.; Bergeron, B. V.; Meyer, G. J.; Searson, P. C. P. *J. Phys. Chem. B* **2001**, *105* (29), 6867–6873.

152. Bergeron, B. V.; Marton, A.; Oskam, G.; Meyer, G. J. *J. Phys. Chem. B* **2005**, *109* (2), 937–943.

153. Zhang, Z.; Chen, P.; Murakami, T. N.; Zakeeruddin, S. M.; Grätzel, M. *Adv. Funct. Mater.* **2008**, *18* (2), 341–346.

154. Wang, M.; Chamberland, N.; Breau, L.; Moser, J. E.; Humphry-Baker, R.; Marsan, B.; Zakeeruddin, S. M.; Grätzel, M. *Nat. Chem.* **2010**, *2* (5), 385–389.

155. Li, D.; Li, H.; Luo, Y.; Li, K.; Meng, Q.; Armand, M.; Chen, L. *Adv. Funct. Mater.* **2010**, *20* (19), 3358–3365.

156. Nevin, K. P.; Hensley, S. A.; Franks, A. E.; Summers, Z. M.; Ou, J.; Woodard, T. L.; Snoeyenbos-West, O. L.; Lovley, D. R. *Appl. Environ. Microbiol.* **2011**, *77* (9), 2882–2886.

157. Daeneke, T.; Kwon, T. H.; Holmes, A. B.; Duffy, N. W.; Bach, U.; Spiccia, L. *Nat. Chem.* **2011**, *3* (3), 211–215.

158. Tsao, H. N.; Yi, C.; Moehl, T.; Yum, J. H.; Zakeeruddin, S. M.; Nazeeruddin, M. K.; Grätzel, M. *ChemSusChem* **2011**, *4* (5), 591–594.

159. Bai, Y.; Yu, Q.; Cai, N.; Wang, Y.; Zhang, M.; Wang, P. *Chem. Commun.* **2011**, *47* (15), 4376.

160. Giribabu, L.; Bolligarla, R.; Panigrahi, M. *Chem. Rec.* **2015**, *15* (4), 760–788.
161. Hamann, T. W. T. *Dalt. Trans.* **2012**, *41* (11), 3111.
162. Yella, A.; Mathew, S.; Aghazada, S.; Comte, P.; Grätzel, M.; Nazeeruddin, M. K. *J. Mater. Chem. C* **2017**, *5* (11), 2833–2843.
163. Koh, T. M.; Nonomura, K.; Mathews, N.; Hagfeldt, A.; Grätzel, M.; Mhaisalkar, S. G.; Grimsdale, A. C. *J. Phys. Chem. C* **2013**, *117* (30), 15515–15522.
164. Kontos, A. G.; Stergiopoulos, T.; Likodimos, V.; Milliken, D.; Desilvesto, H.; Tulloch, G.; Falaras, P. *J. Phys. Chem. C* **2013**, *117* (17), 8636–8646.
165. Likodimos, V.; Stergiopoulos, T.; Falaras, P.; Harikisun, R.; Desilvestro, J.; Tulloch, G. *J. Phys. Chem. C* **2009**, *113* (21), 9412–9422.
166. Gao, J.; Bhagavathi Achari, M.; Kloo, L. *Chem. Commun.* **2014**, *50* (47), 6249–6251.
167. Mozaffari, S.; Nateghi, M. R.; Zarandi, M. B. *Renew. Sustain. Energy Rev.* **2017**, *71*, 675–686.
168. Mehmood, U.; Al-Ahmed, A.; Al-Sulaiman, F. A.; Malik, M. I.; Shehzad, F.; Khan, A. U. H. *Renew. Sustain. Energy Rev.* **2017**, *79*, 946–959.
169. Balasingam, S. K.; Jun, Y. *Isr. J. Chem.* **2015**, 955–965.
170. Mohamad, A. A. *J. Power Sources* **2016**, *329*, 57–71.
171. Li, B.; Wang, L.; Kang, B.; Wang, P.; Qiu, Y. *Sol. Energy Mater. Sol. Cells.* **2006**, 549–573.
172. Cao, Y.; Saygili, Y.; Ummadisingu, A.; Teuscher, J.; Luo, J.; Pellet, N.; Giordano, F.; Zakeeruddin, S. M.; Moser, J.-E.; Freitag, M.; et al. *Nat. Commun.* **2017**, *8*, 15390.
173. Margulis, G. Y.; Lim, B.; Hardin, B. E.; Unger, E. L.; Yum, J. H.; Feckl, J. M.; Fattakhova-Rohlfing, D.; Bein, T.; Grätzel, M.; Sellinger, A. et al. *Phys. Chem. Chem. Phys.* **2013**, *15* (27), 11306–11312.
174. Eisenmenger, N. D.; Delaney, K. T.; Ganesan, V.; Fredrickson, G. H.; Chabinyc, M. L. I. *J. Phys. Chem. C.* **2014**, *118* (26), 14096–14106.
175. Mor, G. K.; Basham, J.; Paulose, M.; Kim, S.; Varghese, O. K.; Vaish, A.; Yoriya, S.; Grimes, C. A. *Nano Lett.* **2010**, *10* (7), 2387–2394.
176. Sahoo, H. *J. Photochem. Photobiol. C Photochem. Rev.* **2011**, *12* (1), 20–30.
177. Mor, G. K.; Basham, J.; Paulose, M.; Kim, S.; Varghese, O. K.; Vaish, A.; Yoriya, S.; Grimes, C. A. H. *Nano Lett.* **2010**, *10* (7), 2387–2394.
178. Menke, S. M.; Holmes, R. J. *Energy Environ. Sci.* **2014**, *7* (2), 499–512.
179. Obeng, E. M.; Dullah, E. C.; Abdul Razak, N. S.; Danquah, M. K.; Budiman, C.; Ongkudon, C. M. *J. Biol. Methods* **2017**, *4* (2), 71.
180. Hardin, B. E.; Yum, J.-H.; Hoke, E. T.; Jun, Y. C.; Péchy, P.; Torres, T.; Brongersma, M. L.; Nazeeruddin, M. K.; Grätzel, M.; McGehee, M. D. *Nano Lett.* **2010**, *10* (8), 3077–3083.
181. Yum, J. H.; Hardin, B. E.; Hoke, E. T.; Baranoff, E.; Zakeeruddin, S. M.; Nazeeruddin, M. K.; Torres, T.; McGehee, M. D.; Gra(a-umlaut)tzel, M. *ChemPhysChem* **2011**, *12* (3), 657–661.
182. Hoke, E. T.; Hardin, B. E.; McGehee, M. D. *Opt. Express* **2010**, *18* (4), 3893–3904.
183. Yum, J. H.; Hardin, B. E.; Moon, S. J.; Baranoff, E.; Nüesch, F.; McGehee, M. D.; Grätzel, M.; Nazeeruddin, M. K. *Angew. Chemie: Int. Ed.* **2009**, *48* (49), 9277–9280.
184. Yum, J.; Baranoff, E.; Hardin, B. E.; Hoke, E. T.; Mcgehee, M. D.; Frank, N.; Grätzel, M. *Energy Environ. Sci.* **2010**, *3*, 434–437.
185. Puntambekar, A.; Chakrapani, V. **2016**, *245301*, 1–7.
186. Freitag, M.; Teuscher, J.; Saygili, Y.; Zhang, X.; Giordano, F.; Liska, P.; Hua, J.; Zakeeruddin, S. M.; Moser, J. E.; Grätzel, M.; et al. *Nat. Photonics* **2017**, *11* (6), 372–378.
187. Scalia, A.; Bella, F.; Lamberti, A.; Bianco, S.; Gerbaldi, C.; Tresso, E.; Pirri, C. F. *J. Power Sources* **2017**, *359*, 311–321.

3 Organic Bulk Heterojunction Solar Cells

Daize Mo, Tianyu Bai, Leilei Tian, and Feng He

CONTENTS

3.1   INTRODUCTION

Organic semiconductors have attracted considerable attention from both the academic and industrial communities due to their numerous applications, such as organic light-emitting diodes (OLEDs), organic field-effect transistors (OFETs), and organic solar cells (OSCs).[1–4] In particular, the bulk heterojunction (BHJ) organic solar cells have the potential for harnessing low-cost solar energy because of their many advantages when compared with their inorganic counterparts (silicon-, CdTe-, and CdInGaSe-based devices), such as simple device structure, low cost, abundant materials, light weight, and easy large area fabrication on flexible substrates.[5–8] Due to these advantages, extensive research efforts around the world have been devoted to understanding and improving the performance of BHJ organic solar cells in the past 20 years.

The BHJ solar cells possess a sandwich structure with a blend active layer containing two components,[9] a conjugated polymer or a small molecule as the electron donor and a fullerene derivative ($PC_{61}BM$ and $PC_{71}BM$) as the electron acceptor between two electrodes. They are known for their outstanding optical properties and their ability to transport charges.[10] In a BHJ structure, donor and acceptor materials are mixed together to form a bicontinuous interpenetrating network with large interfacial areas for efficient exciton dissociation.[4] The first conceptual OSCs were reported by Kearns and Calvin in 1958 and had a pristine organic material (magnesium phthalocyanine) between two electrodes.[11] However, the power conversion efficiency (PCE) stayed in the order of 0.1% or lower for more than 20 years.[11] In 1986,[12] Tang introduced the donor-acceptor bilayer planar heterojunction to the OPV cell and achieved power-conversion efficiencies (PCEs) of around 1%. Later, Heeger and Wudl groups[13,14] observed ultrafast electron transfer from poly[2-methoxy-5-(2-ethylhexyloxy)]-1,4-phenylenevinylene (MEH-PPV) to C_{60}, which suggested the feasibility of using conjugated polymers as electron donors and fullerene derivatives as electron acceptors in PSCs. Heeger and coworkers[9] introduced the BHJ structure to the blends of polymer and fullerene. Friend and coworkers[15] also demonstrated the efficient photogeneration in a BHJ structure based on all polymer blends with not only polymer donor and polymer acceptor. Later, it was realized that domain sizes of donor and acceptor can be further optimized with additives.[16] Since then, the BHJ structure has become the standard architecture for organic solar cells. Thus far, the PCEs of single, double, and triple BHJ organic solar devices using conjugated polymers as the donors and fullerene derivatives as the acceptors have surpassed 10.5%,[8] 11.3%,[17] and 11.7%,[7,18] reaching the dawn of commercialization.

As discussed earlier, the photovoltaic performance of BHJ organic solar devices is closer to the inorganic solar cells (PCE: 15%–20%). Therefore, summarizing current state-of-the-art BHJ organic solar devices is very important for the future development of this field. In this chapter, we describe the bulk heterojunction solar cell in five parts: the basics, device structure, materials design, morphology, and interface engineering. Also, although several excellent and comprehensive reviews by Sariciftci et al.[19] and Frechet et al. have appeared in the past,[20] this chapter will focus especially on more recent advances. We encourage readers to cover these reviews for more of the basis of BHJ organic solar devices.

3.1.1 BULK HETEROJUNCTION SOLAR CELL BASICS

The ratio of the output electric power to the incident solar power is defined as the power conversion efficiency (PCE):

$$\text{PCE} = \frac{P_{\text{out}}}{P_{\text{in}}} = \frac{J_{\text{SC}} \times V_{\text{OC}} \times \text{FF}}{P_{\text{in}}}$$

The PCE is directly proportional to three parameters: open-circuit voltage (V_{OC}) (V), short-circuit current density (J_{SC}) (A/m²), and fill factor (FF) under standard solar irradiation (AM 1.5G 100 mW/cm²) (Figure 3.1). To allow for valid comparison of device performance, an international standard for input power is used. Therefore, there are three major device characteristics that completely determine the efficiency of the device. The following describes the factors that influence these device characteristics for OSCs.

V_{OC} (the maximum voltage during the measurements), is related to the difference between the lowest unoccupied molecular orbital (LUMO) of the acceptor materials and the highest occupied molecular orbital (HOMO) of the donor polymer.[21] Other factors connected to the processes, such as charge recombination in the cell, the morphology of the active layer,[22] and interfaces,[22] can also influence the V_{OC}. It was found that there exists a linear relationship between the HOMO position, which is related to the diagonal bandgap of the heterojunction and the open-circuit voltage.[23]

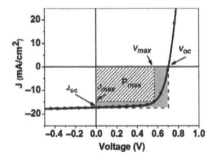

FIGURE 3.1 Current density versus voltage plot characteristic of a solar cell device. (Reproduced with permission from Lu, L. et al., *Chem. Rev.*, 115, 12666–12731, 2015. Copyright 2015 American Chemical Society.)

From this analysis, a simple relationship between the HOMO of the donor material and V_{OC} of the device was derived. This was reported as follows:

$$V_{OC} = \left(\frac{1}{e}\right)\left(\left|E^{Dodor}\ HOMO\right| - \left|E^{PCBM}\ LUMO\right|\right) - 0.3\ V$$

J_{SC} represents the maximum current density of the organic solar cell devices that can be obtained, mainly determined by the number of photons absorbed by the materials within the solar spectrum and also affected by the thickness of the active layer, interface, and the spectral absorption range absorbed by the organic materials. Furthermore, the charge transport properties are also a factor that affected the current density (J_{SC}). The J_{SC} is directly related to the external quantum efficiency (EQE). The relationship can be expressed as follows:

$$J_{SC} = \frac{q}{hc} \int_{\lambda_{min}}^{\lambda_{max}} EQE \times P_{in}\ (\lambda)\lambda \times d\ (\lambda)$$

The EQE is the ratio of the photogenerated electrons collected to the number of incident photons at a specific wavelength.

Fill factor (FF) describes the quality of the solar cell, which is decided by the number of photogenerated carriers and the number of the photogenerated carriers by the electrode. The fill factor of solar cells is determined by

$$FF = \frac{J_m \times V_m}{J_{SC} \times V_{OC}}$$

J_m and V_m as the current and the voltage in the maximum power point of the J/V curve in the 4th quadrant reflect the diode properties of the solar cells. In fact, FF represents the carrier transport and competition complex process.

The molar absorption coefficient of the absorbing molecule is important to obtain high external quantum efficiencies (EQEs), and the HOMO/LUMO energy levels should be adjusted properly to give higher V_{OC} and FF values. The EQE as a function of wavelength (λ) is the ratio between the collected photogenerated charges and the number of incident photons, ultimately being the product of four efficiencies (η): absorption (A), exciton diffusion (ED), charge separation (CS), and charge collection (CC).

$$EQE\ (\lambda) = \eta_A\ (\lambda) \times \eta_{ED}\ (\lambda) \times \eta_{CS}\ (\lambda) \times \eta_{CC}\ (\lambda)$$

In a typical BHJOPV device, a heterojunction consisting of a p-type organic donor and an n-type organic acceptor is the photoactive part for converting solar light to electricity. So far, the most successful architecture to build organic photovoltaic solar cells is the BHJ structure prepared by mixing donors and acceptor to generate nanoscale phase separation.[24] The BHJ structure offers a high density of heterojunction interfaces in the device, and the structure can be easily implemented.[5] It also allows for a quick survey of the best composition of materials in the active layer. The composite active layer can be prepared by solution or vacuum deposition techniques.

Solution-processed BHJ solar cells offer the possibility of manufacturing the composite active layer over a large area in one simple step at room temperature, which can be very effective both in cost and in energy.[25]

As a class of excitonic solar cells, organic solar cells rely on a charge photogeneration mechanism, which is different from that of silicon-based solar cells (Figure 3.2).[26,27] In inorganic solar cells, a free electron-hole pair is formed up on light absorption, whereas in organic solar cells photoexcitation leads to the formation of an exciton, that is, a coulombically bound electron-hole pair.[28] This fundamental difference is caused by the low dielectric constant of organic materials (typically 2–5), which is insufficient to cause immediate electron-hole dissociation.

The exciton is formed in the organic layer, which consists of an organic p-type material (electron donor) blended with an organic n-type material (electron acceptor), upon light absorption. Once the exciton has been formed, it diffuses through the active layer until it reaches the donor-acceptor interface to dissociate into free charge carriers (holes and electrons) that migrate toward the electrodes under the internal field. Unfortunately, not every formed exciton will dissociate into free charge carriers, regardless of whether the exciton reaches the donor-acceptor interface or not. An exciton typically has a lifetime of several nanoseconds and within this time it can diffuse over a distance of 5–10 nm.[29,30] If the exciton does not reach the donor–acceptor interface within its lifetime, it will decay and the absorbed energy is lost by heat release. On the other hand, if the exciton reaches the interface, it does not necessarily lead to electron transfer to the acceptor and the formation of free charge carriers. If the energy offset between the donor's LUMO and the acceptor's LUMO is too small, then no electron transfer will occur. Recombination mechanisms are other counterproductive phenomena to the charge separation process. There are two recombination mechanisms, geminate recombination and bimolecular recombination. In the case of geminate recombination, the bound charges do not separate at the donor-acceptor interface, but they recombine, relaxing to the initial ground state. Bimolecular recombination, on the other hand, results from the recombination of free charge carriers formed from dissociation of different excitons.[31]

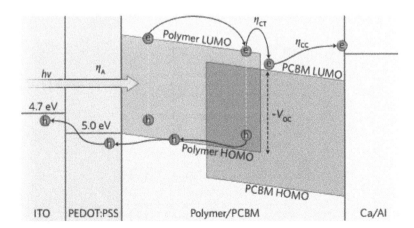

FIGURE 3.2 The operating mechanism of a PSC. (Reproduced from Li, G. et al., *Nat. Photon.*, 6, 153–161, 2012. With permission from Springer Nature.)

3.2 SOLAR CELL ARCHITECTURES

In order to meet the specific requirement for efficient photon to charge conversion, different device architectures have been developed. Figure 3.3 shows a typical bilayer device (p–n diode). Charge separation occurs at the interface between the two layers. Ideally, the donor material should only be in contact with the electrode material with the higher work-function (typically ITO) and the acceptor-material with the lower work-function electrode (typically Al). The different architectures are now given as follows.

3.2.1 BILAYER SOLAR CELL

The formation of the heterojunction by Tang et al.[12] in 1986 was first demonstrated in the form of a bilayer solar cell. As shown in Figure 3.3, the common structure of a bilayer solar cell consists of an anode, hole collection layer, active layer composed of donor and acceptor, electron collection layer, and cathode fabricated sequentially. The hole collection layer and electron collection layer are used to modify the work function of the electrodes to form an ohmic contact. A single, well-defined interface exists between the donor and acceptor at which excitons dissociate. With this structure, the bilayer solar cell is the simplest structure described by the basic operating principle of the solar cell.

A significant drawback for a bilayer solar cell is that the short exciton diffusion length of organic materials limits the thickness of the donor and acceptor layers. If the donor or acceptor layer is too thick, the excitons generated far away from the heterojunction may recombine before reaching the heterojunction. Also, the donor and acceptor layers are limited to tens of nanometers, which lead to weak absorption. To ensure that excitons are generated near the heterojunction, interference effects have to be considered fully during the design of bilayer solar cells. These mutual trade-off factors lead to low EQE and impose challenges in the design of bilayer OSCs.[34]

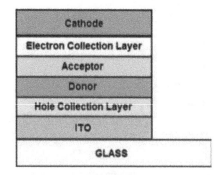

FIGURE 3.3 Structure of a bilayer solar cell. (Reproduced from Fung, D. and Choy, W., *Organic Solar Cells, Green Energy and Technology,* Springer, London, UK, 2013. With permission from Springer Nature.)

3.2.2 BULK HETEROJUNCTION SOLAR CELLS

One of the most important breakthroughs in the field of OSCs is arguably the discovery of the bulk heterojunction (BHJ) in the mid 1990s.[15] (Figure 3.4) The bulk heterojunctions may be achieved by solution casting of donor and acceptor pigments of polymer/ polymer, polymer/molecule, or molecule/moleculedonor-acceptor blends. The most efficient devices today are the solution processed **PBDB-T:IT-M** devices with a high PCE of 12.05% under AM 1.5G, 100 mW cm^{-2}. Often, the bulk heterojunction solar cells are built on a transparent substrate coated with a conductive and transparent electrode material. Due to its excellent transparency and conductivity, ITO (indium tin oxide) is applied in most of the reported devices. In the so-called standard configuration (Figure 3.5a) the ITO is coated with a hole transport layer (HTL). Thin films of doped conjugated polymer such as PEDOT:PSS (poly(3,4-ethylenedioxythiophene)poly(styrenesulfonate)) or a thin oxide layer (e.g., MoO$_3$) have been used as HTLs. On top of the HTL, the photoactive layer, a blend of donor and acceptor material is coated, followed by an optional electron transport layer (ETL) and a low work function electrode. ETL materials are often oxides such as zinc oxide or titanium dioxide. Such a transparent thin layer can also improve

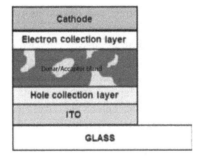

FIGURE 3.4 Structure of a bulk heterojunction solar cell. (Reproduced from Fung, D. and Choy, W., *Organic Solar Cells, Green Energy and Technology*, Springer, London, UK, 2013. With permission from Springer Nature.)

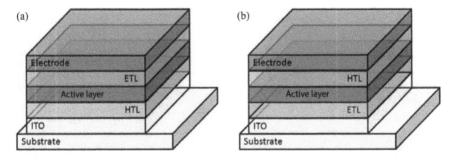

FIGURE 3.5 Different device architectures of bulk heterojunction solar cells. (a) Standard device design with the cathode on top of the device stack and (b) inverted device architecture with the cathode located on the transparent substrate. (Reproduced from Scharber, M.C. and Sariciftci, N.S., *Prog. Polym. Sci.*, 38, 1929–1940, 2013.)

the light absorption in the photoactive layer when used as a so-called optical spacer.[33] In the standard architecture, the top electrode is the cathode and calcium, barium, or aluminum is applied for collecting the electrons generated in the photoactive layer.[20]

In the inverted architecture, the transparent electrode coated on the substrate acts as a cathode. Either by modifying the work function of the electrode material by applying an interfacial layer,[34] or by using transparent oxides such as zinc oxide[35] or titanium dioxide,[36] a selective contact to the acceptor material in the active layer is formed. On top of the active layer an HTL such as PEDOT: PSS or a thin oxide layer (e.g., MoO_3) has been used, and the device is finalized with an air-stable high work-function electrode material such as silver or gold. Both device architectures allow the preparation of high-performance bulk heterojunction solar cells.[37] The inverted design offers processing advantages (no vacuum process is required) and shows improved ambient stability due to the absence of a low work function electrode.

3.2.3 Tandem Solar Cells

Currently, the PCE for single-junction PSCs has reached more than 12% due to synergistic effects through the optimization of energy levels, donor polymer bandgaps, new non-fullerene acceptor, mobilities, and device morphology. To further push PCE beyond 15%, one needs to enhance light absorption without sacrificing V_{OC} and FF. To address this issue, tandem PSCs consisting of two or more single cells with complementary absorption wavelength ranges are stacked together and show impressively improved efficiency. Figure 3.6a depicts a typical polymer tandem cell comprising wide-bandgap and low-bandgap polymer solar cells, with an interconnecting layer (ICL).[38] Each cell is a donor-acceptor (D-A) bulk hetero-junction solar cell. Figure 3.6b shows the solar spectrum, the absorption of wide- and low-bandgap cells. When stacking two complementary cells with a large ($E_g \sim 1.9$ eV) and small bandgap ($E_g \sim 1.4$ eV) polymer, 60% of the photons from the sun can be covered.[39]

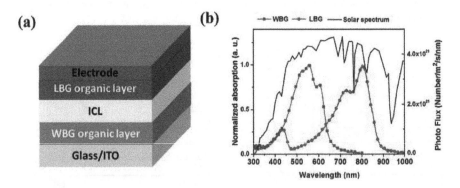

FIGURE 3.6 (a) Tandem polymer device structure including wide-bandgap polymer solar cell (front cell) and low-bandgap polymer solar cell (rear cell); front and rear cells are connected to each other by an interconnecting layer (ICL) and (b) typical wide-bandgap polymer, low-bandgap polymer absorption, and solar spectrum. (Reproduced from *Prog. Polym. Sci.*, 38, You, J. et al., 1909–1928, Copyright 2013, with permission from Elsevier.)

The two subcells in the tandem device may be connected either in series[40] or in parallel[41] by varying the interconnecting scheme. The introduction of the tandem architectures would address two specific issues associated with OPV in relation to the limits of active layer thickness and how the active layer materials absorb light. It has been hypothesized that tandem architectures should be able to produce 30% better efficiencies than their single junction counterparts.[42] Tandem organic solar cell efficiencies have reached a 12% benchmark, as produced by Heliatek, and these devices are expected to exceed 15% efficiency in the near future.[42]

3.3   THE MATERIALS OF THE PHOTOACTIVE LAYERS

Significant achievements have been made in OPV device performance through materials design. There are generally two components in the BHJ structure, donor and acceptor. OSCs have witnessed the accelerated development in these three years, especially the related photovoltaic materials. In this part, we mainly focus on the materials (including conjugated polymer donor, fullerene derivative acceptor, solution processable organic molecule donor and acceptor) that have been used for OPVs and demonstrate the latest progress in this field.

3.3.1   Electron Donor Polymers

Numerous polymer donor materials have been developed in the past decades. It is difficult to categorize these materials. In this section, polymers with 2,1,3-benzothiadiazole, Thieno[3,b]thiophene, and benzo[1,2-b;4,5-b′]dithiophene, etc., were used as the examples for molecular structure design of conjugated materials with D/A structures.

3.3.1.1   Benzothiadiazole (BT)-Based Polymer Donors

2,1,3-Benzothiadiazole (BT) has been widely used as an electron-deficient building block in conjugated polymers with D/A structure. It is widely used to copolymerize with various donor monomers to tune the absorption properties. This category of polymer donors (Figure 3.7) has been extensively studied and shown outstanding photovoltaic performances.

With the very strong electron-withdrawing ability, a very small size of the fluorine atom can lower both the HOMO and the LUMO energy levels without introducing much steric hindrance, which would change the underlying structure. Fluorination has also been applied in the benzothiadiazole moiety. In the case of D-A donor photoactive materials, the difluorobenzothiadiazole-based materials have made great achievements recently. Chen et al.[43] reported a low-bandgap (LBG) D-A conjugated polymer **FBT-Th$_4$(1,4)** based on 5,6-difluorobenzothiadiazole (FBT) as the A-unit and quarterthiophene (Th$_4$) with solubilizing alkyl chains attached on the two terminal thiophene rings as the D-unit. It was found that **FBT-Th$_4$(1,4)** showed good film solution-processing condition, high hole mobility (1.92 cm^2 (V s)$^{-1}$), and the highest PCE of 7.64% was achieved with a 230 nm thick active layer. Inspired by these results, the Yan group developed a series of these similar polymers. In 2014,[8] they reported the achievement of high-performance (efficiencies up to 10.8% and fill factors [FFs]

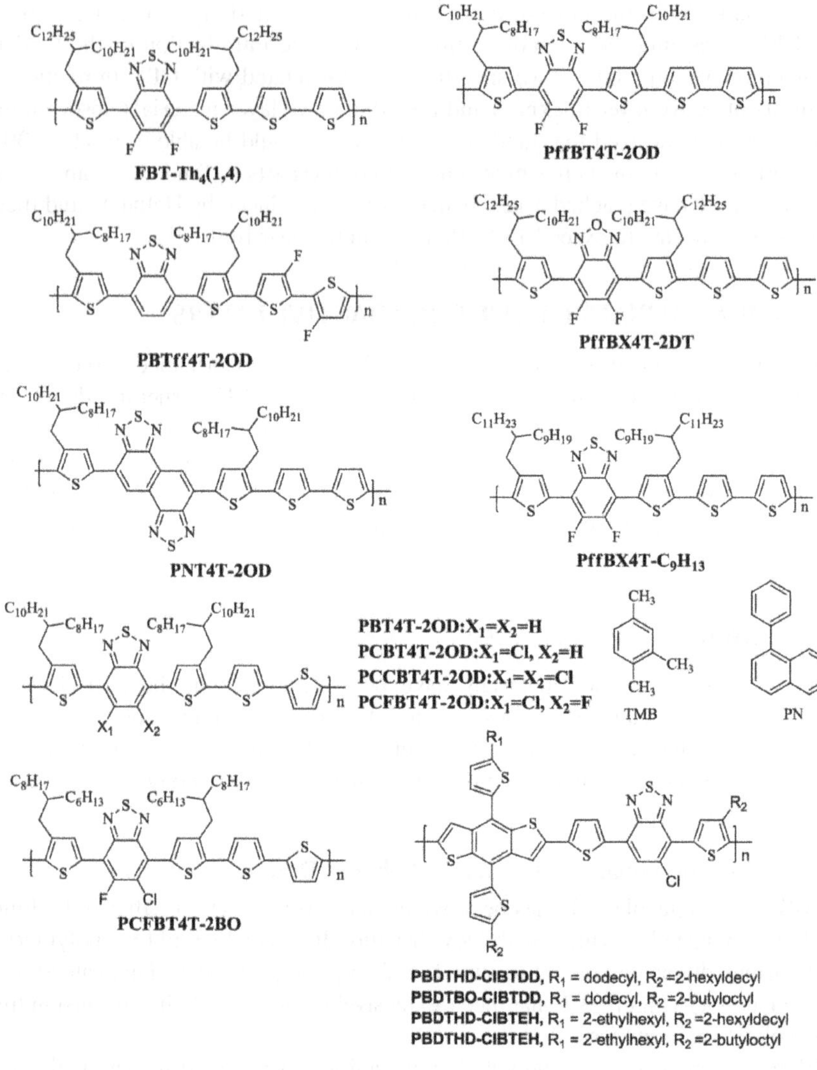

FIGURE 3.7 Molecular structures of difluorobenzothiadiazole-based polymers.

up to 77%) thick-film PSCs based on three different donor polymers (**PffBT4T-2OD**, **PBTff4T-2OD**, and **PNT4T-2OD**) and 10 polymer:fullerene combinations. Among them, **PffBT4T-2OD** enables six cases of high-efficiency (9.6%–10.8%), high FF (73%–77%), and thick-film (250–300 nm) PSCs when combined with traditional PCBM and many nontraditional fullerenes. Very recently, the Yan group also developed a hydrocarbon-based processing system (TMB-PN),[7] which yielded even better OSC morphology and performance (11.7%) than that obtained with conventional halogenated solvents (9.6%). The PN additive was found to play a critical role by introducing multiple beneficial effects (promoting face-on polymer backbone orientation, reducing domain size, and increasing domain purity) and thus enhancing the

PCE of the OSCs from 6.4% to 11.7%. The choice of the host solvent TMB was also important, as it improves the molecular orientation relative to the D/A interfaces in the BHJ film.

Recently, chlorination of BT-based polymers has attracted the researchers' attention. Mo et al. reported a series of chlorinated BT-benzo[1,2-b:4,5-b']dithiophene (BDT) polymers [(**PBDTHD-ClBTDD**)-(**PBDTHD-ClBTEH**)]. These chlorinated polymers showed deep HOMO energy levels, which promoted the efficiency of their corresponding PSCs by increasing the device V_{OC}. Although the introduction of a large Cl atom increased the torsion angle of the polymer backbone, the chlorinated polymers maintained a favorable backbone orientation in blend films for efficient PSC application. The PSC device based on a 250 nm blend film of **PBDTHD-ClBTDD** and $PC_{71}BM$ demonstrated a V_{OC} of 0.76 V, a J_{SC} of 16.79 mA cm^{-2}, and a FF of 71.69%, yielding an overall PCE of 9.11%.[44] Later, Hu et al. explored the relationship between the number of chlorine atoms and the photovoltaic properties BT-based polymers (**PBT4T-2OD, PCBT4T-2OD**, and **PCCBT4T-2OD**).[45] It was found that the best PSCs with PCBT4T-2OD:$PC_{71}BM$ blend film as the active layer showed a PCE of 8.21% with a V_{OC} of 0.73 V, a J_{SC} of 16.18 mA cm^{-2}, and a FF of 68.97%, which was approximately 68% higher than that of its nonchlorine analog **PBT4T-2OD** (4.89%). One-chlorine-and-one-fluorine-substituted BT units were also developed by Hu et al. (**PCFBT4T-2OD** and **PCFBT4T-2BO**). The introduction of fluorine atoms in the polymer **PCFBT4T-2OD** further enhanced the π–π stacking, compared with the one-chlorine substituted **PCBT4T-2BO**, which was helpful for the charge transport in the active layer and to enhance the device performance in PSCs. The **PCFBT4T-2OD**:$PC_{71}BM$ device exhibited the PCE of 8.84% with a V_{OC} of 0.72 V, a J_{SC} of 17.61 mA cm^{-2}, and a FF of 68.85%.[46]

3.3.1.2   Thieno[3,b]thiophene(TT)-Based Polymer Donors

Fluorinated thieno[3,4-b]thiophene was first introduced to OPVs by Liang et al., who found that the fluorination could deep the HOMO level of its conjugated polymer and improve the V_{OC}.[47] After an extensive structural optimization of the PTB family (Figure 3.8), the pioneer polymer **PTB7** was born, which exhibited an excellent photovoltaic effect with a PCE of about 7.4%.[48] Hou et al. demonstrated that the BDT-based polymers (**PTB7-Th**) with 2-alkylthienyl groups [two-dimensional conjugated (2D) structures] exhibited broader absorption bands, higher hole mobilities, and better photovoltaic properties compared to their alkoxyl substituted analogues; enhanced PCEs up to 8.6% have been obtained in the PSC with a conventional device architecture.[49] Therefore, different conjugated side groups 2-alkylfuryl, 2-alkylthienyl, and 2-alkylselenophenyl (**PBDTTT-EFF, PBDTTTEFT**, and **PBDTTT-EFS**) were introduced into the benzodithiophene (BDT) units.[50] Oversized aggregations are formed in the **PBDTTT-EFF**:$PC_{71}BM$ blend, which can be ascribed to the strong interchain π–π stacking due to the low steric hindrance of the conjugated side groups, with a V_{OC} of 0.69 V and a J_{SC} of 11.77 mA/cm^2, which are lower than those in the devices based on the other two polymers.

The introduction of alkylthio substituents onto poly BDT-TT-based conjugated polymers has been proved to be an effective method to improve the photovoltaic properties of the polymers. Hou et al. developed three alkylthiothiophene-substituted

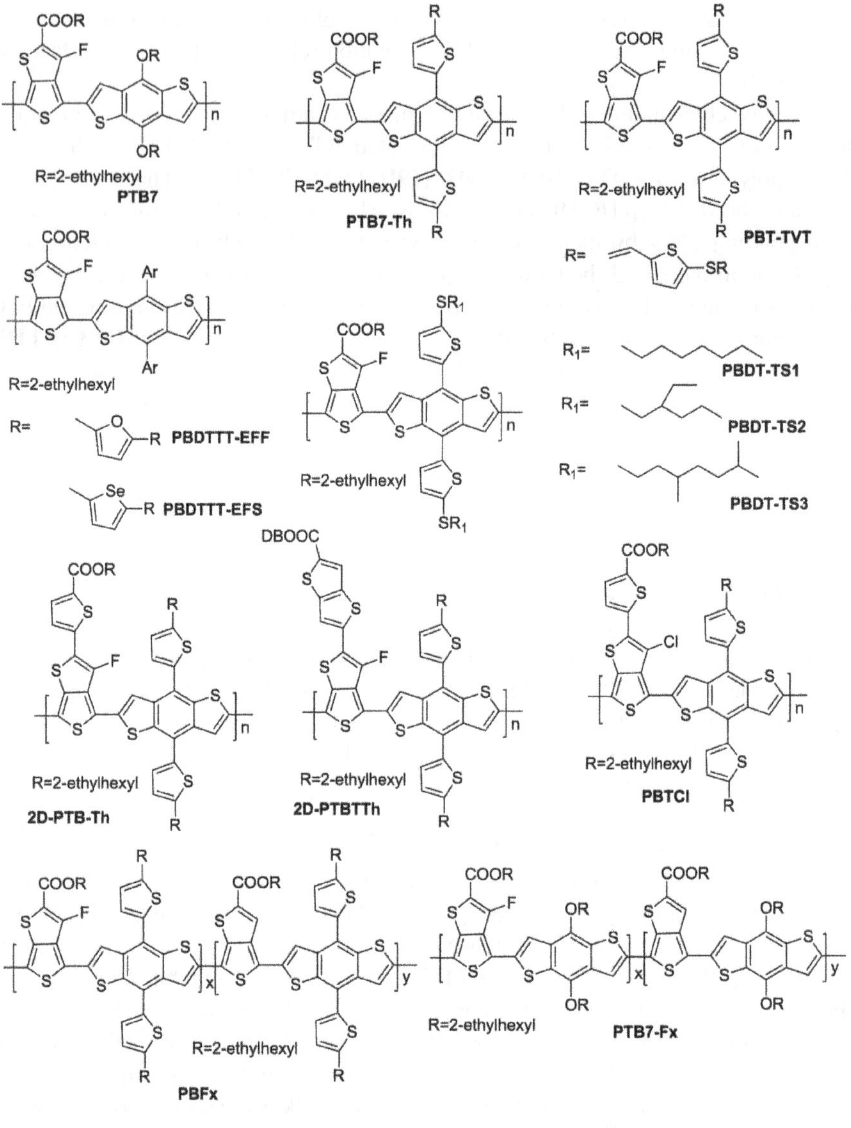

FIGURE 3.8   Molecular structures of thieno[3,b]thiophene-based polymers.

BDT-based polymers (**PBDT-TS1, PBDT-TS2,** and **PBDT-TS3**);[51] the alkyls have little influence on absorption spectra and molecular energy levels of the polymers, but the linear alkyl has stronger and tighter π–π stacking due to the reduced steric hindrance. Finally, the PSC based on PBDT-TS1 shows a higher PCE of 9.52% than the other two polymers. (*E*)-5-(2-(5-(Alkylthio)thiophen-2-yl)vinyl)-thiophene-2-yl functional groups were also introduced onto 4- and 8-positions of BDT units (**PBT-TVT**).[52] Benefiting from the prolonged conjugation of the conjugated side groups, the new polymer shows deeper HOMO level (−5.29 eV), greatly improved optical absorption property, and higher hole mobility. As a result, the PSCs based on it demonstrated better photovoltaic performance than the device of **PBT7**; one of the highest results for PSCs based on $PC_{61}BM$ was obtained with a PCE of 7.67%. The polymer with fully two-dimensional (2D) conjugated side chains (**2D-PTB-Th**, **2D-PTB-TTh**)[53] with enhanced sunlight absorption (PCEs: 9.13%; **PTB7-Th** (8.26%)) and efficient solar energy conversion was developed by us very recently.

Liu et al. investigated the different amounts of fluorine decoration on the photovoltaic performance of polythienothiophene-co-benzodithiophene copolymers (**PBFx**).[54] The best device performance with a PCE of 8.75% was obtained from the polymer with the highest fluorine content due to the decreased size scale of the BHJ morphology and enhanced V_{OC} and FF. Fluorinated polymers **PTB7-Fx**[55] with varied degrees of fluorination used as electron donor materials were also reported by Guo and coworkers. In addition, full fluorination of the third C-atom of thienothiophene was shown to give rise to the highest PCEs due to the different LUMO levels of the polymers instead of the film morphology.

The chlorinated thieno[3,4-b]thiophene applied (**PBTCl**) in the fullerene-free PSCs was reported by Wang et al.[56] The polymer showed blue-shifted absorption due to chlorine compared to the absorption of PTB7-th containing fluorine, but the optical absorption of the chlorinated polymer was more complementary with ITIC. The chlorine substitution also lowered the HOMO level of PBTCl and increased V_{OC} of the devices. The PBTCl-based nonfullerene PSCs exhibited a PCE of 7.57% and a V_{OC} of 0.91 V, 13% increasing to the fluorine-analogue-based device. Qu and coworkers[57] also reported the chlorinated TT-BDT terpolymers to optimize the chlorine/fluorine content. As the content of chlorine is increased in polymers, although the twist angle between the donor and acceptor is increased, the HOMO levels are decreased. This opens a window to constantly modify the V_{OC} values without reducing other factors of the polymer solar cells. When the Cl content was 25%, the optimized device exhibited a PCE of 8.31% with a V_{OC} of 0.82 V, a J_{SC} of 15.31 mA cm^{-2}, and a FF of 66.19%.

3.3.1.3 Benzo[1,2-b:4,5-b']dithiophene-Based Polymer Donors

In 2008, Hou et al. first introduced the benzo[1,2-b:4,5-b']dithiophene (BDT) units in the design of photovoltaic polymers, and the optical and electronic properties of the BDT-based polymers (Figure 3.9) could be easily tuned, suggesting that BDT was a promising unit for conjugated photovoltaic polymers.[1,58] The rigid and planar conjugated structure of BDT makes it attractive for achieving highly tunable molecular energy levels, high optical bandgaps, and high hole motilities.[1] Therefore, numerous photovoltaic polymers have been developed using BDT or its analogues as building blocks.

When a BDT unit combined with the acceptor, benzothiadiazole (BT), the copolymers **PBTBD**[58] showed an optical bandgap of 1.70 eV, and its device based on a structure of ITO/PEDOT:PSS/**PBTBD**:$PC_{71}BM$/Ca/Al showed a J_{SC} of 2.97 mA/cm^2, a V_{OC} of 0.68 V, a FF of 44%, and a *PCE* of 0.90%. Although the PCEs of the PSC devices based on it were still very low, this study introduced the way to modulate the bandgap and the molecular energy level of the photovoltaic polymer by selecting different D-A combinations. **PTB7** was one of the most studied donor materials developed in 2010 by Yu et al.,[48] and numerous impressive

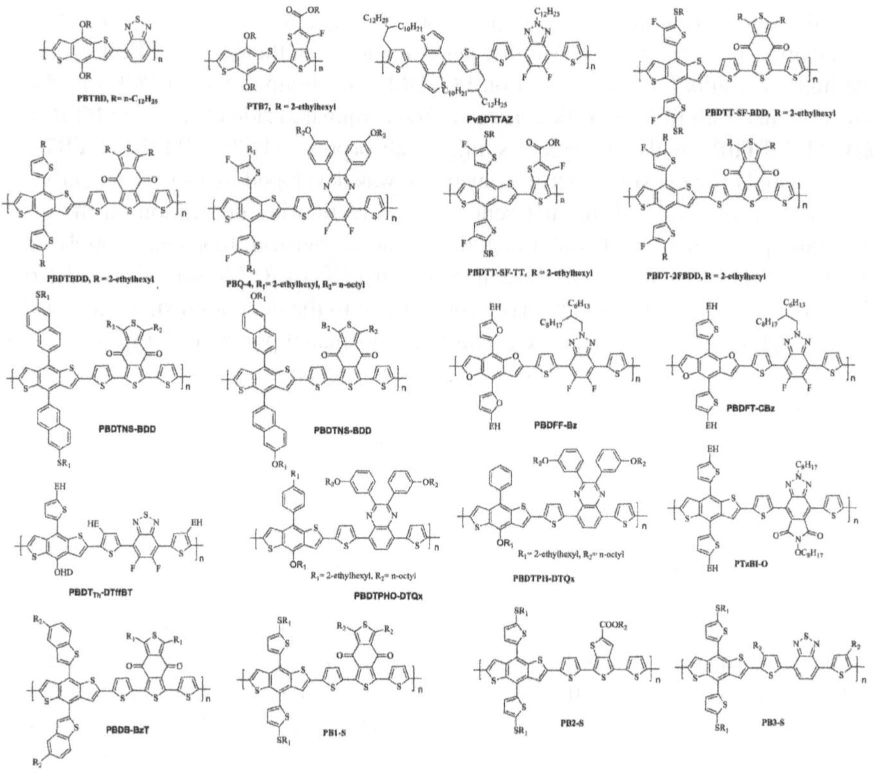

FIGURE 3.9 Molecular structures of BDT-based polymers.

device results were achieved by using it. **PTB7** has a strong absorption from 550 to 750 nm, and the cyclicvoltammetry (CV) measurement indicated that the introduction of the fluorine atom in **PTB7** decreased its HOMO and LUMO to −5.15 and −3.31 eV, respectively. The device ITO/PEDOT:PSS/**PTB7**:PCBM/Ca/Al yielded an impressive *PCE* of 7.4% with a V_{OC} of 0.74 V, a J_{SC} of 14.50 mA/cm², and an FF of 68.97%. Impressively, Wu and coworkers[59] improved the PCE of the **PTB7**-based device to 9.2% by applying an inverted device structure and new interface material. In addition, the combination of BDT and TT units such as **PBDTTT-C-T** and **PTB7-Th** has also been developed and displayed high device performance. Hou et al.[60] synthesized four conjugated polymers composed of BDT-based and 2,3-diphenyl-5,8-di(thiophen-2-yl)quinoxaline (DTQx)-based units. Fluorination of the DTQx units and the conjugated side groups of the BDT unit shows a synergistic effect on molecular energy level modulation of the polymers, and as a result, the polymer **PBQ-4** showed the deepest HOMO level in these polymers, and the device based on **PBQ-4**:PC$_{71}$BM exhibited a high V_{OC} of 0.90 V and a high PCE of 8.55%.

A PCE of 6.67% was obtained from the **PBDTBDD**/PC$_{61}$BM-based PSC,[61] which was a remarkable result for the PSCs using a PC$_{61}$BMas an electron acceptor. An optimal PCE of 6.67% with a high FF of 72% was achieved by manipulating the processing temperature. The photovoltaic efficiency of the **PBDTBDD** was further improved to 8.75% when a novel cathode interface layer of a-ZrAcac was used in the device.[62] As we know, the introduction of fluorine on the backbone has proven to be an effective method to modify the HOMO and LUMO levels and achieved enhanced V_{OC} and higher PCE in PSC devices. Zhang et al. reported a high-performance polymer donor **PBDT-2FBDD** based on a BDT-2F unit,[63] which shows a large bandgap of 1.80 eV, a deep HOMO level of −5.50 eV, strong crystallinity, and a dominant face on packing with a small π–π stacking distance of 3.78 Å. Consequently, the $PC_{71}BM$-based PSCs achieve a high PCE of 9.2% with a V_{OC} of up to 0.98 V. Two years later, the **PBDT-2FBDD**:IDIC-based PSCs without extra treatments also show an outstanding PCE of 11.9%, which was also conducted by Zhang et al.[64] Two novel simultaneously fluorinated and alkylthiolated BDT-based D-A polymers, **PBDTT-SF-TT** and **PBDTT-SF-BDD**, were developed by Du et al.[65] Both fullerene-based **PBDTT-SF-TT** and **PBDTT-SF-BDD** PSCs, high V_{OC} of 1.01 and 0.97 V, and high J_{SC} of 15.17 and 14.70 mA cm^{-2} were obtained, respectively, indicating the synergistic effect of fluorination and alkylthiolation on BDT moiety. Finally, a high PCE of 9.07% for **PBDTT-SF-TT** and PCE of 9.72% for **PBDTT-SF-BDD** were achieved. The alkylthio substituted polymers **PB1-S**, **PB2-S**, and **PB3-S** were synthesized for use as electron donors in fullerene-free PSCs.[66] The **PB1-S**:ITIC active layer exhibited the best photovoltaic performance with a PCE as high as 10.49%.

A new BDT building block containing alkylthio naphthyl as a side chain and the resulting polymer **PBDTNS-BDD** is synthesized by Huang et al., which shows a lower HOMO energy level than that of its alkoxyl naphthyl counterpart **PBDTNO-BDD**.[67] An optimized photovoltaic device using PBDTNS-BDD as a donor exhibits PCE of 8.70% and 9.28% with $PC_{71}BM$ and ITIC as acceptors, respectively. Surprisingly, the ternary blend devices based on **PBDTNS-BDD** and two acceptors ($PC_{71}BM$ and ITIC), shows a PCE of 11.21% much higher than that of **PBDTNO-BDD**-based ternary devices (7.85%). Qin et al. also synthesized a new polymer **PBDB-BzT,** and the THF-processed PBDB-BzT:IT-M blend film resulted in a PCE of 12.10%, the highest value for the NF-PSCs processed using non-chlorinated and non-aromatic solvents.[68] Difuranbenzo[1,2-b:4,5-b′] (BDF), a furan-based derivative, was also developed and applied in the PSCs. Gao et al. designed and synthesized two wide-bandgap two-dimensional conjugated polymers, **PBDFT-Bz** and **PBDFF-Bz**[69] and **PBDFF-Bz**:m-ITIC, which showed a promising PCE of 10.28%, very competitive with the BDT-based counterparts. Zhong et al. developed a novel wide-bandgap conjugated polymer **PTzBI-O** and exhibited an impressive PCE of 7.91% in the all PSCs.[70]

Gu and coworkers proposed a new strategy for introducing an alkylthienyl unit as side chain to fabricate asymmetric BDT-based polymer was efficient in improving the photovoltaic performance of the corresponding polymers.[71] The optimized **PBDTTh-DTffBT**-based photovoltaic device exhibits a V_{OC} of 0.87 V, a J_{SC} of 15.06 mA cm^{-2}, a FF of 70.4% and a high PCE of 9.22%. By taking a similar concept, two novel copolymer donors, **PBDTPH-DTQx** and **PBDTPHO-DTQx**, were also developed.[72] The PCE of **PBDTPH-DTQx**-based polymer solar cells is 5.6%, with balanced V_{OC} = 0.7 V, J_{SC} = 11.89 mA cm^{-2} and FF = 67.3%, which is almost the highest PCE compared with similar BDT unit and fluorine-free substituted DTQx- based polymer. Liu et al. reported a wide-bandgap polymer PvBDTffBT based on a new building block: a vertical-benzodithiophene (vBDT) unit. This polymer modulation strategy significantly improves the PCE from 3% to over 8% due to the more twisted backbone of **PvBDTffBT** when blended with ITIC-Th.[73] Furthermore, when paired with O-IDTBR, a PCE = 11.6% and a small V_{loss} = 0.55 V could be achieved.[74]

3.3.1.4 Isoindigo(ID)-Based Polymer Donors

Owing to its strong electron withdrawing ability and planar backbone, isoindigo (ID) has been shown to be a useful acceptor block that was used to construct conjugated copolymers yielding high-performance organic thin-film transistors. Moreover, ID-based polymers (Figure 3.10) exhibit strong absorption across the visible light region, high extinction coefficients, and deep HOMO energy levels, which makes ID one of the most promising electron-deficient building blocks for constructing D-A type polymers toward high-performance PSCs. Peng et al. synthesized two D-A copolymers based on isoindigo/fluorinated isoindigo and bis(dialkylthienyl)-benzo-dithiophene (**PBDTT–ID** and **PBDTT–FID**).[75] The fluorinated substitution made this type of copolymer prefer a more planar configuration arising from introduced F-H, F-S, and F-π_F interactions. As expected, **PBDTT–FID** has a smaller bandgap, lower energy levels, and better carrier mobility compared to **PBDTT–ID**, and it showed PCEs of 5.52% with high V_{OC} up to 0.94 V due to the deeper HOMO level. Peng et al. also found that both the hole and electron mobilities of the fluorinated isoindigo-based polymer **PDTS-FID** were enhanced in its BHJ blend compared with the nonfluorinated **PDTS-ID**-based one. In another study, Geng and a coworker reported dithienocarbazole (DTC) and isoindigo (IID)- based D-A low-bandgap con-jugated polymers [**P(IID-DTC)**, **P(IID1F-DTC)**, and **P(IID2F-DTC)**][76] for prepar-ing PSCs with a PCE up to 8.2%, and found that introducing one fluorine atom in the IID unit could improve the solubility of the polymer in non-chlorinated solvents such as oxylene and 1,2,4-trimethyl-benzene, allowing the fabrication of 7.5% PSCs with o-xylene as the solvent (**P1-P3**).[77] To improve the mobility, the alternating copoly-mers of IID and bithiophene [**P(1FIID-BT)**] were synthesized,[78] leading to a PCE of 7.46% based on 270 nm thick films and non-chlorinated solvent processability. Yan et al. synthesized a series of isoindigo (ID) and quaterthiophene (T4)-based D-A copo-lymers (**PID-T4**, **PID-ffT4**, and **PffID-T4**),[79] and demonstrated that fluorination has another role to affect the aggregation properties and performance of the resultant polymers. In addition, other polymers (**PIID-5T**, **PFIID-5T**, **PFIID-T-BDT-T**, and **PFIID-2T-BDT-2T**) were also investigated and proved the effectiveness of fluorina-tion in the isoindigo unit.[80]

By contrast with fluorination, chlorination of isoindigo (IID) units has been investigated less. Lei et al.[81] developed the first chlorination isoindigo polymers, which are the first ambipolar polymers that can offer both balanced carrier transport and transport in ambient conditions due to the direct modification of the isoindigo cores with electron-deficient chlorine atoms and can lower both LUMO levels and HOMO levels. In another work,[82] they also demonstrated that chlorinated polymers with reduced polymer backbone planarity will show proper phase separation with acceptors. The chlorinated one leads to higher device performance of 4.60% than fluorinated ones (1.19%). Therefore, chlorination is a powerful strategy to modu-late and balance different factors in D-A conjugated polymers, and its effects are

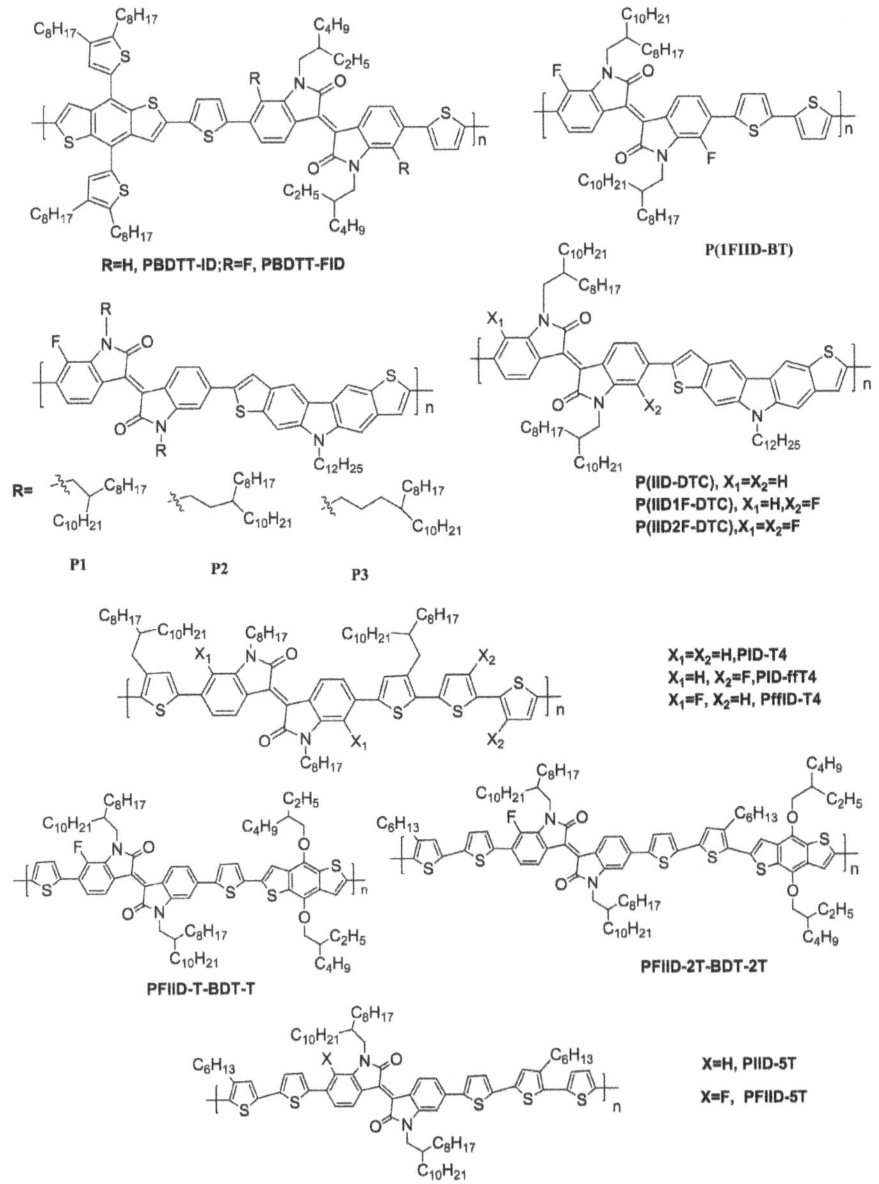

FIGURE 3.10 Molecular structures of ID-based polymers.

far beyond frontier orbital energy-level modulation. Chlorinated thiophene-fused isoindigo, chlorinated benzothiophene-fused isoindigo, and chlorinated benzofuran-fused isoindigo were also developed by Wan and coworkers.[83–85] Solution-processed OFETs based on them also exhibited stable performance in ambient conditions due to their low-lying LUMO level.

3.3.2   Electron Small-Molecule Donors

Compared with the polymer donors, small molecules donors offer potential advantages, such as well-defined molecular structure, definite molecular weight, high purity, tunable electronic structures, mass-scale production, and better device reproducibility. After surveying small-molecule solar cells with promising PCEs, we found it appropriate to catalog them into three groups based on structural features, oligothiophene-based small molecules, dithienosilole (DTS)-based small molecules, and BDT-based small molecules.

3.3.2.1   Oligothiophene-Based Small Molecules

Oligothiophenes (Figure 3.11) are among the best-studied semiconducting materials due to their good transport properties and easy tunable optical and electrochemical properties. However, the OPV performance of general thiophene materials including polymers and small molecules is restricted by their limited absorption in the visible and near infrared regions. Introducing electron-withdrawing units, thus forming an intramolecular D-A structure, is one of the efficient ways to broaden the molecular absorption region.[86] In 2006, Schulze et al. reported a low-bandgap oligothiophene, a,a'-bis(2,2-dicyanovinyl)-quinquethiophene (**DCV5T**). In comparison to thin films of unsubstituted quinquethiophene, the optical bandgap of DCV5T is reduced from around 2.5–1.77 eV because of the introduction of electron-accepting dicyanovinyl (DCV) end groups, high V_{OC} to 1 V, and a PCE of 3.4% was obtained.[87]

In 2009, by controlling the oligomer units, Liu et al. synthesized a series of oligothiophenes with tunable and low bandgap (lowed to 1.68 eV).[88] Coupled with their good solubility and stability, the device ITO/PEDOT:PSS/**DCV7T**:PCBM/LiF/Al exhibits a PCE as high as 3.7%, among the highest efficiency for solution-processed small-molecule BHJ solar cells at that time.[89] By replacing the end-capped with electron-withdrawing group, three new small molecules were synthesized by Liu et al. (**DCAE7T**, **DCAO7T**, and **DCAEH7T**). All these molecules demonstrate high PCEs (4.46%–5.08%) for solution-processed BHJ OSCs, and a PCE of 5.08% was achieved based on **DCAO7T** and $PC_{61}BM$ without any special treatment.[90] Demeter and coworkers synthesized another symmetrical A-D-A donor containing thiobarbituric (TB) acceptor groups (**DER7T**) and combined these two groups to produce the unsymmetrical A-D-A' compound (**ERCV7T**), and showed that breaking the symmetry of the donor structure can significantly increase V_{OC} of the device.[91]

By introducing a new dye unit, 3-ethylrhodanine into the conjugated thiophene backbone, a molecule named **DERHD7T** with a stronger solar absorption was developed. A record-high PCE of 6.10% was obtained by using a blend of **DERHD7T** and $PC_{61}BM$ as the active layer, with a high V_{OC} of 0.92 V and a remarkable J_{SC} of 13.98 mA cm^{-2}.[92] Using 2-(1,1-dicyanomethylene)rhodanine as the terminal unit, DRCN7T was developed.[93] A PCE of 9.30% (certified at 8.995%), with $J_{SC} = 14.87$ mA cm^{-2} and FF = 68.7% was achieved due to the network of highly crystalline donor fibrils with ~10 nm diameters, which is close to the exciton diffusion length in organic materials. Quinquethiophenes (O5T) proved to have a deeper HOMO level than septithiophenes for the decreased conjugations; therefore, higher V_{OC} could be expected to obtain for O5T derivatives. Long et al. synthesized three O5T derivatives

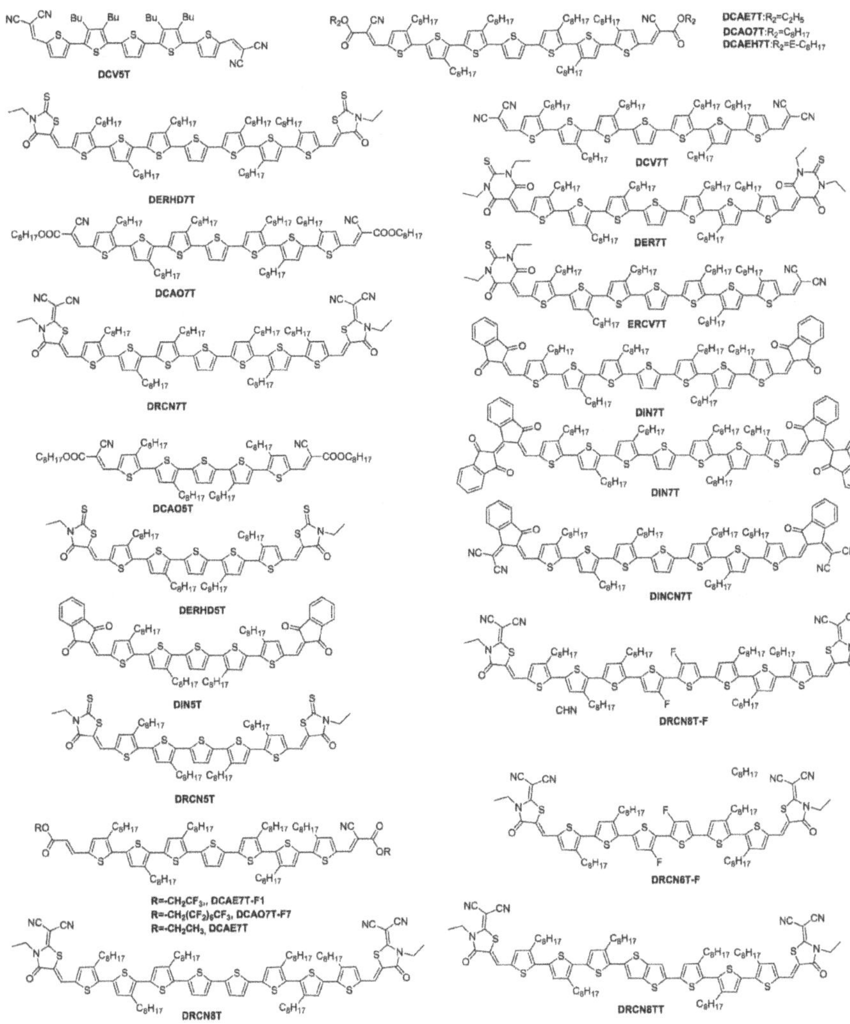

FIGURE 3.11 Chemical structures of oligothiophene-based small molecules.

with different end groups of octyl 2-cyanoacetate (**DCAO5T**), 3-ethylrhodanine (**DERHD5T**), and 2H-indene-1,3-dione (**DIN5T**).[94] Among them, **DERHD5T** shows V_{OC} as high as 1.08 V and PCE of 4.63%. In 2015, Kan et al. reported the devices based on **DRCN5T**/PC$_{71}$BM showed a notable certified PCE of 10.10% using a simple solution spin-coating fabrication process, among the highest PCE for single-junction small-molecule-based OPVs at that time.[95] Three new oligothiophene derivatives with an A-D-A structure incorporating 1,3-indanedione or the derivative of 1,3-indanedione units as the terminal acceptor groups—**DIN7T**, **DINCN7T**, and **DDIN7T**—have been developed by He and coworkers.[96] The acceptor units not only have a huge effect on the bandgaps and energy levels but also have a great impact on the solubility and the packing mode in the film. The **DIN7T**-based BHJ solar cell device achieved a PCE of 4.93%, a high FF of 0.72, and J_{SC} of 8.54 mA cm^{-2}. He and coworkers synthesized two small molecules, **DCAE7T-F1** and **DCAO7T-F7**, by introducing fluorinated alkyl chains into the terminal unit. It has been found that as the fluorinated alkyl length increased, the surface energy decreased and the lipophobicity increased. Due to its high lipophobic property and a problem with its wettability, **DCAO7T-F7** was not able to produce a uniform film by spin coating. A PCE of 2.26% was achieved with a V_{OC} of 0.83 V, J_{SC} of 5.55 mA cm^{-2}, and FF of 0.50 for **DCAE7T-F1**-based solar cells.[97] By replacing the central building block with thieno[3,2-b]thiophene unit and 3,3'-difluoro-2,2,-bithiophene, the new small molecules **DRCN8TT**,[98] **DRCN6T-F**, and **DRCN8T-F**[99] were developed. The **DRCN8T** achieved a PCE of 8.11%, much better than that of **DRCN8T** and very close to the analogue molecules (**DRCN7T**) having a different symmetry. However, PCEs of 2.26% and 5.07% were obtained for **DRCN6T-F** and **DRCN8T-F**, lower than those of non-fluorinated molecules **DRCN6T** and **DRCN8T**. The relatively poor performance for the DRCN6T-F and DRCN8T-F were mainly caused by their low J_{SC}, due to their unfavorable morphologies and low charge carrier mobilities.

3.3.2.2 Dithienosilole (DTS)-Based Small Molecules

Dithieno[3,2-b:20,30-d]silole (DTS, Figure 3.12) have been widely used in synthesizing high-efficiency polymer donor materials. DTS-based copolymers show a broad absorption, relatively lower HOMO energy level, and higher hole mobility,

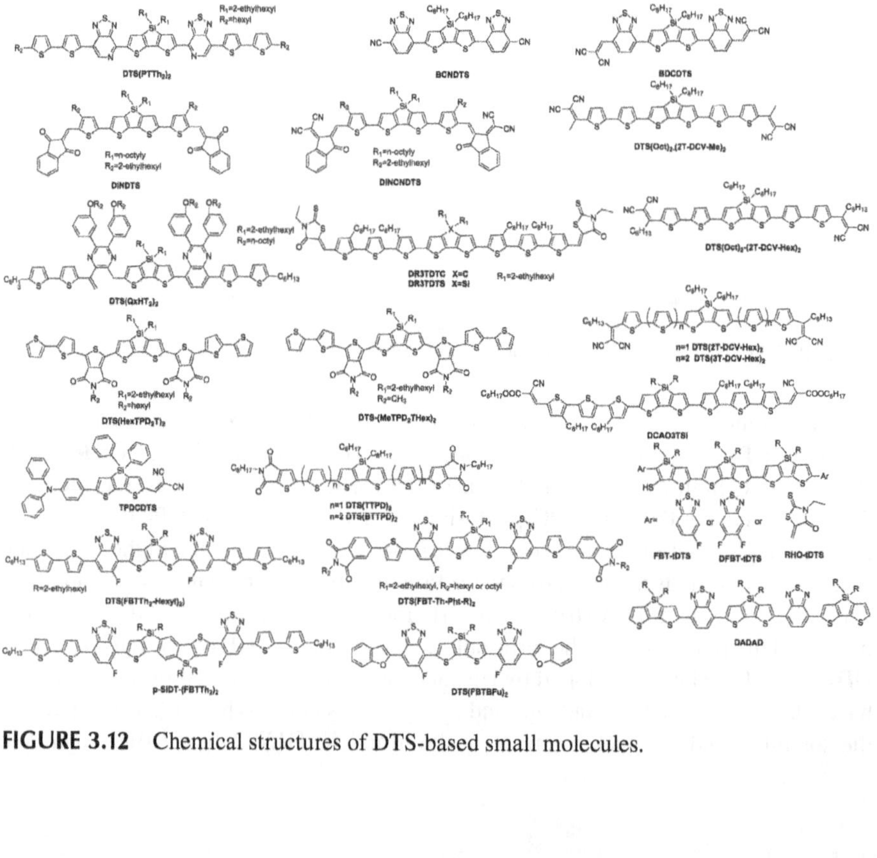

FIGURE 3.12   Chemical structures of DTS-based small molecules.

which are attractive for the application as the donor in PSCs.[100] For example, Lu et al. synthesized a DTS-based copolymer that demonstrated a PCE as high as 7.3% when the polymer was used as the donor blended with $PC_{70}BM$.[101] On the other hand, a new D-π–A molecule (**TPDCDTS**) adopting coplanar diphenylsubstituted DTS as a central π-bridge, a PCE up to 3.82% was achieved when blended with C_{70} as an acceptor.[102]

Lin and coworkers synthesized two A-A-D-A-A-type molecules (**BCNDTS** and **BDCDTS**), where two terminal electron-withdrawing cyano or dicyanovinylene moieties and the bilayer and planar mixed heterojunction devices based on **BCNDTS** exhibited decent PCE of 2.3% and 3.7%, respectively.[103] In 2012, Sun et al. reported efficient solution-processed SM BHJ solar cells based on a new molecular donor, **DTS(PTTh₂)2**; and a record PCE of 6.7% was achieved for the devices from **DTS (PTTh₂)₂**:$PC_{70}BM$.[104] Two new dithienosilole-based molecules, **DINDTS** and **DINCNDTS**, with 1,3-indanedione (IN) or malononitrile derivative 1,3-indanedione (INCN) units as end-capped groups, respectively, have been synthesized by Chen et al.[105] The optimal DINDTS:$PC_{71}BM$-based solar cells showed a J_{SC} of 13.50 mA cm^{-2} and PCE of 6.60%. However, **DINCNDTS**:$PC_{71}BM$ exhibited very poor PCE of 0.58% with a very low J_{SC} of 1.82 mA cm^{-2}. A new linear DTS-based oligo-thiophene end-capped with methyl and electron withdrawing dicyanovinyl groups, **DTS(Oct)₂-(2T-DCV-Me)₂**, was prepared by Luponosov et al.[106] The BHJ OSC based on **DTS(Oct)₂-(2T-DCV-Me)₂**:$PC_{71}BM$ (1:0.8, wt%) shows an initially high PCE of 5.44% without any special treatment needed.[107] Nevertheless, the OSCs based on **DTS(2T-DCV-Hex)₂** exhibited the relatively low PCEs of 2.06% with the J_{SC} val-ues of 6.82 mA cm^{-2}. In 2011, Zhou et al. reported the OPV performance of a small molecule based on a DTS (**DCAO3TSi**) unit, with an outstanding PCE of 5.84%.[108] Further, Ni et al. synthesized two new A-D-A small molecules with **DTC** and **DTS** as the central building block unit and 3-ethyl-rhodanine as the end-capping groups (**DR3TDTC** and **DR3TDTS**). The optimized device based on DR3TDTS exhibited a high PCE of 8.02%, while the device based on DR3TDTC only showed a low PCE of 0.75%, although with only the difference of one atom on the central core units.[109]

A small molecule with D1-A-D2-A-D1 structure denoted as **DTS(QxHT₂)₂** based on quinoxaline acceptor and dithienosilone donor units was synthesized by Keshtov and coworkers. The PCE of the **DTS(QxHT₂)₂**:$PC_{71}BM$ was achieved up to 7.81% based on an active layer processed with solvent additive DIO/chloroform, using CuSCN as a hole transport layer instead of PEDOT:PSS.[110] Two different thienopyrroledione (TPD)-based SMs with different alkyl substitution positions were reported by Choi et al.— (**DTS(HexTPD₂T)₂**, **DTS-(MeTPD2THex)₂**].[111] The **DTS(HexTPD₂T)₂**-based OSC device exhibited a promising PCE of 6.0% with V_{OC} = 0.94 V, J_{SC} = 11.8 mA cm^{-2}, and FF = 0.54, while the DTS(MeTPD₂THex)₂-based one showed a moderate PCE of 3.1% with V_{OC} = 0.93 V, J_{SC} = 6.4 mA cm^{-2}, and FF = 0.52. Two novel small molecules **DTS(TTPD)₂** or **DTS(BTTPD)₂** based on a A-π-D-π-A framework end-capped with a TPD unit were synthesized.[112] The best solar cells using **DTS(TTPD)₂** as a donor and $PC_{61}BM$ as an acceptor demonstrated efficient performance with an obviously high V_{OC} of 0.97 V and a PCE of 1.20% by annealing.

The fluorobenzothiadiazole (FBT) unit was used in the synthesis of DTS-based small molecules. Bazan et al. showed the PCEs of **p-DTS(FBTTh₂)₂**[113] can exceed 8%

by controlling the deposition conditions, modifying the compositions of BHJ blends with fullerene acceptors, and adjusting the device architectures. Introduction of the "weak" SIDT donor fragment into the interior of the $D^1AD^2AD^1$ molecular architecture resulted in a new high-efficiency molecular donor, *p*-**SIDT(FBTTh₂)₂**, being synthesized.[114] PCEs of up to 6.4% with a large V_{OC} of 0.91 V can be observed within *p*-**SIDT(FBTTh₂)₂**:PC₇₁BM bulk heterojunction thin films when the films are processed with 0.4% diiodooctane (DIO) solvent additive. Phthalimide end-capped derivatives of **DTS(FBT-Th-Pth-Hexyl)₂** were synthesized, but only PCEs of 0.74% were achieved.[115] Benzofuran (BFu) end-capping groups were introduced into this series **[DTS(FBTBFu)₂]**, and a PCE up to 2.46% was achieved.[116]

Huang et al. reported a series of D-A type of π-conjugated oligomers based on DTS as the electron donor and BT as the electron acceptor. It was found that the higher molecular weight chromophore exhibited a narrower bandgap compared to lower molecular weight counterparts. The inverted device structure of ITO/PFN-OX/**DADAD**:PCBM/MoO₃/Al achieved the best device performance with a PCE of 1.12%.[117] Three new small molecules, **FBT-tDTS**, **DFBT-tDTS**, and **RHO-tDTS**, were synthesized by using tDTS as the novel donor unit and FBT, DFBT, and RHO as acceptor units, respectively.[118] Compared with **FBT-tDTS** and **DFBT-tDTS**, **RHO-tDTS** with a vinyl linkage has a more rigid backbone, which makes it exhibit a broader absorption as well as higher crystallinity and charge-carrier mobility. As a result, the **RHO-tDTS**-based device achieved the highest PCE of 7.56% after solvent annealing.

3.3.2.3 Benzo[1,2-b:4,5-b']dithiophene (BDT)-Based Small Molecules

Among various small molecules designed for solution-processed solar cells, BDT was as an attractive donor building block (Figure 3.13) for donor molecules in OPVs for the following reasons: (1) its structural symmetry and the rigid fused aromatic system could enhance electron delocalization and promote cofacial π–π stacking in the solid state, thus benefiting charge transport in the devices; (2) as a relatively weak donor, BDT would maintain a low HOMO energy level of the resulting molecules.[119] Currently, solution processed small molecules incorporating BDT units have achieved PCEs over 11%.[120]

In 2011, Liu et al. synthesized a new small molecule, **DCAO3T(BDT)3T**, with BDT as the central unit and electron-withdrawing alkyl cyanoacetate groups as the end-capped group.[121] The highest PCE of 5.44% was obtained by using a blend of **DCAO3T(BDT)3T** and PC₆₁BM as the active layer, combined with a high V_{OC} of 0.93 V, a J_{SC} of 9.77 mA cm⁻², and a notable FF of 59.9%. Later, **DCAO3TBDT** and **DR3TBDT**, with 2-ethylhexoxy substituted BDT as the central building block and octyl cyanoacetate and 3-ethylrhodanine as different terminal units, were developed by Zhou and coworkers.[122] An impressive PCE of 7.38% was obtained from the **DR3TBDT**-based solar cells, which is the highest for any small-molecule-based solar cell at that time. With dialkylthiol-substituted BDT as the central building block, a new small molecule **DR3TSBDT** was synthesized and shown an optimized PCE of 9.95%.[123] A small molecule named **DRBDTCO**, based on BDT with an asymmetric side chain, and its dimer, **dDRBDTCO**, with the octamethylene connector was

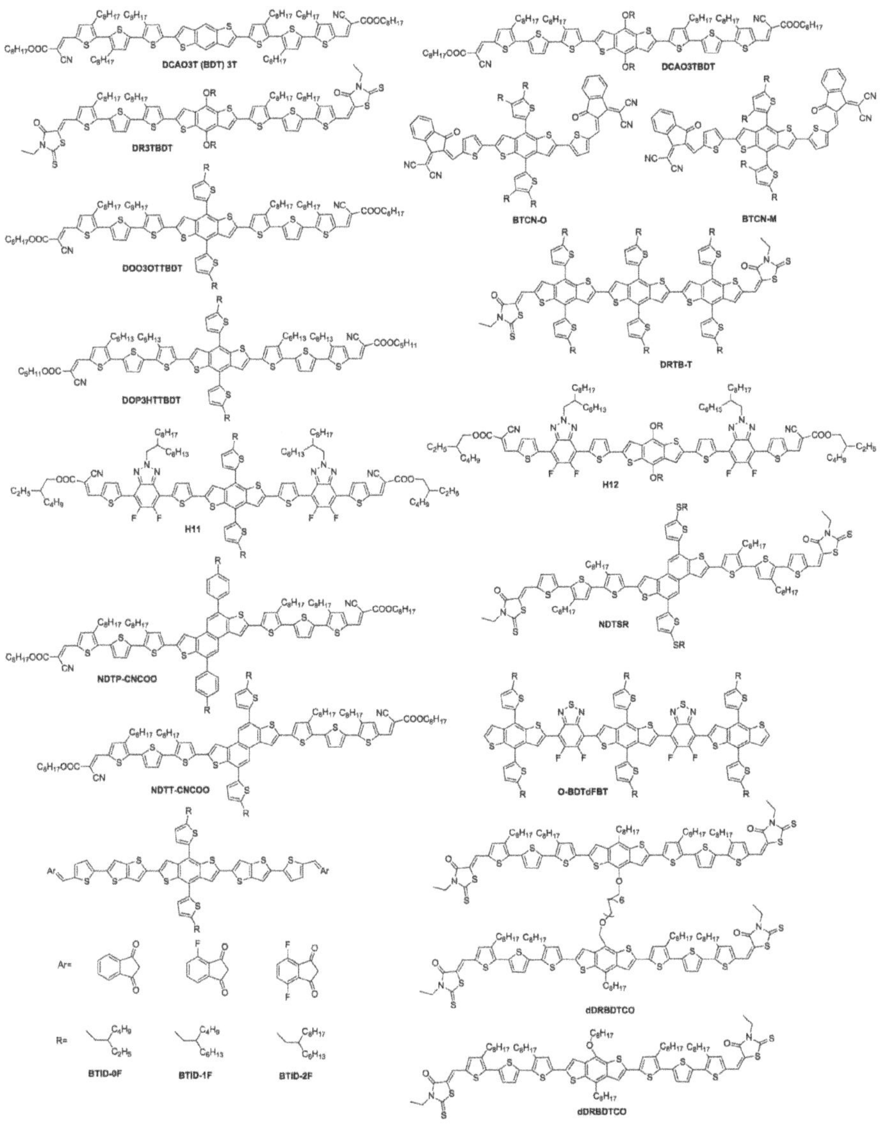

FIGURE 3.13 Chemical structures of BDT-based small molecules.

synthesized.[124] The optimized PCE of a **DRBDTCO**-based device was 8.18%, which is higher than that of its **dDRBDTCO**-based device.

For 2D BDT unit, by introducing thiophene or other π conjugated groups in the orthogonal direction of BDT, the π-electrons could delocalize to the conjugated side groups, resulting in enlarged π-conjugation and thus better interchain π–π stacking, which may be beneficial to exciton diffusion and charge transport. In 2014, Deng et al. synthesized two solution-processable small molecules, **DOO3OTTBDT** and **DOP3HTTBDT**, based on a conjugated backbone with ethylhexyl-thiophene substituted benzodithiophene (TBDT) as the core.[125] The **DOP3HTTBDT** device exhibited a PCE of 5.6% with a V_{OC} of 0.87 V, a J_{SC} of 9.94 mA cm^{-2}, and an impressive FF of 65%; **DOO3OTTBDT** showed a deeper HOMO level with a V_{OC} of 0.94 V but lower J_{SC}. A wide-bandgap molecule, **DRTB-T**, was designed using an alkyl-thienyl-substituted BDT trimer as the central unit and 3-ethylrhodanines as the end-capping groups, and it was synthesized by Yang et al.[126] The NFSMOSCs using DRTB-T and a nonfullerene acceptor (IC-C6IDTIC) exhibited a record 9.08% PCE with a high V_{OC} of 0.98 V. Liu et al. proved that the steric hindrance caused by the nonconjugated alkyls in their central units plays a critical role that affects their electron donating and accepting properties (**BTCN-O** and **BTCN-M**), which suggests a new strategy for the molecular design of OPV materials.[127] A D-A structured medium-bandgap organic small molecule **H11** with BDTT as central donor unit and fluorobenzotriazole as acceptor unit, achieved a PCE of 9.73% for the all organic small molecules OSCs with **H11** as donor and a low-bandgap n-OS IDIC as acceptor.[128] For comparison, a control molecule **H12** without thiophene conjugated side chains on the BDT unit showed only 5.51%. Yuan et al. demonstrated that the oligomer donor **O-BDTdFBT** can be comparable to its polymer analog **P-BDTdFBT**.[129] Although the short conjugation length resulted in a larger bandgap, **O-BDTdFBT** displayed high PCE of 8.10% due to the high-degree molecular ordering and excellent intrinsic phase separation with PC$_{71}$BM.

Two novel small molecules (**NDTT-CNCOO** and **NDTP-CNCOO**) using 2D-conjugated NDT unit as the core were synthesized by Zhu et al.[130] Compared with **NDTT-CNCOO**, **NDTP-CNCOO**-based BHJ solar cells exhibited higher FF, higher J_{SC}, and higher PCE (7.20% with an active layer thickness of 300 nm), the best result reported for NDT-based small molecule solar cells. Encouraged by these results, a new A-D-A small molecule donor named **NDTSR** is synthesized.[131] **NDTSR**:IDIC system exhibits a PCE of 8.05%, while **NDTSR**:ITIC system only shows a low PCE of 1.77%. The solution-processable small molecules with end acceptors substituted with various fluorine atoms (0F, 1F, and 2F, respectively) were synthesized by Deng and coworkers (**BTID-0F**, **BTID-1F**, and **BTID-2F**).[125] The fluorination was beneficial to hierarchical morphology with higher domain purity, enhanced surface enrichment, and more directional vertical phase distribution, which reduced the loss of V_{OC}, J_{SC}, and FF simultaneously. As a result, a record PCE of 11.3% was obtained in inverted OSCs-based BTID-2F: PC$_{71}$BM, with V_{OC} of 0.95 V, J_{SC} of 15.7 mA cm^{-2} and FF of 76%.

3.3.3 ELECTRON FULLERENE ACCEPTORS

Since the discovery of the BHJ, fullerenes are the most used OPV acceptors, and much progress has been made in cell architecture, efficiency, and understanding of the physical principles. PC$_{60}$BM and its corresponding C$_{70}$ derivative (PC$_{70}$BM) have been dominantly used as acceptors in OPVs. PC$_{70}$BM is preferable over the C$_{60}$ derivative for it possesses stronger visible absorption, which is widely used in the fabrication of BHJ PSCs.

Absorption spectra of PC$_{60}$BM and PC$_{70}$BM are shown in Figure 3.14. It can be seen that both the two materials show strong absorption at the ultraviolet region,

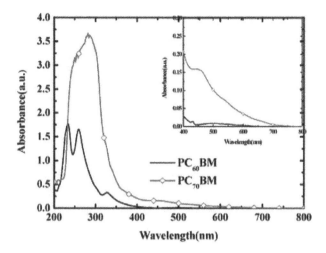

FIGURE 3.14 Absorption spectra of $PC_{60}BM$ and $PC_{70}BM$ in THF solutions (10^{-5} mol L^{-1}): the inset shows the enlarged absorption spectra in the visible region. (Reproduced from Hou, J. and Guo X., *Organic Solar Cells, Green Energy and Technology*, Springer, London, UK, 2013. With permission from Springer Nature.)

from 200 to 400 nm, but $PC_{70}BM$ shows stronger absorption in a visible region compared to $PC_{60}BM$. In the UV-visible region from 200 to 700 nm, the absorbance of $PC_{70}BM$ is much stronger than that of $PC_{60}BM$. In the visible region from 400 to 700 nm, $PC_{70}BM$ shows quite strong absorption, in comparison with the very weak absorption of $PC_{60}BM$ (see inset of Figure 3.14). Since OPV devices using $PC_{70}BM$ as acceptor will harvest more sunlight, many OPVs using $PC_{70}BM$ as acceptor show higher J_{SC} and hence better PCEs than that of $PC_{60}BM$-based devices. However, C_{70} is much more expensive than that of C_{60} due to its complicated, time-consuming process, which limits its application. This could be the problem for future commercial applications in PSCs. The corresponding C_{84} derivative of PCBM, $PC_{84}BM$ was also developed by Hummelen et al.[132] $PC_{84}BM$ possesses a LUMO energy level, a relatively high electron mobility, and a broad visible absorption extending to near infrared. The PSCs based on MDMO-PPV/$PC_{84}BM$ show poorer photovoltaic performance than that of the PSCs with $PC_{60}BM$ and $PC_{70}BM$ as acceptors with a PCE of only 0.3% due to the poorer solubility of the big size.

Indene-fullerene adducts were also used as electron acceptor materials in bulk heterojunction organic solar cells.[133–135] Indene-fullerene multiadduct can be obtained, which can be separated readily through column chromatography. Due to the high LUMO levels of indene-fullerene monoadduct (−3.86 eV) of ICMA and indene-fullerene bisadduct (−3.74 eV) compared with PCBM (−3.91 eV), the devices ICMA/P3HT and ICBA/P3HT showed higher V_{OC} than that of P3HT/PCBM-based devices. Furthermore, the good solubility of ICBA and higher levels than ICMA made the optimized P3HT:ICBA PSC exhibit a PCE of 6.48% with a high V_{OC} of 0.84 V. Therefore, bisadduct fullerene derivatives have emerged as new acceptor materials with higher photovoltaic performance for PSCs.

In addition to the aforementioned fullerene derivative acceptors, there are some other fullerene derivatives for application as acceptors in PSCs reported in litera-ture.[136] These include SIMEF with side chains containing Si atoms, trimetallic nitride endohedral fullerenes, and other C_{60} derivatives with multi side chains, and so on.

3.3.4 ELECTRON NON-FULLERENE ACCEPTORS

Fullerene-based acceptors have some drawbacks, such as weak absorption, limited tunability, batch-to-batch performance variations, high synthetic costs, and morpho-logical instability. Recently, a variety of new non-fullerene acceptors (NFA) have been rapidly developed to further enhance the OPV device performance, and the PCE of single-junction devices has now exceeded 12%.[137] In this part, we highlight and discuss some of the important classes of materials that have shown promise as alternative electron acceptor materials in organic solar cells.

3.3.4.1 PDI-Based Acceptors

The most widely investigated NFA molecules to date were based on the perylene diimide (PDI) core unit, which possesses many desirable features for OPV electron acceptors, such as high electron mobility, high electron affinity (EA; *ca.* 3.9 eV for the unmodified PDI, which is similar to widely used fullerene acceptors), strong inter-molecular π–π interactions, and high absorption coefficients.[138] The PDI molecule also offers two positions for functionalization (β positions of the central perylene ring and the imide nitrogens), which meant the optoelectronic/energy properties and thin film morphologies of it would be easily tuned (Figure 3.15).

The low LUMO, good electron transport, and broad absorption render PDI poly-mers as promising candidates for all-polymer solar cells. An electron-transporting polymer based on PDI and the dithienothiophene unit (**PDI-DTT**) was reported by Zhan et al.[139], which shows a high FET mobility of 1.3×10^{-2} cm^2/(Vs). Zhan et al. also[140] developed a novel all-polymer solar cell containing **PDI-DTT** as the accep-tor and a high-performance copolymer of benzodithiophene and thienothiophene as the donor semiconductor. The optimized cells show a PCE up to 3.45% with a J_{SC} of 8.55 mA/cm^2, a V_{OC} of 0.752 V, and a FF of 52%. M. S. Roy et al.[141] developed a novel alternating phenylenevinylene copolymer, which combined with perylene bisimide units. All polymer solar cells with structure ITO/P3HT:**PDIPLV** (1:1 w/w)/Al were fabricated and exhibit a V_{OC} of 0.60 V, a J_{SC} of 2.98 mA/cm^2, FF of 0.39, and PCE of about 2.32% after the films are thermally annealed.

A series of PDI-based polymers by combination of PDIs with different donor segments—including vinylene, thiophene, dithieno[3,2-b:2′,3′-d]pyrrole, fluorene, dibenzosilole, and carbazole—were developed and utilized as *n*-type polymers for all-PSC applications.[142] Two donor polymers, P3HT and PT1, were used to test the solar cell performance of the PDI-based polymers. Compared to P3HT, PT1 exhibits a lower HOMO energy level and better film morphology in the blends. Among all the devices, the combination between PT1 and the PDI-carbazole-based polymer (**PDI-PC**) gives the best performance with a V_{OC} of 0.70 V, a J_{SC} of 6.35 mA/cm^2, and a FF of 50%, ultimately resulting in a PCE of 2.23%. PDI and oligothiophene copolymers were also synthesized for all-polymer solar cells. **PDI-PT** having a

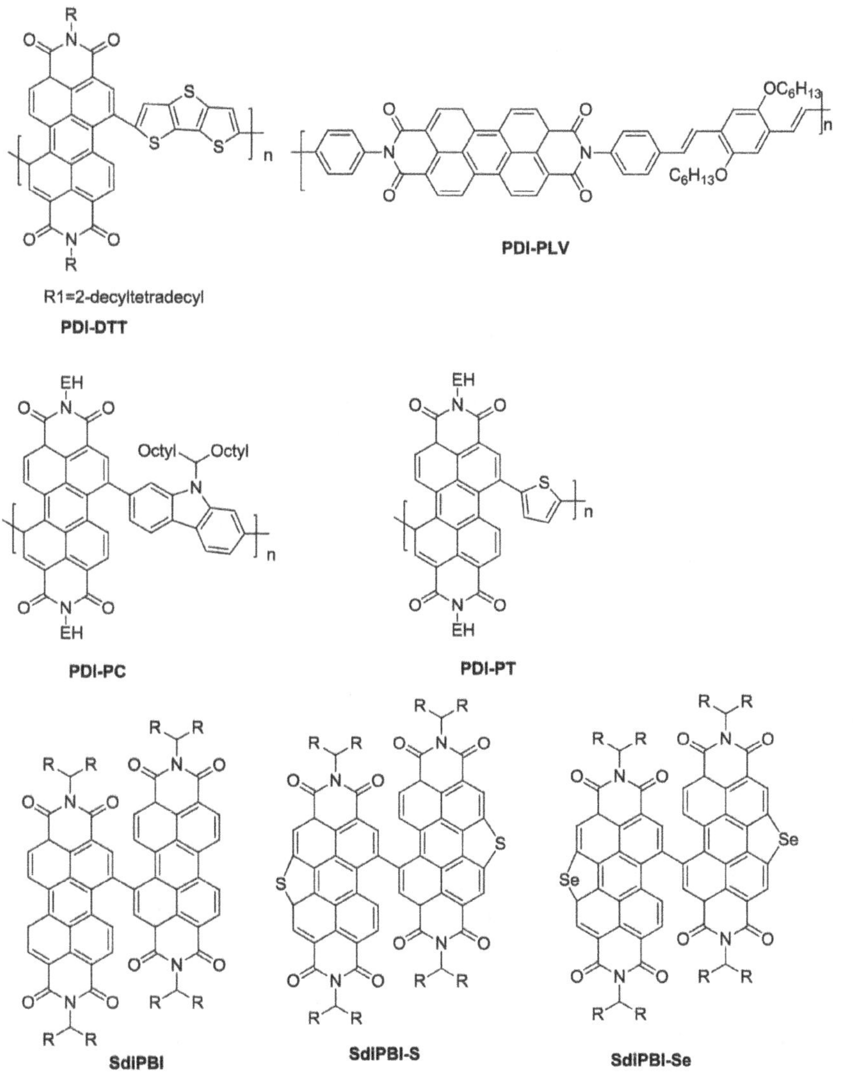

FIGURE 3.15 Chemical structures of PDI-based electron acceptors.

monothiophene donor was synthesized, and an optimal PCE of 0.97% was achieved when **PDI-PT** was blended with a polythiophene derivative.

In addition to the PDI polymers were promising candidates for all-polymer solar cells. The PDI oligomers were also developed to boost and show very impressive device performance. A single bay-linked PDI dimer (**SdiPBI**)[143] with about a 70° angle between two PDI units, demonstrated good OPV performance arising from its flexibly twisted structure. BHJ OPV devices based on the **SdiPBI** acceptor and the (PBDTT-F-TT) polymer donor demonstrated a PCE up to 5.90% by using an inverted cell structure with a fullerene self-assembled monolayer on ZnO. A closely related

PDI dimer (**SdiPBI-S**)[144] with sulfur bridges in the bay positions had a more twisted molecular configuration, a slightly lower electron affinity, and a blue shifted absorption profile providing better spectral complementarity with narrow- bandgap donor polymers. Next, a novel selenophene-containing PBI acceptor, **SdiPBI-Se**,[145] was synthesized. The introduction of a selenium atom to the PBI core results in a high lowest unoccupied molecular orbital (LUMO) level of −3.87 eV, a twisted molecular configuration, and a high electron mobility of 6.4×10^{-3} cm^2 V^{-1} s^{-1}. By incorporating polymer donor PDBT-T1, organic solar cells based on **SdiPBI-Se** show outstanding performance with a PCE of 8.4%, a V_{OC} of 0.96 V, a J_{SC} of 12.49 mA cm^{-2}, and an unprecedented high FF of 70.2%. This is due to the synergistic effects of efficient photon absorption, high and balanced charge carrier mobility, and ultrafast charge generation. Very recently, two kinds of conjugated C$_3$-symmetric perylenedyes, namely triperylene hexaimides (TPH) and selenium-annulated triperylene hexaimides (TPH-Se),[146] are efficiently synthesized. Both TPH and TPH-Se have broad and strong absorption in the region of 300–600 nm together with suitable LUMO levels of about −3.8 eV. TPH and TPH-Se acceptor-based solar cells show PCE of 8.28% and 9.28%, respectively, which are the highest values that have been reported for PDI acceptors (Figure 3.15).

3.3.4.2 NDI-Based Acceptors

Compared to the PDI-based molecules, the smaller fused-ring unit naphthalene diimide (NDI)-based small molecules were less investigated, due to their better planarity and stronger intermolecular interactions than their PDI analogues, along with a larger bandgap and weak absorption in the visible spectrum. To overcome this, usually electron donating groups or strong light absorption groups were introduced to the NDI skeleton through the *N*-position or aromatic position.

The **P(NDI2OD-T2)** is the most thoroughly studied polymer acceptor so far. Composed of NDI and bithiophene moieties, **P(NDI2OD-T2)**[147] was first reported for use in OFETs (Figure 3.16). A high electron mobility of 0.45–0.85 cm^2/(V s) was achieved under ambient conditions in combination with Au contacts and various polymeric dielectrics. Later, it was introduced as an acceptor material to all-polymer photovoltaic devices. Moore et al.[148] demonstrated that the efficiency of theP3HT:**P(NDI2OD-T2)** device was only 0.2% with poor J_{SC} and FF. They found that fast geminate recombination within 200 ps of excitation contributed to the low J_{SC}. This is due to a poor morphology with widely varied and overly large domain sizes up to 1 μm in the blend. However, Fabiano et al. found that due to balanced electron and hole mobility, high FF approaching 70% can be achieved in P3HT:**P(NDI2OD-T2)** devices. Unfortunately, because of the poor morphology, no improvement in PCE was attained. In addition to using P3HT as the donor polymer, several other donor polymer systems have been studied with **P(NDI2OD-T2)** as acceptor. Ito and coworkers[149] used PTQ1 as the donor polymer and achieved a large PCE of 4.1%. When the donor/acceptor weight ratio varies from 20%:80% to 70%:30%, PCE increases. Tang et al.[150] reported all-polymer BHJ PSCs with PTB7 as the donor and **P(NDI2OD-T2)** as acceptor. The two polymers exhibit complementary absorption spectra. Morphology studies revealed that crystalline **P(NDI2OD-T2)** domains dispersed in amorphous PTB7, and a **P(NDI2OD-T2)**-rich top layer is formed in the device. A modest PCE

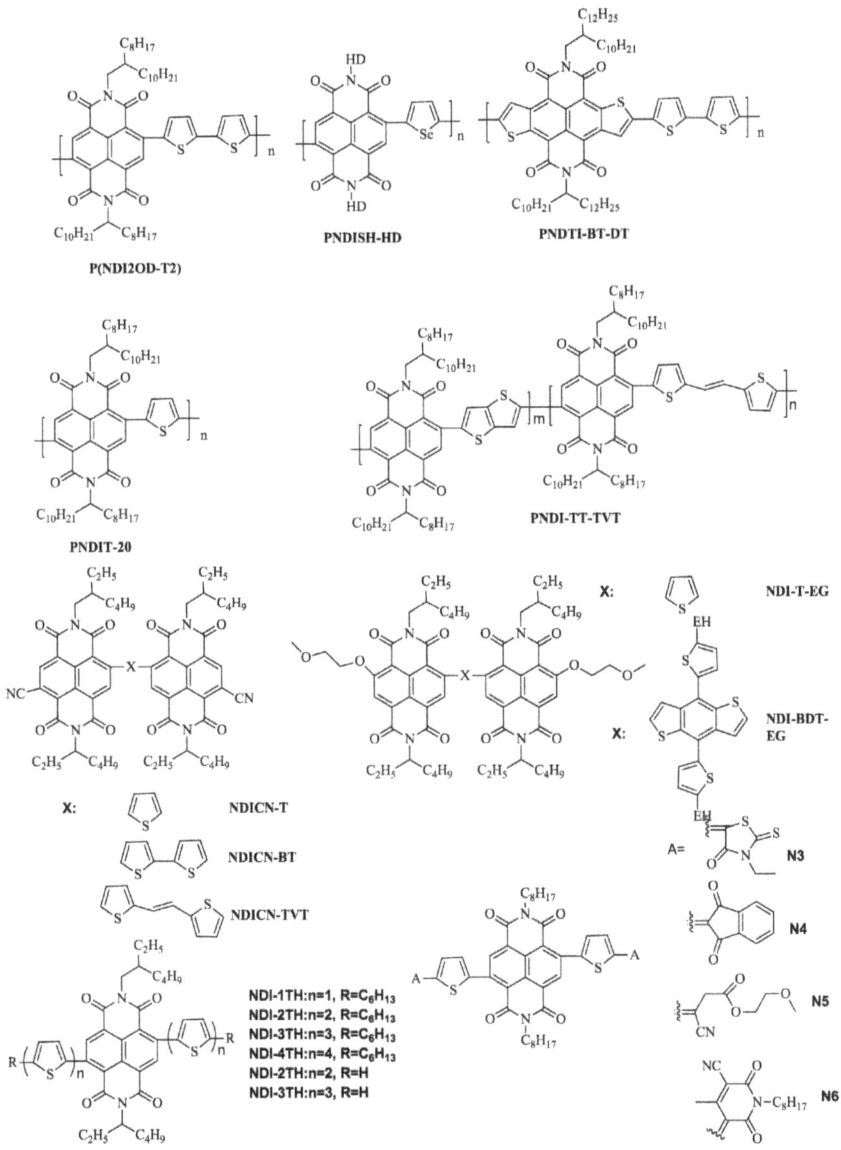

FIGURE 3.16 Chemical structure of various NDI-based polymeric acceptors.

of 1.1% result has been achieved. The crystalline morphology of PNDIS-HD also helps to achieve balanced charge mobility in the blends.

In addition to **P(NDI2OD-T2)**, another polymer containing NDI and seleno-phene units shows great potential toward the application in all-polymer solar cells.[151] Jenekhe and coworkers reported such a cell using a NDI-selenophene copolymer (**PNDIS-HD**) as the acceptor and a thiazolothiazole copolymer (PSEHTT) as the donor, leading to a PCE of 3.3%. Selenophene containing polymers show higher electron mobility than their thiophene counterparts, which is ascribed to better orbital overlapping from the larger π orbitals in the selenium atom. Zhou et al.[152] reported all-polymer solar cells based on PTB7 as donor polymer and an NDI-family copolymer based on naphthodithiophene diimide and bithiophene to produce the polymer (**PNDTI-BT-DT**) as an acceptor material. **PNDTIBT-DT** shows strong absorption in the near-IR region. A PCE of 2.56% is attained with chloroform as the solvent. Shen et al. fabricated all-PSCs based on **PNDIT-20** paired with a donor polymer PTB7-Th and demonstrated PCEs of 3.88% by using non-halogenated solvents.[153] Li et al. reported a polymer solar cell fabricated from blends of PTB7-Th and **PNDI-TT-TVTs** (containing 25% of TT and 75% of TVT), which displayed a PCE of 5.27%, significantly higher than those achieved by devices based on alternating arranged copolymers.[154]

In 2011, Jenekhe et al. reported a homologous series of six novel oligothiophene-**NDI**-based oligomer semiconductors (**NDI-Th**).[155] BHJ solar cells incorporating them as the electron acceptor and P3HT as the electron donor showed a PCE of 1.5% with a V_{OC} of 0.82 V and a bicontinuous nanoscale morphology. Hong et al. synthesized three NDI-based small molecules, **NDICN-T**, **NDICN-BT**, and **NDICN-TVT**.[156] The photovoltaic devices prepared with **DTS-F:NDICN-TVT** gave the highest PCE of 3.01%, with a V_{OC} of 0.75 V, a J_{SC} of 7.10 mA cm^{-2}, and a FF of 56.2%, whereas the DTS-F:NDICN-T and **DTS-F:NDICN-BT** devices provided PCEs of 1.81% and 0.13%, respectively. The solvophobic 2-methoxyle thoxyl (EG) groups are used to end-cap the solvophiphilic NDI to improve the self-organization properties of the NDI dimmers (**NDI-T-EG** and **NDI-BDT-EG**).[157] The devices with PBDTTT-C-T as donor exhibit the champion performance, affording PCE of 1.24% and 1.31%, respectively, with **NDI-BDT-EG** and **NDI-T-EG** as acceptor. To further improve the photovalatic performances of the **NDI**-based acceptor, the utilization of terminal acceptors flanked with an **NDI** unit has also prestend (**N3-N6**).[158,159] The target chromophore-bearing cyanopyridone acceptor units (**N6**) afforded a PCE of 6.10% when paired with **P3HT**, the highest for the NDI core-based non-fullerene acceptors.

3.3.4.3 Calamitic-Shaped Small Molecules-Based Acceptors

The electron-donating extended fused rings—for example, indacenodithiophene (IDT) and indacenodithieno[3,2-b]thiophene (IDTT)—were tailored by end-capping electron-deficient groups and also used as electron acceptors. Now, A-D-A acceptors based on extended fused-rings have made great breakthroughs, demonstrating promising performance with PCEs of ~12%, even higher than those of fullerene counterparts (up to 10%–11%) (Figure 3.17).

Yang et al. reported a series of halogenated ITIC, containing F, Cl, Br, and I. The absorption peak is red-shifted from H- to F-, Cl-, Br-, and I-ITIC due to the inductive effect and π-electrons delocalizing onto empty d-orbitals on the halogens. Halogenated semiconductors possess deep frontier energy levels and high crystallinity and provide high electron mobilities up to 1.3 cm^2 V^{-1} s^{-1} and PCEs over 9% in NFSCs (**F-ITIC**: 8.8%, **Cl-ITIC**: 9.5%, **Br-ITIC**: 9.4%, and **I-ITIC**: 8.9%).[160] For comparison, **H-ITIC** provided an electron mobility of 0.047 cm^2 V^{-1} s^{-1} and a PCE of 6.4%. Dai et al.[161] designed four INIC series based on IBDT end-capped with IC or fluorinated IC (**INIC-INIC-3**). Fluorine substitution downshifts the LUMO energy level (−3.88 eV to −4.02 eV),

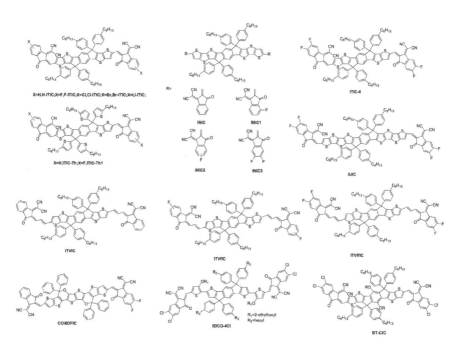

FIGURE 3.17 Structures of fused-ring electron acceptor (FREA) molecules with different end groups.

red-shifts the absorption spectrum (706–744 nm), and enhances electron mobility. The difluorinated **INIC3** exhibit PCEs as high as 11.5% (V_{OC} of 0.852 V, J_{SC} of 19.68 mA cm^{-2}, FF of 68.5%), significantly higher than that of nonfluorinated **INIC** (7.7%). Three n-OS acceptors with narrow E_g values of <1.4 eV were synthesized by introducing double-bond π-bridges into ITIC (**ITVIC**) and ITIC with monofluorine (**ITVfIC**) or bifluorine (**ITVffIC**) substituents on its end groups.[162] The PSCs based on **J71:ITVffIC** demonstrated a PCE of 10.54% with a high J_{SC} of 20.60 mA cm^{-2} and a V_{OC} of 0.81 V, suggesting that **ITVffIC** is a promising narrow-bandgap NIR acceptor for application in tandem/multijunction, semitransparent, and ternary PSCs.

A fused-undecacyclic electron acceptor **IUIC**[163] was also developed and afforded PCEs of up to 10.2% with an average visible transmittance of 31%, higher than PTB7-Th: **ITIC4** (PCEs = 6.42%, AVT = 28%) control in the semitransparent organic solar cells (ST-OSCs). This is the first example of ST-OSCs with PCEs breaking 10%. A new fluorinated nonfullerene acceptor, **ITIC-Th1**, was designed and synthesized by Zhao et al. Nonfullerene OSCs based on a fluorinated **ITIC-Th1**[164] electron acceptor exhibit PCEs as high as 12.1%, significantly higher than the nonfluorinated **ITIC-Th** (8.88%). By increasing the electron-donating capability of D unit and/or the electron-accepting capability of A unit, Xiao et al. developed a low-bandgap A-D-A acceptor, **COi8DFIC**,[165] which exhibits outstanding performance in NFOSCs with a J_{SC} of 26.12 mA cm^{-2} and a decent PCE of 12.16% achieved from PTB7-Th:**COi8DFIC** solar cells. Later, the highest PCE record of 14.08% was achieved in PTB7-Th:**COi8DFIC:PC$_{71}$BM** (1:1.05:0.45) ternary cells.[166]

Fluorination of the acceptor moiety has proved to be an effective method to enhance the ICT effect. However, the fluorination procedure is generally tedious and costly, which is unfavorable for practical applications. Cui and coworkers incorporated high electron affinity chlorine atoms (Pauline electronegativity for Cl: 3.16) into the NF acceptor (**IEICO-4Cl**)[167] to enhance the ICT effect and red-shifted its absorption spectrum compared to **IEICO-4F**,[168] implying that chlorination is more effective than fluorination in enhancing the ICT effect and is more suitable for utilizing NIR solar photons than **IEICO-4F** in the OSCs. The electron acceptor, **BT-CIC**,[169] comprises four chlorine atoms at the 5,6-positions of the 2-(3-oxo-2,3-dihydroinden-1-ylidene)-malononitrile and was developed by Li et al. which has an energy gap of ~1.3 eV leading to an optical absorption edge at ~1000 nm, achieved the highest efficiency reported for NIR organic solar cells (PCE = $11.2 \pm 0.4\%$) and PCE = $7.1 \pm 0.1\%$ with an average visible transmittance of $43 \pm 2\%$ in the semitransparent OPV. Considering the synthetic accessibility and lower cost of chloro-containing precursors compared to the well-developed fluorinated molecules, this work provides new avenues in the design of NIR acceptors with applications to semitransparent and tandem solar cells for building integrated photovoltaics.

3.4 PREPARATION TECHNIQUES

There are two common techniques for thin film production. When evaporation on thermal stability is required, materials for solution processing need to be soluble. Small molecules may be thermally more stable but less soluble than polymers, where solubility often is achieved by side-chain solubilization. Polymers will decompose under excessive heat and have too much molar mass to evaporate. The evaporation is the best choice for small molecules, and polymers are mainly processed from solution.[19]

3.4.1 Evaporation

To grow films by thermal evaporation, usually a vacuum of $<10^{-5}$ mbar is applied. Thus, the mean free path of the evaporated molecule is longer than the distance between the evaporation source and the sample holder. In addition, contaminants such as oxygen and water are reduced and can be eliminated further by a treatment under ultra-high vacuum ($<10^{-9}$ mbar) or evaporation inside of a glove box with inert atmosphere. To create interpenetrating donor-acceptor networks or to achieve molecular doping, co-evaporation techniques can be applied.[170,171]

3.4.2 Wet Processing

Common to all wet processing techniques is the solving of organic materials in an appropriate solvent such as water or any other polar or nonpolar organic solvent. A special case is the solution processing of a soluble monomer coupled with a polymerization reaction during (e.g., electrochemical polymerization) or after (e.g., via heat treatment, UV curing, and so forth) the film forming process (precursor route). This has the advantage that after preparation the resulting polymers are insoluble, and another film can be deposited from solution on top of them. If polymers or polymer/

polymer or polymer/molecule blends are directly processed from solution, several common techniques are applied: (i) spin coating, (ii) doctor blading, (iii) screen printing, (iv) inkjet printing, and many more. This exploitation of existing printing techniques assures an easy upscaling of the production and low-energy consumption during production of solar cells, which is important for the energy amortization (energy delivered by a solar cell during its lifetime as compared to the energy needed to produce the solar cell itself).

3.4.3 Manufacturing Techniques in Large-Area OPV

PCE of the lab-scale OPV devices has reached up to 10%–12% by the development of novel donor materials and device optimization, indicating the bright future for OPV devices in commercial applications. However, the typical laboratory OPV comprises the use of vacuum processing for the electrode deposition on rigid glass substrates with a very small active area of a few square millimeters. Moreover, the thin film deposition of solution results in a limited material usage and low-fabrication cost for OSCs. To evolve from lab-scale demonstrator devices to real large-area deposited photovoltaic modules, the introduction of adequate processing techniques is required. So far, the main five processing techniques, such as spin coating, screen printing, inkjet printing, doctor blading, and R_2R processing have been developed to fabricate polymer solar cell modules on a reasonable scale.[172]

3.5 MORPHOLOGY CONTROL OF THE ACTIVE LAYER

Although all active layers adopt the same general BHJ structure, significant morphological differences exist, especially with regard to domain size and degree of interpenetration between domains. Polymer morphology has also been proven to be extremely important in determining the optoelectronic properties in polymer-based devices. A long-standing generalization is that the ideal active layer morphology will have an interpenetrating network of donor and acceptor materials, with domain sizes on the order of the exciton diffusion length or around 10 nm. Essentially, the active layer should have enough interfacial area to dissociate the greatest possible amount of excitons, while also maintaining continuous charge transport pathways to the electrodes. Numerous methods have been conducted to characterize and control the blend morphology and include the solvent, donor/acceptor concentrations, thermal annealing times and temperatures, solvent annealing conditions, additives, and the interlayer surface energies. Here, several methods have been applied to control the bulk morphology and will be discussed in this section.

3.5.1 Solvents Effects

Solution processing has many advantages over other film fabrication technologies (requiring complicated instruments, costly and time-consuming procedures).[173] Therefore, solution processing has been developed into the most favored methodology for fabricating organic optoelectronic devices. The choice of solvent(s) also has a significant influence on the morphology and thus device performance. In most cases, high boiling solvents such as CB and DCB give better performance than that of low boiling solvents such as chloroform (CF), and the polymer shows good solubility in the solvent chosen. Park et al.[174] reported that PCDTBT:PC$_{71}$BM showed a PCE of 6.1% when processed in DCB, which was higher than the results in both CB and CF. This is because the DCB-processed system results in the formation of much smaller domains in the active layer compared to CB- and CF-processed devices. In 2001, Shaheen et al. reported[175] the nearly threefold improvement of MDMO-PPV/PCBM devices by processing the active layer from chlorobenzene rather than toluene. They found that changing the solvent used for processing allowed for the formation of a more intimately mixed active layer with smaller domain sizes, which can be expected based on the better fullerene solubility in chlorobenzene. In the P3HT system, it has been demonstrated that different solvents result in changes not only in lateral phase separations but also in vertical material distributions.[176] Devices fabricated from toluene, CB, and xylene show a PCBM-enriched top layer that is beneficial to device performance, while films made from CF exhibited a P3HT-enriched top layer. In some cases, CF can also be a good solvent for PSC fabrication, and the resulting PSCs show state-of-the-art performance due to its good solvation capability.[177,178]

Solvent annealing is another effective strategy to control the morphology of BHJ blends by slowing the evaporation rate of the solvent. This is done by placing spin-cast films in contact with solvents or solvent vapors in a closed container, which slows the drying process. Mihailetchi et al. reported that the hole mobility of P3HT in the P3HT:PCBM blend improves 30-fold after solvent annealing of the active layer.[179] Yang and coworkers showed that the combined effects of controlling the P3HT:PCBM growth rate via solvent annealing followed by thermal annealing of the device leads to high hole mobility and balanced charge transport with a PCE of 4.4%.[180]

3.5.2 THERMAL ANNEALING

Thermal annealing has been shown to be an effective method for the modification of the active layer morphology, thereby influencing the overall device performance. This way has been proven by the result of the formation of larger P3HT and PCBM domains, improving P3HT crystallization in P3HT/PCBM devices, resulting in the extension of the optical absorption into the red and improving the charge transport characteristics.

At first, extensive efforts were devoted to optimizing thermal annealing to improve the morphology and performance of P3HT:PCBM devices. Yang and coworkers[270] observed that upon thermal annealing, self-organization occurred and the absorption of the device was red shifted due to the enhanced interchain interaction from the highly ordered, crystalline structure. Erb et al.[181] studied the effect of annealing on the structural and optical properties of P3HT:PCBM films using an X-ray diffraction technique. They found that after thermal annealing, P3HT main chains became oriented in parallel and the side chains perpendicular to the substrate in the polymer crystallites. Simultaneously, thermal annealing was found to exclude PCBM crystallites from the polymer films. Chen et al. used a variety of techniques, including GIXD, NEXAFS, and DSIMS, to determine how preannealing and postannealing affect the active layer morphology.[182] They found that both annealing strategies resulted in the formation of a bicontinuous network of polymer and fullerene with domains on the order of the exciton diffusion length, and they observed increased power conversion efficiencies for both cases (PCEs of 0.61%, 1.10%, and 3.37% for as spun, preannealed, and postannealed, respectively). However, the pre-annealed samples showed an increase in P3HT concentration near the surface of the active layer due to its lower surface energy and a preferential packing of P3HT in an "edge-on" fashion, both of which limited the improvement in device efficiency. In contrast, the post-annealed samples showed an increase in PCBM concentration near the cathode and a reorientation of P3HT to the "face-on" orientation, both of which promote efficient charge transfer and are responsible for the greater improvement in device efficiency with postannealing rather than preannealing. The GIXD spectra highlighting the different propensities for edge-on and face-on polymer organization with the different annealing methods are shown in Figure 3.18. The difference after the post-annealing response is a result of the importance of the difference in interfacial energies between the anode and the cathode.

In addition to the huge success in improving crystallinity, charge transport, and morphology in the P3HT system, thermal annealing is found to enhance the performance of several other donor polymers. Yan et al. investigated the influences of various processing parameters (spin rate, temperature, etc.) on the morphology and properties of PffBT4T-2OD-based solar cells.[183] It was found that the high temperature conditions can significantly reduce polymer crystallinity and change polymer backbone orientation from face-on to edge-on. For the PffBT4T-2OD polymer, PCE increased to 10.3% when annealed at 100°C, giving a PCE value of 7.9% at 80°C, which decreased as the annealing temperature went down.

3.5.3 ADDITIVES EFFECTS

As mentioned earlier, thermal annealing or controlled solvent evaporation after film casting has proved to be critical for optimizing charge separation and transport within the bulk heterojunction morphology. Unfortunately, attempts to improve the

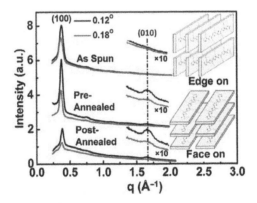

FIGURE 3.18 GIXD curves of P3HT/PCBM blend films at different incident angles. As spun; preannealed 30 min; postannealed 30 min. The insets represent the schemes of edge-on and face-on of P3HT chains. (Reproduced with permission from Chen, D. et al., *Nano Lett.*, 11, 561–567, 2011. Copyright 2011 American Chemical Society.)

performance of PCPDTBT:C_{71}-PCBM solar cells by these methods were not very successful.[184] Adding alkanedithiols to the PCPDTBT:C_{71}-PCBM solution causes the red shifts of the absorption peak and emergency of the absorption peak associated with the π–π* transition, which indicates that the PCPDTBT chains interact more strongly and there is improved local structural order compared with films processed from pure chlorobenzene (Figure 3.19).

Heeger and coworkers clarified the mechanism of how processing additives control the morphology.[16] As shown in Figure 3.20, the alkanedithiol selectively dissolves the PCBM, but P3HT and PCPDTBT are not soluble. Because the fullerenes are selectively dissolved in alkanedithiol, three separate phases are formed during the process of liquid–liquid phase separation and drying: a fullerene-alkanedithiol phase, a polymer aggregate phase, and a polymer-fullerene phase. The alkanedithiol has a higher boiling point than the chlorobenzene host solvent; the PCBM tends to remain

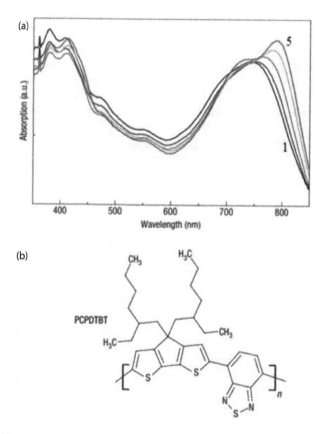

FIGURE 3.19 Ultraviolet-visible absorption. (a) The spectral response indicates a red shift from a pure PCPDTBT:C_{71}-PCBM film (Spectrum 1) to films cast from chlorobenzene containing 24 mg mL^{-1} 1,3-propanedithiol (Spectrum 2), 1,4-butanedithiol (Spectrum 3), 1,6-hexanedithiol (Spectrum 4), and 1,8-octanedithiol (Spectrum 5). (b) The molecular structure of PCPDTBT. (Reproduced from Peet, J. et al., *Nat. Mater.*, 6, 497–500, 2007. With permission from Springer Nature.)

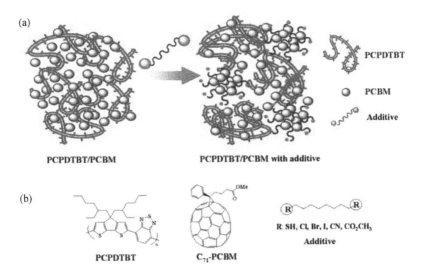

FIGURE 3.20 (a) Schematic depiction of the role of the processing additive in the self-assembly of bulk heterojunction blend materials and (b) structures of PCPDTBT, C_{71}-PCBM, and additives. (Reproduced with permission from Lee, J. K. et al., *J. Am. Chem. Soc.*, 130, 3619–3623, 2008. Copyright 2008 American Chemical Society.)

in solution (during drying) longer than the semiconducting polymer, thereby enabling control of the phase separation and the resulting morphology of the BHJ material. According to this mechanism, Heeger and coworkers developed two general guidelines that have been identified for additive design: (i) selective (differential) solubility of the fullerene component of the BHJ material and (ii) higher boiling point than the host solvent. Chen and coworkers used solution-phase small-angle X-ray scattering to study the effects of the additive DIO on the aggregation of PTB7:PC$_{71}$BM PSCs.[185] Without DIO, the large PCBM aggregates prevented intercalation of PCBM into PTB7 domains. DIO dissolved the PCBM aggregates and resulted in smaller domains with an improved PTB7:PCBM interpenetration network. Energy-filtered TEM (EFTEM) measurement also shows that DIO results in better phase separation in PTB7:PCBM devices with an average distance of 20–40 nm between domains. The use of solvent additives has become one of the most important methods for controlling the development of crystalline domains with low-bandgap polymer solar cells.

3.6 INTERFACIAL ENGINEERING

From a materials design perspective, polymers with high mobilities necessary to efficiently extract and transport free charges to different electrodes are desired. However, there is generally a limited choice of electrode materials available whose work function can exactly match the energy level of the organic semiconductors. In this case, the modification of an organic active layer-electrode interface is critical to achieve high performance in PSCs. The multiple roles served by the interfacial layer include (1) tuning the work function of the electrode to promote Ohmic contact at the active layer and electrode interface, (2) determining the polarity of the device (conventional device or inverted device), (3) improving the selectivity toward holes or electrons while blocking the other and minimizing charge recombination at the interface, (4) enhancing light harvesting by introducing optical spacers, and (5) improving device stability.

Interfacial layers between the electrodes and the active layer are introduced to facilitate this process, which include both a hole-selective layer (HSL) and an electron-selective layer (ESL) in a single-junction PSC device. Poly(3,4-ethylenedioxythiophene):polystyrenesulfonate (PEDOT:PSS) is the most widely used HSL to promote the formation of an Ohmic contact for efficient hole collection combined with the strong advantages of high optical transparency and solution processability.[4] Despite the improvement observed in conventional structure organic photovoltaics (OPVs) when PEDOT:PSS is used as the HSL, the material also has some very significant flaws. Therefore, great effort has been made to develop anodic interlayer materials to replace PEDOT:PSS. So far, p-type transition metal oxides such as NiO and V_2O_5 as HSLs have been widely studied in OPVs. In early studies, these metal oxides were prepared mostly through vacuum deposition processes. These are incompatible with the high-throughput roll-to-roll process and thus are not cost effective. Therefore, various solution-processed methods were developed to prepare metal oxide films that include NiO,[186] V_2O_5,[187] CuO,[188] WO_3,[189] RuO_2,[190] CrOx,[190] and NiAc.[191] Among them, molybdenum oxide (MoO_3) thin films have drawn much attention and been widely used. On the other hand, solution-processed graphene oxide (GO) is another alternative as an efficient HSL.[192] Chhowalla and coworkers used 2 nm GO as the HSL for P3HT:PCBM devices, which achieved comparable PCE to PEDOT:PSS HSL devices. In addition, many organic compounds, such as polyanilines,[193] conjugated polyelectrolyte,[194] and conjugated microporous polymer[195] also have been used as efficient HSLs in PSCs.

In conventional PSC devices, the cathode is always thermally evaporated Al, with Ca or LiF as ESLs for efficient hole blocking and electron collection. However, low work function metals are sensitive to oxidation, which leads to unstability. In addition, vacuum deposition is not compatible with the large-scale roll-to-toll manufacturing. Therefore, various solution-processed methods have been developed with the aim toward preparing stable cathode buffer layers, such as ZnO,[196] tungsten polyoxometalate,[197] and conjugated polyelectrolytes (CPEs).[198] Among them, ZnO is the most widely used inorganic ESL in OPVs due to its environmental friendliness, ambient stability, low cost, high transparency, high conductivity, and good hole-blocking properties. Water- and alcohol-soluble and inexpensive nonconjugated polyelectrolytes (NPEs) are promising cathode modifiers that can reduce the work function of the electrode by the formation of a dipole layer at the interfaces. Water- and alcohol-soluble CPEs composed of a π-conjugated backbone and surfactant-like side groups (such as amine, ammonium, phosphate, sulfonic, and zwitterionic groups) are another class of promising ESL for OPVs. In addition, the fullerene-based ESL materials are another option because they match the LUMO energy level of commonly used acceptor materials such as PCBM and ICBA, while they feature deep HOMO energy levels that endow them with good hole-blocking properties. Recently, many fullerene-based ESL materials have been developed by attaching polar groups such as phosphoric esters,[199] amines,[200] cationic ammonium,[201] and carboxylic acids to fullerenes.[202]

3.7 CONCLUSION

In this chapter, we have briefly described the basics of organic bulk heterojunction solar cells, including conventional structures, basic characterization methods, the materials of the photoactive layers, preparation techniques, etc. We especially paid attention to the photovoltaic materials that have achieved great success in the just a few years. It should be pointed out that the recent developments have led to a rapid increase in power conversion efficiencies for non-fullerene acceptors (NFAs) OSCs, with values now exceeding ~13%–14%, demonstrating the viability of using to replace FAs in next-generation high-performance OSCs. Although PCE of OPV cells has been reached over 14%, the development of active layer materials is still the key to boost the efficiency. Further enhancement in the PCEs of NFA solar cells (to approximately 15%–20% when NFA solar cells are characterized in laboratories) will provide a great opportunity to realize future industrial manufacture.

REFERENCES

1. Yao, H.; Ye, L.; Zhang, H.; Li, S.; Zhang, S.; Hou, J. *Chemical Reviews* 2016, 116, (12), 7397–7457.
2. Wang, C.; Dong, H.; Hu, W.; Liu, Y.; Zhu, D. *Chemical Reviews* 2012, 112, (4), 2208–2267.
3. Dou, L.; Liu, Y.; Hong, Z.; Li, G.; Yang, Y. *Chemical Reviews* 2015, 115, (23), 12633–12665.
4. Lu, L.; Zheng, T.; Wu, Q.; Schneider, A.; Zhao, D.; Yu, L. *Chemical Reviews* 2015, 115, (23), 12666–12731.
5. Günes, S.; Neugebauer, H.; Sariciftci, N. *Chemical Reviews* 2007, 107, (4), 1324–1338.
6. Li, G.; Zhu, R.; Yang, Y. *Nature Photonics* 2012, 6, (3), 153–161.
7. Zhao, J.; Li, Y.; Yang, G.; Jiang, K.; Lin, H.; Ade, H.; Ma, W.; Yan, H. *Nature Energy* 2016, 1 (2),15027–15033.
8. Liu, Y.; Zhao, J.; Li, Z.; Mu, C.; Ma, W.; Hu, H.; Jiang, K.; Lin, H.; Ade, H.; Yan, H. *Nature Communications* 2014, 5, (5), 5293–5300.
9. Yu, G.; Gao, J.; Hummelen, J. C.; Wudl, F.; Heeger, A. J. *Science* 1995, 5243, (270), 1789–1791.
10. Heeger, A.; Sariciftci, N.; Namdas, E. *Semiconducting and Metallic Polymers.* Oxford, UK: Oxford University Press; 2010, p. 278.
11. Kearns, D.; Calvin, M. *The Journal of Chemical Physics* 1958, 950, (29), 950–951.
12. Tang, C. *Applied Physics Letters* 1986, 183, (48), 183–185.
13. Sariciftci, N.; Smilowitz, L.; Heeger, A.; Wudl, F. *Science* 1992, 5087, (258), 1474–1476.
14. Kraabel, B.; Lee, C.; McBranch, D.; Moses, D.; Sariciftci, N.; Heeger, A. *Chemical Physics Letters* 1993, 213, (3–4), 389–394.
15. Halls, J.; Walsh, C.; Greenham, N.; Marseglia, E.; Friend, R.; Moratti, S.; Holmes, A. *Nature* 1995, 376, (6540), 498–500.
16. Lee, J.; Ma, W.; Brabec, C.; Yuen, J.; Moon, J; Kim, J.; Lee, K.; Bazan, G.; Heeger, A. *Journal of the American Chemical Society* 2008, 130, (11), 3619–3623.
17. Zhou, H.; Zhang, Y.; Mai, C.; Collins, S.; Bazan, G.; Nguyen, T.; Heeger, A. *Advanced Materials* 2015, 27, (10), 1767–1773.
18. Yusoff, A.; Kim, D.; Kim, H; Shneider, F; Silva, W; Jang, J. *Energy & Environmental Science* 2015, 8, (1), 303–316.
19. Hoppe, H.; Sariciftci, N. *Journal of Materials Research* 2004, 19, (7), 1924–1945.
20. Scharber, M. C.; Sariciftci, N. S. *Progress in Polymer Science* 2013, 38, (12), 1929–1940.

21. Brabec, D. J.; Cravino, A.; Meissner, D.; Sariciftci, N. S.; Fromherz, T.; Minse, M.; Sanchez, L.; Hummelen, J. C. *Advanced Functional Materials* 2001, 11, (5), 374–380.

22. Van Duren, J.; Loos, J.; Morissey, F.; Leewis, C.; Kivits, K.; Vanzendoorn, L.; Rispens, M.; Hummelen, J.; Janssen R. *Advanced Functional Materials* 2002, 12, (10), 665–669.

23. Scharber, M.; Muhlbacher, D.; Koppe, M.; Denk, P.; Waldauf, C.; Heeger, A.; Brabec, C. *Advanced Materials* 2006, 18, (3), 789–794.

24. Liang, Y.; Yu, L. *Accounts of Chemical Research* 2010, 43, (9), 1227–1236.

25. Brabec, C.; Sariciftci, N.; Hummelen, J. *Advanced Functional Materials* 2001, 11, 15–26.

26. Gregg, B. *Journal of Physical Chemistry B* 2003, 107, (20), 4688–4698.

27. Clarke, T.; Durrant, J. *Chemical Reviews* 2010, 110, (11), 6736–6767.

28. Ohkita, H.; Cook, S.; Astuti, Y.; Duffy, W.; Tierney, S.; Zhang, W.; Heeney, M. et al. *Journal of the American Chemical Society* 2008, 130, (10), 3030–3042.

29. Halls, J.; Pichler, K.; Friend, R.; Moratti, S.; Holmes, A. *Applied Physics Letters* 1996, 68, (22), 3120–3122.

30. Markov, D.; Amsterdam, E.; Blom, P.; Sieval, A.; Hummelen, J. *Journal of Physical Chemistry A* 2005, 109, (24), 5266–5274.

31. Schroeder, B.; Ashraf, R.; McCulloch, I. *Thiophene-Based High-Performance Donor Polymers for Organic Solar Cells.* Weinheim, Germany: John Wiley & Sons; 2014.

32. Fung, D., Choy, W. Introduction to Organic Solar Cells. In: Choy W. (Ed.) *Organic Solar Cells, Green Energy and Technology*, London, UK: Springer; 2013.

33. Andersson, B.; Huang, D.; Moulé, A.; Inganäs, O. *Applied Physics Letters* 2009, 94, (4), 21–23.

34. Zhou, Y.; Fuentes-Hernandez, C.; Shim, M.; Dindar, A.; Haske, W.; Najafabad, E.; Khan, T. et al. *Science* 2012, 336, (6079), 327–332.

35. White, M., Olson, D., Shaheen, S., Kopidakis, N., Ginley, D. *Applied Physics Letters* 2006, 89, (14), 143517.

36. Kim, J.; Kim, S.; Lee, H.; Lee, K.; Ma, W.; Gong, X.; Heeger, A. *Advanced Materials* 2010, 18, (5), 572–576.

37. Waldauf, C.; Morana, M.; Denk, P.; Schilinsky, P.; Coakley, K.; Choulis, S.; Brabec, C. *Applied Physics Letters* 2006, 89, (23), 233517.

38. You, J.; Dou, L.; Hong, Z.; Li, G.; Yang, Y. *Progress in Polymer Science* 2013, 38 (12), 1909–1928.

39. Sista, S.; Hong, Z.; Chen, L.; Yang, Y. *Energy & Environmental Science* 2011, 4 (5), 1606–1620.

40. Sista, S.; Hong, Z.; Park, M.; Xu, Z.; Yang, Y. *Advanced Materials* 2010, 22, (8), E77–E80.

41. Ameri, T.; Dennler, G.; Lungenschmied, C.; Brabec, C. *Energy & Environmental Science*, 2009, 2, (4), 347–363.

42. Heliatek Press release. January 16, 2013, http://www.heliatek.com/newscenter/latest_news/ neuer-weltrekord-fur-organischesolarzellen-heliatek-behauptet-sich-mit-12-zelleffizienz-als technologiefuhrer/?lang=en

43. Chen, Z.; Cai, P.; Chen, J.; Liu, X.; Zhang, L.; Lan, L.; Peng, J.; Ma. Y.; Cao, Y. *Advanced Materials* 2014, 26, (16), 2586–2591.

44. Mo, D.; Wang, H.; Chen, H.; Qu, S.; Chao, P.; Yang, Z.; Tian, L. et al. *Chemistry of Materials* 2017, 29, (7), 2819–2830.

45. Hu, Z.; Chen, H.; Qu, J.; Zhong, X.; Chao, P.; Xie, M.; Lu, W. et al. *ACS Energy Letters* 2017, 2, (4), 753–758.

46. Hu, Z.; Chen, H.; Zhong, X.; Qu, J.; Chen, W.; Liu, A.; He, F. *Acat Polymerica Sinica* 2018, 2, 273–283.

47. Liang, Y.; Feng, D.; Wu, Y.; Tsai, S.; Li, G.; Ray, C.; Yu, L. *Journal of the American Chemical Society* 2009, 131, (22), 7792–7799.

48. Liang, Y.; Xu, Z.; Xia, J.; Tsai, S.; Wu, Y.; Li, G.; Ray, C.; Yu, L. *Advanced Materials* 2010, 22, (20), 135–138.

49. Zhang, M.; Guo, X.; Zhang, S.; Hou, J. *Advanced Materials* 2014, 26 (7), 1118–1123.

50. Zhang, S.; Ye, L.; Zhao, W.; Liu, D.; Yao, H.; Hou, J. *Macromolecules* 2014, 47 (14), 4653–4659.

51. Zhang, S.; Uddin, M.; Zhao, W.; Ye, L.; Woo, H.; Liu, D.; Yang, B.; Yao, H.; Cui, Y.; Hou, J. *Polymer Chemistry* 2015, 6, (14), 2752–2760.

52. Yao, H.; Zhang, H.; Ye, L.; Zhao, W.; Zhang, S.; Hou, J. *Macromolecules* 2015, 48, (11), 3493–3499.

53. Chao, P.; Wang, H.; Qu, S.; Mo, D.; Meng, H.; Chen, W.; He, F. *Macromolecules* 2017, 50, (24), 9617–9625.

54. Liu, P.; Zhang, K.; Liu, F.; Jin, Y.; Liu, S.; Russe, T.; Yip, H.; Huang, F.; Cao, Y. *Chemistry of Materials* 2014, 26, (9), 3009–3017.

55. He, X.; Mukherjee, S.; Watkins, S.; Chen, M.; Qin, T.; Thomsen, L.; Ade, H.; McNeill, C. *Journal of Physical Chemistry C* 2014, 118, (19), 9918–9929.

56. Wang, H.; Chao, P.; Chen, H.; Mu, Z.; Chen, W.; He, F. *ACS Energy Letters* 2017, 2, (9), 1971–1977.

57. Qu, S.; Wang, H.; Mo, D.; Chao, P.; Yang, Z.; Li, L.; Tian, L.; Chen, W.; He, F. *Macromolecules* 2017, 50, (13), 4962–4971.

58. Hou, J.; Park, M.; Zhang, S.; Yao, Y.; Chen, L.; Li, J.; Yang, Y. *Macromolecules* 2008, 41, (16), 6012–6018.

59. He, Z.; Zhong, C.; Su, S.; Xu, M.; Wu, H.; Cao, Y. *Nature Photonics* 2012, 6, (9), 593–597.

60. Liu, D.; Zhao, W.; Zhang, S.; Ye, L.; Zheng, Z.; Cui, Y.; Chen, Y.; Hou, J. *Macromolecules* 2015, 48, (15), 5172–5178.

61. Qian, D.; Ye, L.; Zhang, M.; Liang, Y.; Li, L.; Huang, Y.; Guo, X.; Zhang, S.; Tan, Z.; Hou, J. *Macromolecules* 2012, 45, (24), 9611–9617.

62. Tan, Z.; Li, S.; Wang, F.; Qian, D.; Lin, J.; Hou, J.; Li, Y. *Scientific Reports* 2014, 4, (8), 4691–4699.

63. Zhang, M.; Guo, X.; Ma, W.; Ade, H.; Hou, J. *Advanced Materials* 2015, 27 (31), 4655–4660.

64. Fan, Q.; Wang, Y.; Zhang, M.; Wu, B.; Guo, X.; Jiang, Y.; Li, W. et al. *Advanced Materials* 2018, 30, (6), 1704546–1704553.

65. Du, Z.; Bao, X.; Li, Y.; Liu, D.; Wang, J.; Yang, C.; Wimmer, R.; Städe, L.; Yang, R.; Yu D. *Advanced Energy Materials* 2017, 1701471–1701482.

66. Wang, Q.; Zhang, S.; Xu, B.; Li, S. S.; Yang, B.; Yuan, W. X.; Hou, J. H. *Journal of Physical Chemistry C* 2017, 121, (9), 4825–4833.

67. Huang, G. Y.; Zhang, J.; Uranbileg, N.; Chen, W. C.; Jiang, H. X.; Tan, H.; Zhu, W. G.; Yang, R. Q. *Advanced Energy Materials* 2017, 1702489–1702494.

68. Qin, Y. P.; Ye, L.; Zhang, S. Q.; Zhu, J.; Yang, B.; Ade, H.; Hou, J. H. *Journal of Materials Chemistry A* 2018, 6, 4324–4330.

69. Gao, Y. Y.; Wang, Z.; Zhang, J. Q.; Zhang, H.; Lu, K.; Guo, F. Y.; Yang, Y. L.; Zhao, L. C.; Wei, Z. X.; Zhang, Y. *Journal of Materials Chemistry A* 2018, 6, 4023–4031.

70. Zhong, W. K.; Li, K.; Cui, J.; Gu, T. Y.; Ying, L.; Huang, F.; Cao, Y. *Macromolecules* 2017, 50, (20), 8149–8157.

71. Gu, C. T.; Liu, D. Y.; Wang, J. Y.; Niu, Q. F.; Gu, C. Y.; Shahid, B.; Yu, B.; Cong, H. L.; Yang, R. Q. *Journal of Materials Chemistry A* 2018, 6, (5), 2371–2378.

72. Liu, Z.; Liu, D. Y.; Chen, W. Y.; Wang, J. Y.; Li, F.; Wang, D.; Li, Y. H.; Sun, M. L.; Yang, R. Q. *Journal of Materials Chemistry C* 2017, 5, (27), 6798–6804.

73. Liu, Y. H.; Chen, S. S.; Zhang, G. Y.; Chow, P. C. Y.; Yan, H. *Journal of Materials Chemistry A* 2017, 5, (29), 15017–15020.

74. Chen, S. S.; Liu, Y. H.; Zhang, L.; Chow, P. C. Y.; Wang, Z.; Zhang, G. Y.; Ma, W.; Yan, H. *Journal of the American Chemical Society* 2017, 139, (18), 6298–6301.

75. Yang, Y. C.; Wu, R. M.; Wang, X.; Xu, X. P.; Li, Z. J.; Li, K.; Peng, Q. *Chemical Communications* 2013, 50, (4), 439–441.

76. Liu, J.; Wang, J. T.; Liu, L. H.; Tian, H. K.; Zhang, X. J.; Xie, Z. Y.; Geng, Y. H.; Wang, F. S. *Advanced Materials* 2014, 26, (3), 471–476.

77. Deng, Y. F.; Li, W. L.; Liu, L. H.; Tian, H. K.; Xie, Z. Y.; Geng, Y. H.; Wang, F. S. *Energy & Environmental Science* 2015, 8, (2), 585–591.

78. Dong, X.; Deng, Y. F.; Tian, H. K.; Xie, Z. Y.; Geng, Y. H.; Wang, F. S. *Journal of Materials Chemistry A* 2015, 3, (39), 19928–19935.

79. Hu, H. W.; Jiang, K.; Kim, J. H.; Yang, G. F.; Li, Z. K.; Ma, T. X.; Lu, G. H.; Qu, Y. Q.; Ade, H.; Yan, H. *Journal of Materials Chemistry A* 2016, 4, (14), 5039–5043.

80. Tomassetti, M.; Ouhib, F.; Wisle, A.; Duwe, A. S.; Penxten, H.; Dierckx, W.; Cardinaletti, I. et al. *Polymer Chemistry* 2015, 6, (33), 6040–6049.

81. Lei, T.; Dou, J. H.; Ma, Z. J.; Liu, C. J.; Wang, J. Y.; Pei, J. *Chemical Science* 2013, 4, (6), 2447–2452.

82. Zheng, Y. Q.; Wang, Z.; Dou, J. H.; Zhang, S. D.; Luo, X. Y.; Yao, Z. F.; Wang, J. Y.; Pei, J. *Macromolecules* 2015, 48, (16), 5570–5577.

83. Xu, S. L.; Ai, N.; Zheng, J.; Zhao, N.; Lan, Z. G.; Wen, L. R.; Wang, X.; Pei, J.; Wan, X. B. *RSC Advances* 2015, 5, (11), 8340–8344.

84. Zhao, N.; Ai, N.; Cai, M.; Wang, X.; Pei, J.; Wan, X. B. *Polymer Chemistry* 2015, 7, 1, 235–243.

85. Zhang, H. R.; Zhao, Z. Y.; Zhao, N.; Xie, Y.; Cai, M.; Wang, X.; Liu, Y. Q.; Lan, Z. G.; Wan, X. B. *RSC Advances* 2017, 7, (40), 25009–25018.

86. Wang, N.; Wan, X. J.; Li, M. M.; Wang, Y. C.; Chen, Y. S. *Chemical Communications* 2015, 51, (24), 4936–4950.

87. Schulze, K.; Uhrich, C.; Schüppel, R.; Leo, K.; Pfeiffer, M.; Brier, E.; Reinold, E.; Bäuerle, P. *Advanced Materials* 2006, 18, (21), 2872–2875.

88. Liu, Y. S.; Zhou, J. Y.; Wan, X. J.; Chen, Y. S. *Tetrahedron* 2009, 65, (27), 5209–5215.

89. Yin, B.; Yang, L. Y.; Liu, Y. S.; Chen, Y. S.; Qi, Q. J.; Zhang, F. L.; Yin, S. G. *Applied Physics Letters* 2010, 97, (2), 023303.

90. Liu, Y. S.; Wan, X. J.; Wang, F.; Zhou, J. Y.; Long, G. K.; Tian, J. G.; You, J. B.; Yang, Y.; Chen, Y. S. *Advanced Energy Materials* 2011, 1, (5), 771–775.

91. Demeter, D.; Rousseau, T.; Leriche, P.; Cauchy, T.; Po, R.; Roncali, J. *Advanced Functional Materials* 2011, 21, (22), 4379–4387.

92. Li, Z.; He, G. R.; Wan, X. J.; Liu, Y. S.; Zhou, J. Y.; Long, G. K.; Zuo, Y.; Zhang, M. T.; Chen, Y. S. *Advanced Energy Materials* 2012, 2, (1), 74–77.

93. Zhang, Q.; Kan, B.; Liu, F.; Long, G. K.; Wan, X. J.; Chen, X. Q.; Zuo, Y. et al. *Nature Photonics* 2015, 9, (1), 35–41.

94. Long, G. K.; Wan, X. J.; Kan, B.; Liu, Y. S.; He, G. R.; Li, Z.; Zhang, Y. W.; Zhang, Y.; Zhang, Q.; Zhang, M. T.; Chen, Y. S. *Advanced Energy Materials* 2013, 3, (5), 639–646.

95. Kan, B.; Li, M. M.; Zhang, Q.; Liu, F.; Wan, X. J.; Wang, Y. C.; Ni, W. et al. *Journal of the American Chemical Society* 2015, 137, (11), 3886–3893.

96. He, G. R.; Li, Z.; Wan, X. J.; Zhou, J. Y.; Long, G. K.; Zhang, S. Z.; Zhang, M. T.; Chen, Y. S. *Journal of Materials Chemistry A* 2013, 1, (5), 1801–1809.

97. He, G. R.; Wan, X. J.; Li, Z.; Zhang, Q.; Long, G. K.; Liu, Y. S.; Hou, Y. H.; Zhang, M. T.; Chen, Y. S. *Journal of Materials Chemistry C* 2014, 2, (7), 1337–1345.

98. Zhang, Q.; Wang, Y. C.; Kan, B.; Wan, X. J.; Liu, F.; Ni, W.; Feng, H. R.; Russell, T. P.; Chen, Y. S. *Chemical Communications* 2015, 51, (83), 15268–15271.

99. Kan, B.; Zhang, Q.; Wan, X. J.; Ke, X.; Wang, Y. C.; Feng, H. R.; Zhang, M. T.; Chen, Y. S. *Organic Electronics* 2016, 38, 172–179.

100. Cui, C. H.; Fan, X.; Zhang, M. J.; Zhang, J.; Min, J.; Li, Y. F. *Chemical Communications* 2011, 47, (40), 11345–11347.
101. Chu, T.; Lu, J.; Beaupre, S.; Zhang, Y.; Pouliot, J.; Wakim, S.; Zhou, J.; Leclerc, M.; Li, Z.; Ding, J.; Tao, Y. *Journal of the American Chemical Society* 2011, 133, (12), 4250–4253.
102. Lin, H. W.; Lin, Li. Y.; Chen, Y. H.; Chen, C. W.; Lin, Yu. T.; Chiu, S. W.; Wong, K. T. *Chemical Communications* 2011, 47, (27), 7872–7874.
103. Lin, L. Y.; Lu, C. W.; Huang, W. C.; Chen, Y. H.; Lin, H. W.; Wong, K. T. *Organic Letters* 2011, 13, (18), 4962–4965.
104. Sun, Y. M.; Welch, G. C.; Leong, W. L.; Takacs, C. J.; Bazan, G. C.; Heeger, A. *Nature Materials* 2012, 11, (1), 44–48.
105. Chen, X. J.; Feng, H. H.; Lin, Z. J.; Jiang, Z. W.; Tian, H.; Yin, S. C.; Wan, X. J.; Chen, Y. S.; Zhang, Q.; Qiu, H. *Dyes and Pigments* 2017, 147, 183–189.
106. Luponosov, Y. N.; Min, J.; Ameri, T.; Brabec, C. J.; Ponomarenko, S. A. *Organic Electronics* 2014, 15 (12), 3800–3804.
107. Luponosov, Y. N.; Min, J.; Bakirov, A. V.; Dmitryakov, P. V.; Chvalun, S. N.; Peregudova, S. M.; Ameri, T.; Brabec, C. J.; Ponomarenko, S. A. *Dyes and Pigments* 2015, 122, 213–223.
108. Zhou, J. Y.; Wan, X. J.; Liu, Y. S.; Long, G. K.; Wang, F.; Li, Z.; Zuo, Y.; Li, C. X.; Chen, Y. S. *Chemistry of Materials* 2011, 23, (21), 4666–4668
109. Wang, N.; Li, M. M.; Liu, F.; Wan, X. J.; Feng, H. R.; Kan, B.; Zhang, Q.; Zhang, H. T.; Chen, Y. S. *Chemistry of Materials* 2015, 27, (17), 6077–6084.
110. Keshtov, M. L.; Godovsky, D. Y.; Kuklin, S. A.; Nicolaev, A.; Lee, J.; Lim, B.; Lee, H. K.; Koukaras, E. N.; Sharma, G. D. *Organic Electronics* 2016, 39, 361–370.
111. Choi, Y. S.; Shin, T. J.; Jo, W. H. ACS *Applied Materials & Interfaces* 2014, 6, (22), 20035–20042.
112. Fu, L.; Pan, H. B.; Larsen-Olsen, T. T.; Andersen, T. R.; Bundgaard, E.; Krebs, F. C.; Chen, H. Z. *Dyes and Pigments* 2013, 97, (1), 141–147.
113. Love, J. A.; Proctor, C. M.; Liu, J.; Takacs, C. J.; Sharenko, A.; van der Poll, T. S.; Heeger, A. J.; Bazan, G. C.; Nguyen, T. Q. *Advanced Functional Materials* 2013, 23, (40), 5019–5026.
114. Love, J. A.; Nagao, I.; Huang, Y.; Kuik, M.; Gupta, V.; Takacs, C. J.; Coughlin, J. E. et al. *Journal of the American Chemical Society* 2014, 136, (9), 3597–606.
115. Juan, R. R. S.; Payne, A. J.; Welch, G. C.; Eftaiha, A. F. *Dyes and Pigments* 2016, 132, 369–377.
116. Moon, M. J.; Walker, B.; Lee, J.; Park, S. Y.; Ahn, H.; Kim, T.; Lee, T. H.; Heo, J.; Seo, J. H.; Shin, T. J.; Kim, J. Y.; Yang, C. *Advanced Energy Materials* 2015, 5, (9), 1402044–1402054.
117. Huang, X. L.; Zhang, G. C.; Zhou, C.; Liu, S. J.; Zhang, J.; Ying, L.; Huang, F.; Cao, Y. *New Journal of Chemistry* 2015, 39, (5), 3658–3664.
118. Li, W.; Deng, W. Y.; Wu, K. L.; Xie, G. H.; Yang, C. L.; Wu, H. B.; Cao, Y. *Journal of Materials Chemistry C* 2016, 4, (10), 1972–1978.
119. Li, M. M.; Wang, N.; Wan, X. J.; Zhang, Q.; Kan, B. *Journal of Materials Chemistry A* 2015, 3, (9), 4765–4776.
120. Deng, D.; Zhang, Y. J.; Zhang, J. Q.; Wang, Z. Y.; Zhu, L. Y.; Fang, J.; Xia, B. Z.; Wang, Z.; Lu, K.; Ma, W.; Wei, Z. X. *Nature Communications* 2016, 7, 13740–13748.
121. Liu, Y. S.; Wan, X. J.; Wang, F.; Zhou, J. Y.; Long, G. K.; Tian, J. G. *Advanced Materials* 2011, 23, (45), 5387–5391.
122. Zhou, J. Y.; Wan, X. J.; Liu, Y. S.; Zuo, Y.; Li, Z.; He, G. R.; Long, G. K.; Wang, N.; Li, C. X.; Su, X. C. *Journal of the American Chemical Society* 2012, 134 (39), 16345–16351.
123. Kan, B.; Zhang, Q.; Li, M. M.; Wan, X. J.; Wang, N.; Long, G. K.; Wang, Y. C.; Yang, X.; Feng, H. R.; Chen, Y. S. *Journal of the American Chemical Society* 2014, 136, (44), 15529–15532.

124. Guo, Y. Q.; Wang, Y. C.; Song, L. C.; Liu, F.; Wan, X. J.; Zhang, H. T.; Chen, Y. S. *Chemistry of Materials* 2017, 29, (8), 29, 3694–3703.

125. Deng, D.; Zhang, Y.; Yuan, L.; He, C.; Lu, K.; Wei, Z. X. *Advanced Energy Materials* 2015, 4, (17), 1400538–1400546.

126. Yang, L. Y.; Zhang, S. Q.; He, C.; Zhang, J. Q.; Yao, H. F.; Yang, Y.; Zhang, Y.; Zhao, W. C.; Hou, J. H. *Journal of the American Chemical Society* 2017, 139, (5), 1958–1966.

127. Liu, D. L.; Yang, L. Y.; Wu, Y.; Wang, X. H.; Zeng, Y.; Han, G. C.; Yao, H. F. et al. *Chemistry of Materials* 2018, 30, (3), 619–628.

128. Bin, H. J.; Yang, Y. K.; Zhang, Z. G.; Ye, L.; Ghasemi, M.; Chen, S. S.; Zhang, Y. D. et al. *Journal of the American Chemical Society* 2017, 139, (14), 5085–5094.

129. Yuan, L.; Zhao, Y. F.; Zhang, J. Q.; Zhang, Y. J.; Zhu, L. Y.; Lu, K.; Yan, W.; Wei, Z. X. *Advanced Materials* 2015, 27, (28), 4229–4233.

130. Zhu, X. W.; Xia, B. Z.; Lu, K.; Li, H.; Zhou, R. M.; Zhang, J. Q.; Zhang, Y. J.; Shuai, Z. G.; Wei, Z. X. *Chemistry of Materials* 2016, 28, (3), 943–950.

131. Li, H.; Zhao, Y. F.; Fang, J.; Zhu, X. W.; Xia, B. Z.; Lu, K.; Wang, Z.; Zhang, J. Q.; Guo, X. F.; Wei, Z. X. *Advanced Energy Materials* 2018, 1702377–1702384.

132. Kooistra, F.; Mihailetchi, V.; Popescu, L.; Kronholm, D.; Blom, P. W. M.; Hummelen, J. C. *Chemistry of Materials* 2006, 18, (13), 3068–3073.

133. He, Y. J.; Chen, H.; Hou, J.; Li, Y. F. *Journal of the American Chemical Society* 2010, 132, (4), 1377–1382.

134. Zhao, G. J.; He, Y. J.; Li, Y. F. *Advanced Materials* 2010, 22, (39), 4355–4358.

135. He, Y. J.; Zhao, G. J.; Peng, B.; Li, Y. F. *Advanced Functional Materials* 2010, 20 (19), 3383–3389.

136. Hou, J.; Guo X. Active layer materials for organic solar cells. In: Choy W. (Ed.) *Organic Solar Cells, Green Energy and Technology*, 2013, Springer, London, UK.

137. Li, S. S.; Ye, L.; Zhao, W. C.; Zhang, S. Q.; Mukherjee, S.; Ade, H.; Hou, J. H. *Advanced Materials* 2016, 28, (42), 9423–9429.

138. Kozma, E.; Catellani, M. *Dyes and Pigments* 2013, 98, (1), 160–179.

139. Zhan, X.; Tan, Z.; Domercq, B.; An, Z.; Zhang, X.; Barlow, S.; Li, Y.; Zhu, D.; Kippelen, B.; Marder, S. R. *Journal of the American Chemical Society* 2007, 129, (23), 7246–7247.

140. Cheng, P.; Ye, L.; Zhao, X.; Hou, J.; Li, Y.; Zhan, X. *Energy & Environmental Science* 2014, 7, (4), 1351–1356.

141. Mikroyannidis, J. A.; Stylianakis, M. M.; Sharma, G. D.; Balraju, P.; Roy, M. S. *Journal of Physical Chemistry C* 2009, 113, (18), 7904–7912.

142. Zhou, E. J.; Cong, J. Z.; Wei, Q. H.; Tajima, K.; Yang, C. H.; Hashimoto, K. *Angewandte Chemie International Edition* 2011, 50, (12), 2799–2803.

143. Zang, Y.; Li, C. Z.; Chueh, C. C.; Williams, S. T.; Jiang, W.; Wang, Z. H.; Yu, J. S.; Jen, A. K. Y. *Advanced Materials* 2014, 26, (32), 5708–5714.

144. Sun, D.; Meng, D.; Cai, Y.; Fan, B. B.; Li, Y.; Jiang, W.; Huo, L. J.; Sun, Y. M.; Wang, Z. H. *Journal of the American Chemical Society* 2015, 137, (34), 11156–11162.

145. Meng, D.; Sun, D.; Zhong, C. M.; Liu, T.; Fan, B. B.; Huo, L. J.; Jiang, W.; Choi, H.; Kim, T.; Kim, J. Y.; Heeger, A. J. *Journal of the American Chemical Society* 2015, 138, (1), 375–380.

146. Meng, D.; Fu, H. T.; Xiao, C. Y.; Meng, X. Y.; Winands, T.; Ma, W.; Wei, W. et al. *Journal of the American Chemical Society* 2016, 138, (32), 10184–10190.

147. Yan, H.; Chen, Z.; Zheng, Y.; Newman, C.; Quinn, J. R.; Dotz, F.; Kastler, M.; Facchetti, A. *Nature* 2009, 457, (7230), 679–686.

148. Moore, J. R.; Albert-Seifried, S.; Rao, A.; Massip, S.; Watts, B.; Morgan, D. J.; Friend, R. H.; McNeill, C. R.; Sirringhaus, H. *Advanced Energy Materials* 2011, 1, (2), 230–240.

149. Mori, D.; Benten, H.; Okada, I.; Ohkita, H.; Ito, S. *Advanced Energy Materials* 2014, 4, (3), 1301006.
150. Tang, Y.; McNeill, C. R. *Journal of Polymer Science Part B: Polymer Physics* 2013, 51, (6), 403–409.
151. Earmme, T.; Hwang, Y. J.; Murari, N. M.; Subramaniyan, S.; Jenekhe, S. A. *Journal of the American Chemical Society* 2013, 135, (40), 14960–14963.
152. Zhou, E.; Nakano, M.; Izawa, S.; Cong, J.; Osaka, I.; Takimiya, K.; Tajima, K. *ACS Macro Letters* 2014, 3, (9), 872–875.
153. Shen, G. R.; Li, X. Z.; Wu, X.; Wang, Y. L.; Shan, H. Q.; Xu, J. J.; Liu, X. Y.; Xu, Z..X.; Chen, F.; Chen, Z. K. *Organic Electronics* 2017, 46, 203–210.
154. Li, X. Z.; Sun, P.; Wang, Y. L.; Shan, H. Q.; Xu, J. J.; You, C.; Xu, Z. X.; Chen, Z. K. *Polymer Chemistry* 2016, 7, (12), 2230–2238.
155. Ahmed, E.; Ren, G. Q.; Kim, F. S.; Hollenbeck, E. C.; Jenekhe, S. A. *Chemistry of Materials* 2011, 23 (20), 4563–4577.
156. Hong, J. S.; Ha, Y. H.; Cha, H. J.; Kim, R.; Kim, Y. J.; Park, C. E.; Durrant, J. R.; Kwon, S. K.; An, T. K.; Kim, Y. H. *ACS Applied Materials & Interfaces* 2017, 9, (51), 44667–44677.
157. Wang, X.; Huang, J. H.; Niu, Z. X.; Zhang, X.; Sun, Y. X.; Zhan, C. L. *Tetrahedron* 2014, 70, (32), 4726–4731.
158. Srivani, D.; Gupta, A.; Bhosale, S. V.; Puyad, A. L.; Xiang, W. C.; Li, J. L.; Evansf, R. A.; Bhosale, S. V. *Chemical Communications* 2017, 53, (52), 7080–7083.
159. Srivani, D.; Agarwal, A.; Bhosale, S. V.; Puyad, A. L.; Xiang, W. C.; Evans, R. A.; Gupta, A.; Bhosale, S. V. *Chemical Communications* 2017, 53, (81), 11157–11160.
160. Yang, F.; Li, C.; Lai, W. B.; Zhang, A. D.; Huang, H.; Li, W. W. *Materials Chemistry Frontiers* 2017, 1, 1389–1395.
161. Dai, S. X.; Zhao, F. W.; Zhang, Q. Q.; Lau, T. K.; Li, T. F.; Liu, K.; Ling, Q. D.; Wang, C. R.; Lu, X. H.; You, W.; Zhan, X. W. *Journal of the American Chemical Society* 2017, 139, (3), 1336–1343.
162. Li, X. J.; Huang, H.; Bin, H. J.; Peng, Z. X.; Zhu, C. H.; Xue, L. W.; Zhang, Z. G.; Zhang, Z. J.; Ade, H.; Li, Y. F. *Chemistry of Materials* 2017, 29, (23), 10130–10138.
163. Jia, B. Y.; Dai, S. X.; Ke, Z. F.; Yan, C. Q.; Ma, W.; Zhan, X. W. *Chemistry of Materials* 2017, 30, (1), 239–245.
164. Zhao, F. W.; Dai, S. X.; Wu, Y.; Zhang, Q. Q.; Wang, J. Y.; Jiang, L.; Ling, Q. D. et al. *Advanced Materials* 2017, 29 (18), 1700144–1700150.
165. Xiao, Z.; Jia, X.; Li, D.; Wang, S. Z.; Geng, X. J.; Liu, F.; Chen, J. W.; Yang, S. F.; Russell, T. P.; Din, L. M. *Science Bulletin* 2017, 62, 1494–1496.
166. Xiao, Z.; Jia, X.; Ding, L. M. *Science Bulletin* 2017, 62, 1562–1564.
167. Cui, Y.; Yang, C. Y.; Yao, H. F.; Zhu, J.; Wang, Y. M.; Jia, G. X.; Gao, F.; Hou, J. H. *Advanced Materials* 2017, 29, 1703080–1703086.
168. Yao, H. F.; Cui, Y.; Yu, R. N.; Gao, B. W.; Zhang, H.; Hou, J. H. *Angewandte Chemie International Edition* 2017, 56, (11), 3045–3049.
169. Li, Y. X.; Lin, J. D.; Che, X. Z.; Qu, Y.; Liu, F.; Liao, L. S.; Forrest, S. R. *Journal of the American Chemical Society* 2017, 139, (47), 17114–17119.
170. Geens, W.; Aernouts, T.; Poortmans, J.; Hadziioannou, G. *Thin Solid Films* 2002, 403–404, (1), 438–443.
171. Peumans, P.; Uchida, S.; Forrest, S. R. *Nature* 2003, 425, (6954), 158–162.
172. Ge, Z. Y.; Chen, S. J.; Peng, R. X.; Islam, A. *Organic and Hybrid Solar Cells* 2014, 275–300.
173. Chen, L. M.; Hong, Z. R.; Li, G.; Yang, Y. *Advanced Materials* 2009, 21, (14–15), 1434–1449.
174. Park, S. H.; Roy, A.; Beaupre, S.; Cho, S.; Coates, N.; Moon, J. S.; Moses, D.; Leclerc, M.; Lee, K.; Heeger, A. J. *Nature Photonics* 2009, 3, (5), 297–302.

175. Shaheen, S. E.; Brabec, C. J.; Sariciftci, N. S.; Padinger, F.; Fromherz, T.; Hummelen, J. *Applied Physics Letters* 2001, 78, (6), 841–843.
176. Ruderer, M. A.; Guo, S.; Meier, R.; Chiang, H. Y.; Körstgens, V.; Wiedersich, J.; Perlich, J.; Roth, S. V.; Müller-Buschbaum, P. *Advanced Functional Materials* 2011, 21, (17), 3382–3391.
177. Guo, X.; Zhou, N.; Lou, S. J.; Smith, J.; Tice, D. B.; Hennek, J. W.; Ortiz, R. P. et al. *Nature Photonics* 2013, 7, (10), 825–833.
178. Huo, L.; Liu, T.; Sun, X.; Cai, Y.; Heeger, A. J.; Sun, Y. *Advanced Materials* 2015, 27, (18), 2938–2944.
179. Mihailetchi, V. D.; Xie, H.; de Boer, B.; Popescu, L. M.; Hummelen, J. C.; Blom, P. W. M.; Koster, L. J. A. *Applied Physics Letters* 2006, 89, (1), 012107.
180. Li, G.; Shrotriya, V.; Huang, J.; Yao, Y.; Moriarty, T.; Emery, K.; Yang, Y. *Nature Materials* 2015, 4, (11), 864–868.
181. Erb, T.; Zhokhavets, U.; Gobsch, G.; Raleva, S.; Stühn, B.; Schilinsky, P.; Waldauf, C.; Brabec, C. J. *Advanced Functional Materials* 2005, 15, (7), 1193–1196.
182. Chen, D.; Nakahara, A.; Wei, D.; Nordlund, D.; Russell, T. P. *Nano Letters* 2011, 11, (2), 561–567.
183. Ma, W.; Yang, G. F.; Jiang, K.; Carpenter, J. H.; Wu, Y.; Meng, X. Y.; McAfee, T. et al. *Advanced Energy Materials* 2016, 5, (23), 1501400–1501409.
184. Peet, J.; Kim, J. Y.; Coates, N. E.; Ma, W. L.; Moses, D.; Heeger, A. J.; Bazan, G. C. *Nature Materials* 2007, 6, (7), 497–500.
185. Lou, S. J.; Szarko, J. M.; Xu, T.; Yu, L.; Marks, T. J.; Chen, L. X. *Journal of the American Chemical Society* 2011, 133, (51), 20661–20663.
186. Steirer, K. X.; Ndione, P. F.; Widjonarko, N. E.; Lloyd, M. T.; Meyer, J.; Ratcliff, E. L.; Kahn, A.; Armstrong, N. R.; Curtis, C. J.; Ginley, D. S. *Advanced Energy Materials* 2011, 1, (5), 813–820.
187. Chen, C. P.; Chen, Y. D.; Chuang, S. C. *Advanced Materials* 2011, 23 (33), 3859–3863.
188. Xu, Q.; Wang, F.; Tan, Z.; Li, L.; Li, S.; Hou, X.; Sun, G.; Tu, X.; Hou, J.; Li, Y. *ACS Applied Materials & Interfaces* 2013, 5, (21), 10658–10664.
189. Chen, L.; Xie, C.; Chen, Y. *Advanced Functional Materials* 2014, 24, (25), 3986–3995.
190. Tu, X.; Wang, F.; Li, C.; Tan, Z.; Li, Y. *Journal of Physical Chemistry C* 2014, 118, (18), 9309–9317.
191. Tan, Z.; Zhang, W.; Qian, D.; Cui, C.; Xu, Q.; Li, L.; Li, S.; Li, Y. *Physical Chemistry Chemical Physics* 2012, 14, (41), 14217–14223.
192. Li, S.-S.; Tu, K. H.; Lin, C. C.; Chen, C. W.; Chhowalla, M. *ACS Nano* 2010, 4, (6), 3169–3674.
193. Gustafsson, G.; Cao, Y.; Treacy, G. M.; Klavetter, F.; Colaneri, N.; Heeger, A. J. *Nature* 1992, 24, (2), 477–479.
194. Zhou, H.; Zhang, Y.; Mai, C.-K.; Collins, S. D.; Nguyen, T.-Q.; Bazan, G. C.; Heeger, A. J. *Advanced Materials* 2014, 26, (5), 780–785.
195. Gu, C.; Chen, Y.; Zhang, Z.; Xue, S.; Sun, S.; Zhong, C.; Zhang, H.; Lv, Y.; Li, F.; Huang, F. *Advanced Energy Materials* 2014, 4, (8), 1289–1295.
196. Sun, Y.; Seo, J. H.; Takacs, C. J.; Seifter, J.; Heeger, A. J. *Advanced Materials* 2011, 23, (14), 1679–1683.
197. Palilis, L. C.; Vasilopoulou, M.; Douvas, A. M.; Georgiadou, D. G.; Kennou, S.; Stathopoulos, N. A.; Constantoudis, V.; Argitis, P. *Solar Energy Materials & Solar Cells* 2013, 114, (7), 205–213.
198. He, Z.; Zhong, C.; Huang, X.; Wong, W.-Y.; Wu, H.; Chen, L.; Su, S.; Cao, Y. *Advanced Materials* 2011, 23, (40), 4636–4643.

199. Duan, C.; Zhong, C.; Liu, C.; Huang, F.; Cao, Y. *Chemistry of Materials* 2012, 24, (9), 1682–1689.
200. Hong, D.; Lv, M.; Lei, M.; Chen, Y.; Lu, P.; Wang, Y.; Zhu, J.; Wang, H.; Gao, M.; Watkins, S. E. *ACS Applied Materials & Interfaces* 2013, 5, (21), 10995–11003.
201. Jiao, W.; Ma, D.; Lv, M.; Chen, W.; Wang, H.; Zhu, J.; Lei, M.; Chen, X. *Journal of Materials Chemistry A* 2014, 2, (35), 14720–14728.
202. Yi, C.; Yue, K.; Zhang, W. B.; Lu, X.; Hou, J.; Li, Y.; Huang, L.; Newkome, G. R.; Cheng, S. Z. D.; Gong, X. *ACS Applied Materials & Interfaces* 2014, 6, (16), 14189–14195.

4 Reaction Centers as Nanoscale Photovoltaic Devices

Michael R. Jones

CONTENTS

4.1 INTRODUCTION—A BLUEPRINT FOR A PHOTOCHEMICAL REACTION CENTER

Reaction centers are membrane-embedded complexes of pigment and protein that are found in all organisms capable of chlorophyll-based photosynthesis.[1-5] They work together with light-harvesting complexes to capture solar energy and trap it in the form of a metastable separation of electrical charge across the photosynthetic membrane. Ensuing reduction/oxidation reactions are coupled to proton translocation to establish a transmembrane proton electrochemical gradient that can power a variety of reactions including the synthesis of adenosine triphosphate (ATP). In oxygenic photosynthetic organisms, plants, algae, and cyanobacteria, two types of reaction center operate in series to transfer electrons along a linear pathway from water to nicotinamide adenine dinucleotide phosphate ($NADP^+$), thus also generating reducing power for biosynthesis.[6-10] These reaction centers form part of Photosystem I (PSI) and Photosystem II (PSII). In anoxygenic purple photosynthetic bacteria, a single type of reaction center powers a cyclic flow of electrons that reduces $NADP^+$ indirectly.[1,11-16] The high ATP/ADP and NADPH/$NADP^+$ ratios resulting from the capture of solar energy power biosynthesis including, in photoautotrophic organisms, the fixation of carbon. An excellent, in-depth, and comprehensive treatise covering the primary events of photosynthesis has been written by Blankenship.[5]

Despite huge diversity in their host organisms and considerable diversity at the level of individual proteins, all photosynthetic reaction centers derive from a common structural and mechanistic blueprint.[2,4,8-10,17] The principal photosynthetic pigment in oxygenic phototrophs is chlorophyll and in anoxygenic phototrophs is bacteriochlorophyll; both are magnesium tetrapyrroles and have a number of variants.[18,19] These remarkable pigment molecules provide much of the solar energy capture definitive of photosynthetic organisms, functioning alongside carotenoid and bilin pigments. A diversity of light harvesting or "antenna" pigment proteins exist and much is known about their structures and the mechanisms of energy capture, excited state migration, and energy trapping by reaction centers.[19–27]

Chlorophylls and bacteriochlorophylls also participate in electron transfer as both anions and cations. Some reaction centers also use a (bacterio)pheophytin as an electron carrier, this being a demetallated (bacterio)chlorophyll in which the central Mg is replaced by two protons. In the following, for the sake of simplicity, the catch-all description chlorophyll is used. In all reaction centers characterized to date, membrane-spanning electron transfer takes place along a chain (or "branch" or "wire") that consists of three closely-spaced chlorophyll species and a fourth non-chlorophyll acceptor (Figure 4.1a). The term "species" is used to acknowledge that the electron carrier at the donor end of the chain can sometimes be a pair of chlorophyll molecules. The key photochemical event within the reaction center protein is the separation of charge between two chlorophyll species in response to the formation of a singlet excited electronic state (denoted RC* in Figure 4.1b). This can be created by direct absorbance of a photon of suitable energy but will usually arise from the transfer of excited state energy from chlorophyll and other pigments in an extensive light-harvesting system that surrounds the reaction center. In response to the change

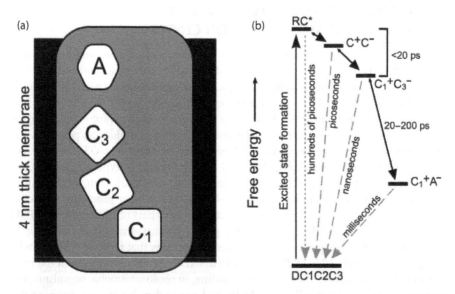

FIGURE 4.1 A blueprint for photochemical charge separation in photosynthesis: (a) Membrane-spanning charge separation occurs in three steps, involving chlorophyll (squares C_1, C_2, and C_3) and non-chlorophyll (hexagon A) charge carriers. (b) Charge separation proceeds through three radical pairs of decreasing free energy. At each step the forward reaction is significantly faster than competing recombination reactions and more thermodynamically favorable than competing reverse reactions.

in the free energy of the system (Figure 4.1b), photochemical charge separation happens within a few picoseconds and produces a radical pair between two of the three chlorophyll species (denoted C^+C^- in Figure 4.1b). Either the positive or negative charge is then very rapidly moved to the third chlorophyll, producing a metastable radical pair $C_1^+C_3^-$ in which the anion and cation are no longer in immediate contact. The lifetime of this second transfer is sometimes shorter than the initial separation, such that the first intermediate becomes challenging to resolve experimentally.

Following the initial charge separation to form C^+C^-, the system comprises a positive and negative charge localized on two chlorophyll species that, although not covalently bound to one another, are in direct edge-to-edge contact or very nearly so. Two processes have the potential to interfere with productive solar energy conversion at this point—recombination of the positive and negative radicals to reform the ground state (Figure 4.1b, dashed arrows) or reversal of the charge separation reaction to re-form the initiating excited state RC* (Figure 4.1b, small reverse arrows). The second electron transfer stabilizes the charge separation in two ways. First, it moves the positive and negative charges further apart such that the distance for direct recombination is greatly increased; this slows the lifetime for direct recombination into the nanosecond regime (Figure 4.1b) and makes the reaction uncompetitive with onward, piosecond timescale electron transfer to the non-chlorophyll acceptor. Second, the drop in free energy on formation of the second radical pair $C_1^+C_3^-$, in particular, disfavors thermal repopulation of the initial excited state (Figure 4.1b). The result is that this second radical pair forms with a very high quantum yield, defined as charges separated per initiating photoexcitation. Two-step formation of this metastable $C_1^+C_3^-$ radical pair through an effectively irreversible process with an overall lifetime of several picoseconds also disfavors "detrapping" of excited state energy back into the large number of light-harvesting chlorophyll pigments surrounding the reaction center.

Membrane-spanning charge separation is completed by a third step of electron transfer to a non-chlorophyll acceptor (A) that occurs with a lifetime of tens to a few hundreds of picoseconds. This also occurs with a high quantum yield because the rate of A reduction is fast relative to nanosecond recombination of $C_1^+C_3^-$ or energetically-uphill reformation of RC*. This third step further stabilizes charge separation through an additional loss of free energy to prevent back reactions and an increase in the distance separating the positive and negative charges, which moves the lifetime for direct recombination into the millisecond regime (Figure 4.1b).

Different types of reaction centers implement this overall blueprint for photochemical charge separation in different ways. Some of this variation comes from the possibility of the initial excited state being delocalized over two (or more) excitonically coupled chlorophylls, the possibility of the cation being shared between two chlorophylls, and the option of hole transfer in the opposite direction to electron transfer. Figure 4.2 illustrates four mechanisms for producing a $C_1^+C_3^-$ state that are thought to operate in photochemical reaction centers. This variation is enabled by differences in the properties and interactions of the cofactors in different reaction centers that stem, in part, from the intrinsic properties of chlorophyll, bacteriochlorophyll, pheophytin, and bacteriopheophytin. The remaining variation is attributable to the protein scaffold that not only dictates the positions and relative orientations

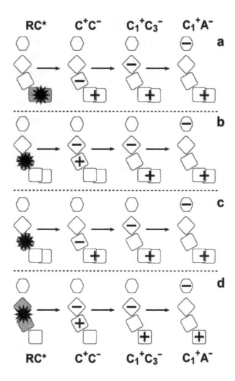

FIGURE 4.2 Implementation of the blueprint for charge separation: (a) An excited state shared between two chlorophylls initiates three-step electron transfer across the membrane. In the initial charge separation the excited species donates an electron to an adjacent acceptor. (b) An excited state localized on a chlorophyll within the electron transfer chain initiates two steps of electron transfer and one of hole transfer. Again, the initial excited state acts as an electron donor to an adjacent acceptor. (c) Formation of an excited state on the same chlorophyll initiates electron transfer from a neighboring chlorophyll to convert the excited state into an anion, with two subsequent steps of electron transfer. Here, the initiating excited state acts as an electron acceptor from an adjacent donor. (d) An excited state distributed over two chlorophylls within the electron transfer chain relaxes to a charge separated state between the same chlorophylls, followed by hole transfer and then electron transfer. Here, charge separation occurs between the two chlorophylls that also participate in the excited state. In all cases the final radical pair has an anion located on a non-chlorophyll acceptor on one side of the membrane and a cation localized on a single chlorophyll, or shared between two chlorophylls, on the opposite side of the membrane.

of the cofactors but also tunes their redox and optical properties through specific protein-cofactor interactions.

The scheme in Figure 4.2a represents the charge separation process that operates in purple bacterial reaction centers (see Section 4.3) where the initiating excited state is shared between two excitonically coupled bacteriochlorophylls, as is the cation formed by charge separation. The schemes in Figure 4.2b and c have also been observed to operate in purple bacterial reaction centers when the middle of the three bacteriochlorophyll species in the electron transfer chain is excited directly.[28] The two differ in the nature of the initial radical pair state formed and then converge after either hole transfer (Figure 4.2b) or electron transfer (Figure 4.2c). The scheme in Figure 4.2d is proposed to operate in PSII reaction centers (see Section 4.4) with the initial excited state shared between the C_3 and C_2 chlorophylls, charge separation between these being followed by hole transfer to a single chlorophyll at the C_1 position.

A final observation on the general blueprint for solar energy conversion by photosynthetic organisms concerns the way sunlight is harvested and trapped by charge separation. Photosynthetic organisms harvest light across the visible spectrum and, in the case of anoxygenic photosynthetic bacteria, into the near-infrared up to about 1200 nm. Different pigments, chlorophylls, bacteriochlorophylls, carotenoids, and bilins absorb in different spectral regions through multiple ground to excited state transitions that give rise to multiple absorbance bands. However, charge separation in the reaction center is initiated by formation of the lowest energy excited singlet state of the initiating (bacterio)chlorophyll species, corresponding to an optical transition at the low energy end of the range of absorbed wavelengths in any given system. For reaction centers containing chlorophyll *a*, this is at around 680–700 nm whereas for reaction centers containing bacteriochlorophyll *a*, this is at around 870 nm. This means that a proportion of the energy absorbed at shorter wavelengths is lost through a combination of internal conversion from higher electronic states to the first singlet state within individual pigments and energy transfer from higher energy pigments to lower energy pigments (e.g., carotenoid → chlorophyll). In addition, as illustrated in Figure 4.1b for the first three steps in charge separation, energy is also sacrificed to ensure that forward electron transfer is strongly favored. The consequence is that although light harvesting and charge separation are widely regarded as operating (under optimal conditions) with a very high quantum yield, the efficiency with which the initially absorbed energy is conserved is not high. Attempts have been made to estimate the efficiency of photosynthetic energy conversion, and the precise values arrived at—typically a few percent—depend on what is considered to be the final state in the highly complex sunlight-to-biomass conversion process.[29–31] From the perspective of photovoltaics, a useful parameter is the potential difference between the final carriers at the oxidizing and reducing ends of the electron transfer chain within each type of reaction center, as outlined in the following.

4.2   PHOTOSYSTEM I—LIGHT, ELECTRONS, AND REDUCING POWER

PSI is one of two membrane-embedded pigment-protein photosystems found in the plants, algae, and cyanobacteria that constitute the oxygenic phototrophs. It is a solar-powered oxidoreductase, using the energy of a single photon to transfer a single electron from a water-soluble redox protein, usually plastocyanin, on one side of the photosynthetic membrane to a second water-soluble redox protein, ferredoxin, on the opposite side of the membrane. Light energy is required to power this transfer because plastocyanin is considerably more oxidizing than ferredoxin, so the membrane-spanning electron transfer takes place against an overall gradient of reduction potential. The electrons that emerge from PSI are sufficiently electronegative to be able to reduce $NADP^+$ to NADPH, a reaction carried out by a ferredoxin:$NADP^+$ oxidoreductase. This NADPH is then used to power biosynthetic reactions. In-depth reviews of the composition, structure, and mechanism of PSI are available.[3,6–10,32–38]

PSI is classified as an "iron-sulphur type" or "Type I" reaction center because the terminal electron acceptor is an iron-sulphur cluster.[1,39] Type I reaction centers are also found in anoxygenic green sulphur bacteria (*Chlorobi*)[40–43] and heliobacteria (*Firmicutes*).[44,45] These reaction centers are simpler than PSI but are less well characterized due to their host organisms being strict anaerobes that are challenging to culture under laboratory conditions. Perhaps their most intriguing feature is that their core structure is formed from a homodimer of a single polypeptide rather than a heterodimer of two distinct but related polypeptides. This feature is of particular interest to researchers attempting to uncover the evolutionary relationships between extant reaction centers and the intermediates through which these evolved from a common ancestor (see Hohmann-Marriott and Blankenship,[46] Nelson and Junge[10] and Cardona[47] for reviews). Shortly before completion of this chapter, a high-resolution X-ray crystal structure was published for the Type-I reaction center from *Heliobacterium (H.) modesticaldum*.[48] This shows considerable structural similarity to the PSI reaction center but also some differences, most notably a lower density of light-harvesting pigments, fewer Fe_4S_4 centers, and a lack of tightly bound quinones (see the following).

Our initial understanding of the structural and mechanistic basis of light-powered, membrane-spanning electron transfer in PSI developed gradually through a combination of spectroscopy, biochemistry, and genetic manipulation. This understanding received a significant boost in 2001 through the publication of an X-ray crystal structure for the naturally trimeric PSI complex from the cyanobacterium *Synechococcus elongatus* at a resolution of 2.5 Å.[49,50] The structure comprised, per monomer, twelve protein subunits and a total of 123 pigment or redox center cofactors, the latter comprising 96 chlorophylls, 22 carotenoids, three iron-sulphur clusters, and two phylloquinones. Between 2003 and 2017, a series of structures were then published for the naturally monomeric PSI from *Pisum sativum* (pea) complexed with four attendant light-harvesting complexes,[51–55] most recently at 2.6 Å resolution.[56] The pea PSI also comprises twelve polypeptide subunits, which together with the four light-harvesting polypeptides, scaffold 156 chlorophyll and 136 carotenoid pigments. Comparison reveals a very high degree of conservation of the core structure between the cyanobacterial PSI and its higher plant counterpart.

The majority of the chlorophyll cofactors of PSI play a light-harvesting role. However, at the heart of the PSI complex, six chlorophylls are found together with the two phylloquinones and three iron-sulphur centers in the reaction center domain. As depicted in Figure 4.3a, these chlorophylls and quinones are arranged in two "branches" or "wires" that span the membrane and are arranged around an axis of twofold pseudosymmetry. The term "pseudosymmetry" is used here to acknowledge that there are differences in sequence between the two related polypeptides, termed PsaA and PsaB, which provide the heterodimeric scaffold that holds the chlorophyll and phylloquinone cofactors in place. As a result, despite the overall backbone folds of PsaA and PsaB being similar, there are subtle differences in the positions and mutual orientations of the cofactors that form the two membrane-spanning wires,

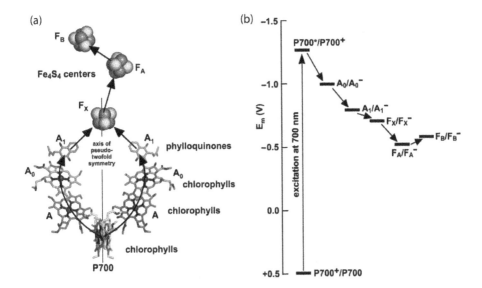

FIGURE 4.3 Structure of the electron transfer chain and the energetics of charge separation in PSI: (a) Initial charge separation can proceed along either membrane-spanning branch of chlorophyll and phylloquinone cofactors. (b) One photon powers the transfer of one electron from the P700 donor to the F_B acceptor, producing the final charge-separated state $P700^+F_B^-$. Figure drawn using Protein Data Bank entry 1JBO.[50]

as well as in the interactions between these cofactors and their protein surroundings that can tune their electronic and electrical properties.

Close to one side of the membrane is a pair of chlorophylls that straddle the pseudosymmetry axis; one is a chlorophyll a and the second an epimer denoted chlorophyll a'.[57] These form the primary electron donor, referred to as P700 because one electron oxidation of these chlorophylls produces a characteristic bleach of their absorbance band at 700 nm.[57–59] Each cofactor branch is then formed from two chlorophylls, termed A and A_0 and a phylloquinone termed A_1, where A refers to "acceptor" (Figure 4.3a). Each of A, A_0, and A_1 is capable of undergoing a one-electron reduction/oxidation reaction and forms a wire to conduct an electron liberated from the P700 electron donor to the opposite side of the membrane. Both wires terminate in a chain of three Fe_4S_4 iron-sulphur centers, the first of which is termed F_X and sits on the pseudosymmetry axis that runs across the membrane and bisects P700. These iron-sulphur centers also engage in one-electron reduction/oxidation chemistry.

The mechanism of charge separation in PSI is reasonably well understood, although not all points are agreed on.[3,9,32,38,60–62] In the most widely discussed description, photochemical charge separation in the PSI reaction center is initiated by conversion of the P700 chlorophylls from their ground electronic state to their first singlet excited state, denoted P700*. This is achieved by picosecond timescale migration of singlet excited state energy from the large number of light-harvesting chlorophylls bound to PSI.[24] The simplest view is this happens by Förster resonance energy transfer (FRET) between adjacent pigments, energy migrating from the site of absorption to P700 by a random walk of pigment-to-pigment hops. However, a detailed description of the process has to take into account additional factors including variations in electronic coupling between different pigments, the possibility of excited states being shared between adjacent pigments, and variations in excited state energies between individual pigments or groups of pigments.[24]

Once excited state energy has arrived in the reaction center, the energy is "trapped" by ultrafast photochemical charge separation to form the radical pair $P700^+A_0^-$, with a lifetime of around 1 ps. This charge separation may occur along either of the two cofactor wires (Figure 4.3a). Charge separation is then further stabilized by transfer of the electron from A_0^- to A_1 with a lifetime of around 30 ps. Intraprotein charge separation is then completed by further transfer of the electron from A_1^- to F_X, then to F_A, and then to F_B. The net result is the separation of a positive and negative charge across a distance of around 48 Å, powered by the energy of one photon (Figure 4.3b). The large separation of $P700^+$ and F_B^- prevents recombination of these charges to the ground state, such that there is time for reduction of $P700^+$ by a diffusing, water-soluble plastocyanin and oxidation of F_B^- by a water-soluble, diffusing ferredoxin.

As indicated earlier, the primary photochemical event is the formation of $P700^+A_0^-$. There is ongoing research on the precise mechanism through which this radical pair is formed as, due to its intervening position, the A chlorophyll must also be involved in this very rapid process. In addition, due to the lack of a strong gradient for localization of excited state energy on P700, there are open questions concerning the nature of the chlorophyll excited state that initiates charge separation. This is explored further in Section 4.5. For the sake of simplicity, in the rest of this section it is assumed that P700* is the initiating excited state.

As illustrated in Figure 4.3a, a feature of PSI that distinguishes it from the two other reaction centers described in this chapter is its use of either of its two cofactor wires to conduct electrons across the membrane.[63-76] There is evidence that the partition of transferring electrons between the two available wires is not necessarily 50:50 and may vary between species,[67,69,74,76] and that the rate at which A_1^- reduces F_X is faster on one wire than on the other by a factor of 10 lifetimes of ~200 ns on the more heavily-used wire and ~20 ns on the less heavily used wire.[63,77,78] The functional relevance of this difference, if any, is not fully understood (see Kargul et al.[38] for a review).

At this point it is convenient to make reference to the very recent X-ray crystal structure for the Type-I RC from *H. modesticaldum*.[48] Perhaps the most intriguing feature of this structure is the absence of quinones in the regions between the bacteriochlorophyll electron transfer chains and the F_X Fe_4S_4 center (which is the terminal acceptor as this reaction center also lacks F_A and F_B). Not only are quinones absent from this structure but also the quinone-binding sites seen in PSI reaction centers are not structurally conserved. The F_X center is closer to the bacteriochlorophyll electron transfer chains than is the case in PSI, supporting the suggestion that electron transfer between the two is direct.[48] This feature places the *H. modesticaldum* reaction center apart from the PSI, PSII, and purple bacterial reaction centers described in detail in this chapter, all of which use a quinone as the electron acceptor.

Returning to PSI, an appreciation of the photovoltaic basis for its function comes from a plot of the reduction potentials of the redox pairs formed during photochemical charge separation (Figure 4.3b). Although light energy can be collected across the visible spectrum by the chlorophyll and carotenoid cofactors of the light-harvesting system, a combination of internal conversion from higher electronic states to the first singlet state within individual pigments, and energy transfer from higher energy pigments to lower energy pigments, results in transfer to the reaction center of an excited state whose energy is equivalent to the direct absorption of a 700 nm photon ($\approx$1.77 eV). The resulting reaction center singlet excited state, P700*, has a reduction potential of around −1.26 V (Figure 4.3b). Its formation triggers a series of six sequential electron transfer reactions that culminate in the reduction of the F_B iron-sulphur center, at a potential of around −0.5 V. The resulting P700$^+$ cation has a potential of around +0.49 V, and thus something over 40% of the energy initially transferred into the reaction center domain is dissipated as heat during the charge separation process, leaving a ~1.0 V potential difference between the positive (P700$^+$/P700) and negative (F_B/F_B^-) terminals of PSI. This is of course a "ballpark" figure as, for example, there is species variation in the measured P700$^+$/P700 reduction potential, similar variations are likely in the exact potentials of the various electron acceptors, and actual potentials depend on experimental conditions. Nevertheless, it is reasonable to conclude that the electrical potential difference between the oxidizing and reducing ends of PSI is likely to be in the region of 1.0 V.

In nature, the particular role of PSI is to produce electrons that are sufficiently electronegative to reduce NADP$^+$ to NADPH, at a potential of around −0.32 V. This is achieved initially by using chlorophyll and phylloquinone as electron carriers within the body of the membrane and Fe_4-S_4 centers at the membrane surface. With regard to exploitation of PSI for biohybrid photovoltaics, the potentials of electrons entering and emerging from PSI have guided the choice of electrode materials and mediators.[79–83] Of particular note, the electrons produced by PSI are sufficiently electronegative to reduce hydrogen ions to molecular hydrogen, and there has been considerable interest in achieving light-powered hydrogen production by coupling preparations of PSI to catalysts such as platinum[84–87] or to hydrogenase enzymes.[88–97] Hence, there are prospects for the use of PSI for solar fuel synthesis in addition to pure photovoltaics.

Studies of the photovoltaic capacity of purified PSI have used the complex from cyanobacteria,[98–108] or the eukaryotic complex from spinach,[109–112] pea,[113] or *Arabidopsis thaliana*.[114] A PSI-LHCI complex from *Cyanidioschyzon merolae*, a red microalga, has also been used in recent work[115,116] as have thylakoid membranes from spinach.[117] A minority of studies have utilized genetically modified PSI complexes, particularly those from cyanobacteria where genetic modification is more accessible. In addition to the general approach of poly-histidine tagging for the purposes of protein purification, genetically-engineered cysteine residues have been introduced to the PSI from *Synechocystis* in order to adhere it with a specific orientation to a gold electrode through the formation of a strong sulphur-gold covalent bond.[118] Using specific molecular linkers, engineered cysteines have also been used to bind PSI to gallium arsenide[119] or carbon nanotubes.[120]

Advantage has also been taken of the possibility of removing or exchanging the extra-membrane PsaE subunit of PSI in order to genetically encode a propensity to bind to a specific protein or material. To construct a hybrid electron transfer system, a genetically modified *Synechocystis* PSI lacking an extra-membrane PsaE subunit was interacted with a hybrid protein in which the PsaE subunit was genetically fused to a membrane-bound hydrogenase from *Ralstonia eutropha*, and the resulting hybrid complex was assessed for light-induced hydrogen evolution when bound to a gold electrode.[90] Binding to the electrode was achieved by coating the gold surface with a Ni-NTA terminated self-assembled monolayer to enable vectoral PSI binding via an extra-membrane poly-histidine tag also used for protein purification. This dual use of the poly-histidine tag for purification and oriented binding to a modified electrode has been exploited in a variety of studies using PSI, PSII, or purple bacterial photoproteins. Binding of PSI to zinc oxide nanowires has also been directed by exchanging the native PsaE subunit with a 50-fold molar excess of an engineered PsaE modified by a "ZnO tag" protein sequence that directs binding to zinc oxide surfaces (sequence RSNTRMTARQHRSANHKSTRARS).[99,121] The same approach has also been used with the extra-membrane PsaD subunit.[99] Finally, PSI has been modified for binding to a gold electrode modified with a layer of a cysteine-terminated triglycine (GGGC) peptides by adding the amino sequence LPETG to the C-terminus of the PsaE subunit.[105] Covalent binding of PSI to the electrode was achieved through the action of the enzyme Sortase A from the bacterium *Staphylococcus aureus*, which forms a peptide bond between the LPET and GGG sequences.

4.3 PURPLE BACTERIAL REACTION CENTERS—LIGHT, ELECTRONS, AND PROTONS

Purple photosynthetic bacteria are the most heavily studied of the oxygenic phototrophs. These are prokaryotes that carry out chlorophyll-based photosynthesis but which do not use water as an electron source and do not produce oxygen as a waste product. Research on the molecular basis for photosynthetic energy transduction in general experienced a step change in the mid-1980s following the publication of a high-resolution X-ray crystal structure for the reaction center from *Blastochloris viridis* (named at the time *Rhodopseudomonas viridis*).[122–124] This was followed by determination of the X-ray crystal structure of the reaction center from *Rhodobacter* (*Rba.*) *sphaeroides*,[125–132] and this organism has subsequently dominated research into the detailed mechanism of photochemical charge separation using a combination of steady-state and time-resolved spectroscopy, site-directed mutagenesis, and X-ray crystallography.[1,4,13,15,16,133]

The *Rba. sphaeroides* reaction center is a cytochrome c_2:ubiquinone oxidoreductase, using the energy of a single photon to transfer a single electron across the bacterial inner membrane from a molecule of cytochrome c_2 in the bacterial periplasmic space to a molecule of ubiquinone in the membrane interior close to the cytoplasmic side. As with PSI, this electron transfer is achieved using a wire of cofactors that span the membrane, but unlike PSI, which uses phylloquinone and chlorophyll as its membrane-embedded redox cofactors, the *Rba. sphaeroides* reaction center uses ubiquinone, bacteriochlorophyll, and bacteriopheophytin (a demetallated bacteriochlorophyll). The arrangement of these cofactors in the *Rba. sphaeroides* reaction center is shown in Figure 4.4a. As with PSI, the proteins that form the scaffold for the electron transfer cofactors, PufL and PufM, are arranged in a heterodimeric

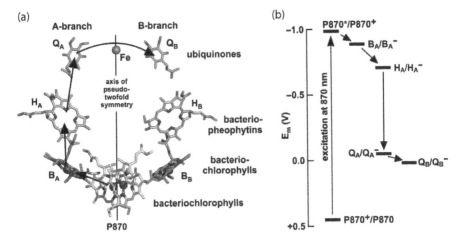

FIGURE 4.4 Structure of the electron transfer chain and the energetics of charge separation in the *Rba. sphaeroides* reaction center: (a) Charge separation proceeds along only one of the two membrane-spanning branches of bacteriochlorophyll, bacteriopheophytin, and ubiquinone cofactors. (b) One photon powers the transfer of one electron from the P870 donor to the Q_B ubiquinone, producing the final charge separated state $P870^+Q_B^-$. A second light-powered charge separation results in double reduction and double protonation of the Q_B ubiquinone to produce Q_BH_2. Figure drawn using PDB entry.

fashion around an axis of twofold pseudosymmetry that runs perpendicular to the membrane plane. Close to the periplasmic side of the membrane are a pair of bacteriochlorophyll molecules that straddle the pseudosymmetry axis. These comprise the primary electron donor and are referred to as P870 (or sometimes P865). Each wire of cofactors is then formed by a "monomeric" bacteriochlorophyll (B_A or B_B), a bacteriopheophytin (H_A or H_B), and a ubiquinone (Q_A or Q_B).

Charge separation is initiated in the *Rba. sphaeroides* reaction center by conversion of the P870 pair of BChls from their ground state to their first singlet excited state, P870*. The first clearly resolved radical pair is $P870^+H_A^-$, formed with a lifetime of 3–5 ps, with no significant formation of the equivalent $P870^+H_B^-$ radical pair. This strong functional asymmetry has led to the distinction of an "active" and an "inactive" branch of cofactors, also referred to as A- and B-branches, respectively.[134,135] Membrane-spanning electron transfer is completed by reduction of the A-branch ubiquinone (Q_A) by H_A^- with a lifetime of around 200 ps. After much debate it is now generally agreed that the reduction of H_A by P870* is a two-step reaction in which $P870^+B_A^-$ is formed prior to $P870^+H_A^-$.[15] This intermediate does not build up and is therefore difficult to detect spectroscopically, as the lifetime for the second step is shorter than that of the first step.[15] Further observations on the fastest phases of charge separation in the *Rba. sphaeroides* reaction center are made in Section 4.5. Formation of $P870^+$ initiates microsecond timescale one-electron oxidation of a water-soluble cytochrome c_2 transiently docked to the periplasmic face of the reaction center, resetting the primary electron donor for the next photooxidation (see Axelrod and Okamura,[136] Pogorelov et al.[137] for reviews).

The strong functional asymmetry exhibited by the pseudosymmetrical cofactor system in the *Rba. sphaeroides* reaction center (Figure 4.4a) is in marked contrast to the functional symmetry observed in the PSI reaction center (Figure 4.3a). The reason becomes apparent when considering the fate of the electrons delivered to the quinone components of the electron transfer wires in the two systems. In PSI, regardless of which of the two available routes the electron takes in crossing the membrane, the role of both quinone cofactors is to pass the electron to the F_X iron-sulphur center that sits on the symmetry axis (Figure 4.3a). In achieving this, each quinone is operating as a single electron relay; although quinones in solution can undergo a two-electron/two-proton chemistry, electron flow through PSI is not linked to proton translocation across the photosynthetic membrane. In contrast, one role of the purple bacterial reaction center is to achieve proton uptake on the cytoplasmic side of the membrane, and this is done using the Q_B ubiquinone at the cytoplasmic end of one of its two membrane-spanning electron transfer chains (Figure 4.4a). Although in the *Rba. sphaeroides* reaction center the two quinones are chemically identical, the structure of the protein scaffold that forms each of the Q_A and Q_B binding sites has evolved to confer specialized functions on its resident quinine.[138–140] At the Q_A site, the ubiquinone head group is locked into the protein structure and its protein environment is relatively hydrophobic. In contrast, the binding pocket for the Q_B ubiquinone is open to the membrane, enabling exchange with the intra-membrane quinone pool, and it is lined with polar amino acids that act as the termini of hydrogen bond networks that can be traced to the extra-membrane protein surface. Accordingly, the Q_A ubiquinone acts as a one-electron relay, oxidizing H_A^- and passing the electron on to the Q_B ubiquinone. In contrast, the Q_B ubiquinone engages in a charge accumulation reaction, forming a stably bound semiquinone after a first photochemical charge separation along the active branch and the doubly reduced/doubly protonated form (ubiquinol, or dihydroubiquinone) after a second photochemical charge separation. Presumably, this asymmetric arrangement where the active branch is specialized for highly efficient picosecond timescale charge separation, and the inactive branch is specialized for slower ubiquinol formation, is more efficient than the symmetrical alternative where Q_A and Q_B would both be responsible for both stabilizing charge separation and accumulating a doubly reduced and doubly protonated state.

The principal cause of this functional asymmetry is thought to be that the free energies of the potential inactive branch radical pairs $P870^+B_B^-$ and $P870^+H_B^-$ are significantly higher than their active branch counterparts, such that the energy of $P870^+B_B^-$, in particular lies above that of $P870^*$.[134,135] Other factors such as small differences in distance and electronic coupling between cofactors, the dielectric environment, and static intra-protein electric fields on the two branches may also be relevant (see Wakeham and Jones[141] for a review). In a series of publications extending over more than twenty years, Kirmaier and Holten have described *Rba. sphaeroides* and *Rba. capsulatus* reaction centers engineered to conduct "wrong-way" electron transfer through a combination of mutations that discourage electron transfer along the active branch and encourage electron transfer along the inactive branch.[135,142,143]

As indicated earlier, at the periplasmic side of the membrane the *Rba. sphaeroides* reaction center oxidizes cytochrome c_2 in a one-electron redox reaction. As a result, acting in isolation the reaction center is not capable of coupling electron transfer to proton translocation across the photosynthetic membrane. To achieve this, the reaction center works in partnership with a cytochrome bc_1 complex that uses as substrates the ubiquinol and oxidized cytochrome c_2 produced by the reaction center.[144–146] Ubiquinol is reoxidized on the periplasmic side of the membrane, liberating protons into the bacterial periplasmic space. One in every two of the electrons released from ubiquinol is used to reduce oxidized cytochrome c_2 to complete a cycle of electron flow between the cytochrome bc_1 complex and the reaction center. The second passes back across the membrane to reduce more ubiquinone on the cytoplasmic side of the membrane in a mechanism known as the Q-cycle.[145,147–149] The net effect is that light energy is used to power formation of an electrochemical gradient of protons across the photosynthetic membrane, which can then be used drive a variety of processes including solute uptake, synthesis of ATP, and rotation of the bacterial flagellum.

To achieve reduction of P870$^+$, the *Rba. sphaeroides* reaction center has a binding site for cytochrome c_2 on the protein surface exposed to the periplasmic space. In many species of purple bacteria, including *Blastochloris viridis*, the reaction center has an additional subunit at this location that encases four heme cofactors.[122–124,150,151] In these species, reduction of the equivalent of P870$^+$ is carried out by the nearest heme cofactor, with subsequent oxidation of cytochrome c_2. The overall strategy of light-powered cyclic electron transfer and coupled proton translocation is therefore preserved, but oxidation of cytochrome c_2 by the photooxidized primary electron donor is indirect. Some studies of photocurrent generation have employed reaction centers with this additional tetraheme cytochrome subunit, as it provides a different way of wiring the reaction center module to an electrode (e.g., see den Hollander et al.[152]).

The energetic basis on which the *Rba. sphaeroides* reaction center operates is shown in Figure 4.4b. The redox potential of the P870 primary electron donor is transformed by ~1.45 eV on conversion to the P870* singlet excited state, triggering sequential reduction of B_A, H_A, Q_A, and Q_B. As with PSI, a fraction of the energy of the initiating excited state is released as heat in order to very strongly favor, at each step, the forward reaction over the competing reverse reaction. In addition, the strategy of rapidly separating the positive and negative charges on opposite sides of the membrane minimizes charge recombination to the ground state. The result is solar energy conversion that has a high quantum efficiency (charges separated per photon absorbed) but a relatively low energy efficiency. At its positive terminus, the *Rba. sphaeroides* reaction center generates an oxidizing potential that is close to that produced by PSI, but the electrons that emerge from the negative terminus are around 0.5 V less reducing as the energy of the excited state that triggers charge separation is lower by a similar amount.

Turning from electron transfer to solar energy capture, the four bacteriochlorophyll and two bacteriopheophytin pigments of the *Rba. sphaeroides* reaction center are each capable of fulfilling a light-harvesting role in addition to any role they may play in electron transfer or photoprotection. As the first singlet excited states of the bacteriopheophytins and monomeric bacteriochlorophylls are located at significantly higher energies than that of the P870 pair, energy absorbed by these pigments is passed on a femtosecond timescale to form P870* and trigger charge separation.[153–155] However, in nature the bulk of solar energy capture by purple photosynthetic bacteria is carried out by light-harvesting pigment proteins that surround the reaction center in the photosynthetic membrane. The structure, organization, and function of these membranes and their component pigment proteins have been extensively reviewed.[27,156–165] The process of energy capture and migration through the purple bacterial light-harvesting system has also been characterized in depth.[20,27,166]

In all species that have been investigated to date, the reaction center is encased in a cylindrical "LH1" light-harvesting pigment protein to form the so-called "RC-LH1 core" complex.[167–171] This LH1 protein is formed from multiple copies of two membrane-spanning proteins that bind bacteriochlorophyll and carotenoid light-harvesting pigments. In some species this cylinder of LH1 protein forms a complete ring around the reaction center whereas in other species there is a break in its continuity.[162] In *Rba. sphaeroides,* the RC-LH1 complex can assemble in a dimeric form in which two reaction centers are surrounded by an S-shaped LH1,[172–176] complete closure of an individual LH1 around its reaction center being prevented by an additional protein called PufX.[177] Removal of PufX by gene deletion produces monomeric RC-LH1 complexes in which the LH1 completely surrounds the reaction center.[174] For the native PufX-containing version of the *Rba. sphaeroides* RC-LH1 complex, the amount of the dimeric form that can be isolated from photosynthetic membranes seems to depend on its carotenoid content. RC-LH1 complexes purified from cells grown under illuminated/anaerobic conditions, where the principal carotenoid is spheroidene, are mostly dimeric whereas RC-LH1 complexes purified from cells grown under dark/semiaerobic conditions, where the principal carotenoid is spheroidenone, are mostly monomeric (but with an incomplete ring of LH1 pigment protein surrounding the reaction center due to the presence of PufX).[178]

The most detailed structural information on a RC-LH1 to date was published in 2014 for the complex from *Thermochromatium tepidum*.[171] This structure shows the electron transfer chain in the central reaction center domain surrounded by a ring of 32 light- harvesting bacteriochlorophylls and 16 light-harvesting carotenoids. An obvious feature of this structure is the physical separation of the electron transfer bacteriochlorophylls from the chemically identical light-harvesting bacteriochlorophylls of the LH1 ring (Figure 4.5). Although this separation means that the transfer of excited state energy from the LH1 bacteriochlorophylls to the P870 bacteriochlorophylls in the reaction center is a relatively slow process (lifetime of 35–50 ps), it is necessary to avoid oxidation of the LH1 bacteriochlorophylls during charge separation (as the potentials for one-electron oxidation of the P870 and LH1 bacteriochlorophylls are similar).[179,180] The reaction center and LH1 protein residing between the electron transfer and light-harvesting cofactors can therefore be viewed as insulation that prevents unwanted redox reactions that could reduce the quantum yield of charge separation. A similar separation is seen in PSII, where electron transfer from the light-harvesting chlorophylls to the highly oxidizing cofactors within the reaction center domain is highly energetically favorable but to a lesser extent in PSI where such transfer is unfavorable.[179,180] This control of electron flow is an important feature of photosynthetic reaction centers, ensuring productive charge separation happens with a high quantum yield and effective electrical connections to external electron donors and acceptors.

The majority of studies of the photovoltaic capacities of purple bacterial proteins have utilized the heavily studied reaction center complex from *Rba. sphaeroides*[181–189]

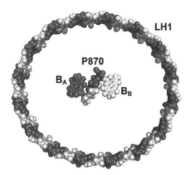

FIGURE 4.5   Arrangement of the reaction center and LH1 bacteriochlorophylls in the RC-LH1 complex from *Thermochromatium tepidum*: The protein that holds these bacterio-chlorophylls in place acts to insulate the electron transfer chain from the cofactors of the light-harvesting system. View is perpendicular to the membrane from the periplasmic side. To distinguish them, neighboring bacteriochlorophylls are colored alternating light and dark grey. Figure drawn using Protein Data Bank entry 3WMM.[171]

or the larger RC-LH1 complex.[190,191] Work by Tan, Jones, and coworkers has used a variant of this RC-LH1 complex that lacks the PufX protein and has an expanded LH1 antenna[192–196] including PufX-deficient complexes that have the green carot-enoid neurosporene in place of the native red carotenoid spheroidenone.[197] In addi-tion to widespread use of His-tags to facilitate purification, some studies have utilized this tag to orient RCs or RC-LH1 complexes on Ni-NTA coated electrodes.[198–201] Alongside *Rba. sphaeroides* proteins, studies have also explored the photovol-taic properties of RC-LH1 complexes from *Rhodopseudomonas acidophila*,[152,202] *Rhodopseudomonas palustris*,[203–205] and *Rhodospirillum rubrum*[203,206,207] and intact photosynthetic membranes from *Rba. sphaeroides*[208] and *Rhodospirillum rubrum*.[209]

As with PSI, engineered cysteine residues have been used to orient *Rba. sphaer-oides* reaction centers on gold or highly oriented pyrolytic graphite electrodes.[210] Multiple mutations in the vicinity of the reaction center quinone and bacteriopheophy-tin sites have also been used to investigate the mechanism of photocurrent generation with quinone charge carriers[211] and the route of electron tunneling through reaction centers under an applied bias.[212] Biochemical modification has also been applied to *Rba. sphaeroides* reaction centers to replace the native bacteriopheophytin with plant pheophytin.[213,214]

4.4   PHOTOSYSTEM II—LIGHT, ELECTRONS, PROTONS, AND OXIDIZING POWER

PSII is the second membrane-embedded reaction center pigment protein found in the plants, algae, and cyanobacteria and, from the point of view of electron transfer, is the most complex of the three reaction centers considered in this chapter.[3,6,8–10,62,215–222] PSII is also a solar-powered oxidoreductase, using the energy of a single photon to transfer a single electron from a water molecule on one side of the photosynthetic membrane to a plastoquinone on the opposite side. The electron transfer chain that links the primary electron donor, P680, to the site of plastoquinone reduction has strong similarities to that in the *Rba. sphaeroides* reaction center, the most marked difference being the use of chlorophyll, pheophytin, and plastoquinone as cofactors rather than bacteriochlorophyll, bacteriopheophytin, and ubiquinone. The principal difference between the two reaction centers concerns the so-called "donor side" where PSII has an additional apparatus for the oxidation of water, a four-electron/four-proton process that requires a very high oxidation potential. This capacity for solar-powered water splitting sets PSII apart and makes it of great interest from the point of view of solar fuel synthesis.

As with the other reaction centers, our understanding of the mechanism of light-powered water oxidation and plastoquinone reduction by PSII has developed from a combination of spectroscopic studies and structural biology, augmented by biochemical and genetic manipulation. The first series of X-ray crystal structures for PSII were deposited in the Protein Data Bank over a four-year period at resolutions of 3.8 Å,[223] 3.7 Å,[224] 3.5 Å,[225] 3.2 Å,[226] and 3.0 Å.[227] These illuminated many aspects of PSII structure and mechanism but also, largely due to the limited resolution, left a great many questions unanswered and much scope for vigorous debate, particularly with regard to the mechanism of water oxidation. The next major step forward was the publication in 2011 of a structure for the PSII complex from a thermophilic cyanobacterium at 1.9 Å resolution,[228] which was followed in 2015 by a structure at a similar resolution, determined the use of femtosecond X-ray pulses to limit radiation damage.[229] At the time of writing, there are 36 Protein Data Bank entries for the PSII complex from the cyanobacteria *Thermosynechococcus elongatus*[223,225–227,230–235] or *Thermosynechoccus vulcanus*,[224,228,229,236–239] plus one structure for PSII from the red alga *Cyanidium caldarium*.[240]

PSII shows some similarities in overall architecture to PSI, in that it comprises a central reaction center domain that is flanked by light-harvesting domains.[2,17,241] The X-ray crystal structure for the dimeric PSII from *Thermosynechoccus vulcanus* reported in 2011 revealed a protein comprising, per monomer, 19 polypeptide subunits, 35 chlorophylls, 11 carotenoids and 2 plastoquinones.[228] Some of these proteins and pigments comprise two proximal light-harvesting complexes, termed CP43 and CP47, that flank the central reaction center domain, and in turn are surrounded by a larger LHCII antenna responsible for light harvesting.[242] Within the central reaction center domain are two membrane-spanning wires of cofactors that are arranged around an axis of twofold pseudosymmetry in a similar fashion to the architectures seen in the *Rba. sphaeroides* reaction center and PSI,[2] the cofactors being held in place by a protein scaffold formed from two related polypeptides termed D1 and D2. Each wire of cofactors comprises two chlorophylls, two pheophytins, and a plastoquinone (Figure 4.6a), the structural arrangement of which has strong similarities to that seen in the *Rba. sphaeroides* reaction center (Figure 4.4a). One notable exception to this is a decreased overlap between the two chlorophylls at the positions corresponding to the P870 bacteriochlorophylls in the *Rba. sphaeroides* reaction center, such that these chlorophylls (labeled P_{D1} and P_{D2} in Figure 4.6a) do not function as an excitonically coupled pair.

Initiation of charge separation in PSII is caused by formation of an excited electronic state among the four chlorophylls of the reaction center, the primary electron

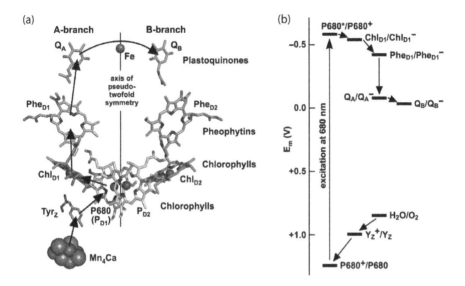

FIGURE 4.6 Structure of the electron transfer chain and energetics of charge separation in PSII: (a) Charge separation proceeds along only one of the two membrane-spanning branches of chlorophyll, pheophytin, and plastoquinone cofactors. The resulting P680$^+$ species oxidized a tyrosine side-chain (Tyr$_Z$), which in turn removes an electron from the OEC. (b) One photon powers the transfer of one electron from the OEC donor to the Q$_B$ plastoquinone. At the acceptor side, a second light-powered charge separation results in double reduction and double protonation of the Q$_B$ plastoquinone to produce Q$_B$H$_2$. At the donor side, the oxidation of two waters requires a total of four sequential light-powered charge separations. Figure drawn using Protein Data Bank entry 3WU2.[228]

donor being given the name P680.[243] Due to similar degrees of coupling between these four chlorophylls there is not a single, well-defined mechanism for the initial step of charge separation in PSII, and it may well be that two or more mechanisms operate in parallel. This point is expanded on a little in Section 4.5. The first clearly resolved intermediate in charge separation is the radical pair P680$^+$Phe$_A^-$, where Phe$_A$ is the pheophytin on the "active" branch adjacent to the Q$_A$ plastoquinone (Figure 4.6a). Membrane-spanning electron transfer then proceeds through formation of P680$^+$Q$_A^-$ and P680$^+$Q$_B^-$.[3,8,10,62,215,217–222]

Unlike in P870$^+$ and P700$^+$, where the cation is shared between two bacteriochlorophylls or chlorophylls, in P680$^+$ the cation is localized on a single chlorophyll, thought to be that labeled P$_{D1}$ in Figure 4.6a.[244,245] P680$^+$ has a redox potential of ~+1.25 V, making it one of the most oxidizing species in biology. It removes an electron from a tyrosine side chain in the D1 protein, which is then re-reduced by an electron derived from one of two water molecules bound to a cluster of oxo-bridged manganese and calcium atoms known as the oxygen-evolving complex (OEC). Full oxidation of two waters to one molecule of oxygen requires the removal of four electrons, powered by four photooxidations of P680. Four protons are released as electrons and are removed sequentially from the OEC.

High-resolution X-ray crystal structures for PSII have brought new insights into the structure of the OEC, revealing it as a Mn_4CaO_5 cluster.[223–230,235–239] Three of the manganese, one calcium, and four oxygen atoms form a distorted cube in which each manganese is bound to three oxygen atoms, and the calcium is bound to two oxygen atoms and the oxygens of two water molecules. The fourth manganese is connected to the cube via one of the cube oxygens and indirectly to one of the cube manganese via a fifth oxo bridge. This latter manganese also binds two water molecules. In this arrangement, the calcium is linked to all four manganese by an oxo bridge. The Mn_4CaO_5 cluster is held in place by several interactions with the surrounding protein such that each manganese has six ligands and the calcium has seven ligands. In the most recent structural study, femtosecond X-ray pulses were coordinated with two-flash visible light excitation in a bid to understand the mechanism of O=O bond formation during water oxidation.[215] This study implicated one of the oxygens linking the cube to the fifth manganese as the site of dioxygen formation.

The energetic basis of charge separation in PSII is shown in Figure 4.6b. On the acceptor side, the reduction potentials of P680* and the subsequent pheophytin and plastoquinone electron carriers are similar to those observed for the *Rba. sphaeroides* reaction center. However, photooxidation of P680 produces an extremely oxidizing cation in order extract electrons from water via the Tyr_Z radical. The ~0.35 V gap between water oxidation and P680$^+$ means that the final gap in potential between the oxidizing and reducing terminals of PSII is of the order of ~0.8 V, which means that around 1 V of energy is expended per 680 nm photon to achieve water oxidation and quinone reduction. An unavoidable consequence of the use of water as a source of electrons is the production of oxygen, and the heady mix of this precursor of reactive oxygen species, excited pigments, and highly oxidizing species renders PSII particularly vulnerable. In addition to photoinhibition of electron transport, PSII proteins are prone to photooxidative damage, particularly the D1 protein that scaffolds P680 and the OEC and contains Tyr_Z. As a result, oxygenic phototrophs exhibit multiple molecular mechanisms for photoprotection and for the repair of PSII.[246–252]

The vulnerability of PSII to damage during turnover is one reason why exploration of its use in photovoltaic devices has been less extensive than has been the case for PSI or purple bacterial reaction center. Studies involving PSII have employed purified reaction centers from cyanobacteria[103,253–265] or PSII-enriched membrane preparations from spinach.[266–268] The only example to date of the use of protein engineering other than His-tagging is a study of a PSII with a single lysine to glutamic acid substitution in the D1 polypeptide.[269]

The OEC is the distinctive feature of PSII, and an enormous effort has been put into understanding its structure and the mechanism of water oxidation through a variety of approaches including X-ray crystallography and extended X-ray absorption fine structure spectroscopy.[270–274] From the point of view of applications, there is of course a great deal of interest in the development of catalysts for solar water splitting that take varied amounts of inspiration from nature.[272,273,275,276] PSII is sometimes erroneously described as being able to split water into oxygen and hydrogen, but of course this is misleading. In addition to oxygen, PSII produces protons that are released on one side of the membrane and electrons that are moved to the opposite side of the membrane. At the point at which those electrons leave PSII they are insufficiently reducing to convert protons into molecular hydrogen. Therefore, on its own, PSII is not capable of producing hydrogen. PSI, on the other hand, is able to shunt the reduction potential of electrons to sufficiently negative values to reduce hydrogen, and so proposals have been made that systems where PSII and PSI work together could be developed that use sunlight to split water into oxygen and hydrogen.[103,258,277]

4.5   NUANCES OF THE FASTEST STEPS OF PHOTOCHEMICAL CHARGE SEPARATION

Although most general textbooks give simple and clear explanations of the mechanism of photochemical charge separation in reaction centers, many aspects of this process are still not fully understood, and the textbook descriptions are sometimes not entirely accurate or up to date. One area of ongoing research and debate is the mechanism of the first step (or two steps) of charge separation.

The most clearly understood mechanism is that operating in the *Rba. sphaeroides* reaction center. As it is possible to separate this protein from its attendant light-harvesting complexes, using biochemical or genetic techniques, it is feasible to investigate the mechanism of ultrafast charge separation by applying time-resolved pulsed laser spectroscopy in which the P870 bacteriochlorophylls are excited directly. This technique initially established that formation of P870* led, within a few picoseconds, to the radical pair $P870^+H_A^-$. After further investigation, and much debate, it was established that $P870^+B_A^-$ forms as a short-lived intermediate in this process (see Zinth and Wachtveitl[15] for a detailed review). This produces the following scheme:

$$P870^* \rightarrow P870^+B_A^- \rightarrow P870^+H_A^-$$

This charge separation characterized in purified reaction centers is the end product of energy harvesting and transport processes in the intact photosystem. In these, energy absorbed by the carotenoid and bacteriochlorophyll cofactors of the core and peripheral light-harvesting proteins produces, as the lowest energy excited state in the antenna, the first excited singlet state of the LH1 BChls absorbing at 875 nm.[12,20,27] This "B875*" state is essentially isoenergetic with the P870 bacteriochlorophyll pair in the reaction center, and so the full energy harvesting and trapping scheme up to $P870^+H_A^-$ can be described as:

$$antenna^* \rightarrow B875^* \rightarrow P870^* \rightarrow {}^{\mathsf{I}}P870^+B_A^- \rightarrow P870^+H_A^-$$

Although in nature the majority of excited state energy would be expected to enter the *Rba. sphaeroides* reaction center via P870, in the laboratory it is possible to directly excite the accessory bacteriochlorophylls, B_A and B_B, in purified reaction centers. This initiates femtosecond timescale energy transfer to P870, but in addition there is evidence from experiments with wild-type and mutated reaction centers that alternative charge separation mechanisms can take place in which the excited state B_A^* can produce $P870^+H_A^-$ without forming $P870^*$ (see van Brederode and van Grondelle[28] for a review). These can be summarized as:

$$P870\ B_A^*H_A \rightarrow P870\ B_A^+H_A^- \rightarrow P870^+B_AH_A^-$$

$$P870\ B_A^*H_A \rightarrow P870^+B_A^-H_A \rightarrow P870^+B_AH_A^-$$

In the first, the initial charge separation takes place between the active branch monomeric bacteriochlorophyll and bacteriopheophytin, with subsequent hole transfer to P870. In the second, the initial event is oxidation of P870 by B_A^*, followed by electron transfer to the bacteriopheophytin. These mechanisms are also illustrated in Figure 4.2b and c.

Although these alternative mechanisms for charge separation are likely to be of limited physiological relevance for purple bacteria *in vivo*, they highlight the possibility that the initial photochemical event in a reaction center may not be a single process but rather multiple parallel processes. These alternative mechanisms could be of greater relevance to isolated reaction centers in a photoelectrochemical cell, where the six bacteriochlorins and one carotenoid of the reaction center are the only light-harvesting pigments present. They are also of greater significance to PSI and PSII where the distinct energy gradient seen in the purple bacterial reaction center is not present.

The first steps of charge separation have also been studied in depth in PSII, where it is also possible to separate the reaction center domain from the attendant light-harvesting pigment proteins. As indicated earlier, in the PSII reaction center the two chlorophylls at the same locations as the P870 bacteriochlorophylls in the purple bacterial reaction center (P_{D1} and P_{D2} in Figure 4.6a) do not form a strongly excitonically coupled "special pair" due to differences in protein structure that decrease their overlap and reduce the strength of the coupling between the two.[218–220] In marked contrast to the multicomponent absorbance spectrum of the *Rba. sphaeroides* reaction center, the absorbance spectrum of the PSII reaction center domain shows very little structure even at cryogenic temperatures indicating that the excited singlet states of the four chlorophylls and two pheophytins are isoenergetic. The consequence is that there isn't a unique focus for excitation energy entering the reaction center, leading to the questions: (1) What is the $P680^*$ state that triggers charge separation? (2) What is the initial radical pair formed? (3) Which chlorophyll forms the $P680^+$ cation? (4) Are $P680^*$ and $P680^+$ the same species?

The structural arrangement of the four chlorophylls and two pheophytins of PSII, and their strongly overlapping absorbance properties, have led to proposals that the excitonic couplings between nearest neighbors are similar in strength and that the singlet excited state that triggers charge separation is delocalized over two or more of these pigments.[244,278] Extensive ultrafast spectroscopic studies, augmented by modeling and computation, have provided evidence for the following mechanisms for charge separation in PSII, with involvement of charge transfer character in the initiating excited states:

$$P_{D1}(Chl_{D1}Pheo_{D1})^* \rightarrow P_{D1}Chl_{D1}^+Pheo_{D1}^- \rightarrow P_{D1}^+Chl_{D1}Pheo_{D1}^-$$

$$(P_{D2}P_{D1})^*\ Chl_{D1}Pheo_{D1} \rightarrow P_{D2}^+P_{D1}^-Chl_{D1}Pheo_{D1} \rightarrow$$

$$P_{D2}P_{D1}^+Chl_{D1}^-Pheo_{D1} \rightarrow P_{D1}^+Chl_{D1}Pheo_{D1}^-$$

In the first, an exciton state delocalized over the active branch chlorophyll and pheophytin produces a charge separation between these cofactors before hole transfer to the P_{D1} chlorophyll.[279–281] In the second, an exciton state delocalized mainly on P_{D1} and P_{D2} produces a charge separation between these chlorophylls before migration of the electron along the active branch and migration of the hole to P_{D1}.[282,283] Both mechanisms end with the state $P_{D1}^+Chl_{D1}Pheo_{D1}^-$, and it is generally agreed that the P680$^+$ radical is indeed localized on the P_{D1} chlorophyll.[284] Thus, P680* and P680$^+$ are not the same species, and in some recent publications the term RC* has been used to avoid confusion on this point. An alternative model has also been proposed in which initial charge separation produces $P680^+Chl_{D1}^-$, with subsequent electron transfer to $Pheo_{D1}$[285,286] (reviewed in Semenov et al.[61]; Nadtochencko et al.[287]; Mamedov et al.[62]).

In PSI, investigation of the first few picoseconds of charge separation is complicated by an inability to biochemically separate the central RC domain from the surrounding antenna. In PSII and the purple bacterial reaction center, the polypeptides that provide the scaffold for the electron transfer chain (D1/D2 and PufL/PufM) are distinct from those that bind the bulk of the light-harvesting pigments, and so the RC pigment protein can be separated from the surrounding antenna. However, in PSI the much larger PsaA and PsaB polypeptides that scaffold the two-electron transfer chains also bind large numbers of light-harvesting chlorophylls and carotenoids. As a result, it is not possible to remove these antenna regions through biochemical treatments or genetic manipulation. As there is strong overlap of the absorbance bands of the light-harvesting and RC chlorophylls in PSI, it is problematic to directly excite the latter in order to study charge separation and problematic to distinguish energy transfer from charge separation.[288,289]

Despite the challenges, it has been proposed on the basis of ultrafast spectroscopy of wild-type and mutated PSI complexes that the initial radical pair formed on each branch is between the two chlorophylls that are not part of the P700 pair, labeled A and A_0.[76,289,290] These studies indicated that this charge separation is a sub-ps process and is followed by a slower (6–20 ps) transfer of the cation to P700. The scheme, therefore, is on either cofactor branch:

$$RC^* \rightarrow P700\ A^+A_0^- \rightarrow P700^+A A_0^-$$

What is not clear in this system is whether the excited state that initiates the process is localized on the P700 chlorophylls or on one or both of the monomeric chlorophylls on the two cofactor branches. Alternative schemes have also been proposed in which the cation is initially formed on P700,[61] or charge separation occurs from a highly delocalized excited state.[62,291,292]

4.6 CONCLUSIONS

Biochemistry, spectroscopy, and structural biology have brought increasingly detailed pictures of the main mechanisms through which photosynthetic organisms harvest solar energy through ultrafast charge separation. Although many of the general principles and basic strategies are now understood, given the complexity, diversity, and sophistication of photosynthetic systems, our understanding is far from complete.

The technical challenge associated with understanding processes occurring in nanoscale objects on ultrafast timescales is considerable, as is the need to be able to relate observations made on single pigments or proteins to photosystems comprising hundreds of proteins and thousands of pigments. Nevertheless, studies of the photophysics of diverse light-activated photosynthetic processes such as energy harvesting, charge separation, electron transfer, and photoprotection have brought unique insights into how nature works at the most fundamental of levels. As an illustration, research on light-harvesting proteins and reaction centers has been at the forefront of efforts to understand the roles played by quantum coherence in biological mechanisms[25,293–299] and how this understanding may influence future solar cell design.[300,301]

The aim of this chapter has been to provide a basic introduction to the three types of photochemical RC that have been utilized for bio-photovoltaics. Between them they cover a major part of the useable solar spectrum and span the range of reduction potential that living systems occupy. These natural materials have many attractive attributes but also present challenges for use in a device setting. As an example, photosystems that operate at extremes of redox potential are prone to photooxidative damage; as they are integral membrane proteins, they also can exhibit limited stability following isolation from the host organism. This is a particular issue for PSII, which generates extremes of oxidizing potential to convert water to oxygen and which is continually repaired by replacement of the D1 protein. It is noticeable that the bulk of studies into RC photovoltaics have concerned PSI or purple bacterial photoproteins, and the limited photostability of PSII *in vitro* has been a factor in this. Although stability is an issue at present, the field of RC photovoltaics is still in its infancy and is developing rapidly, and it will be fascinating to see where the exploitation of natural photosynthetic materials in biohybrid devices leads.

REFERENCES

1. Allen, J. P.; Williams, J. C. *FEBS Lett.* **1998**, *438* (1–2), 5–9.
2. Heathcote, P.; Fyfe, P. K.; Jones, M. R. *Trends Biochem. Sci.* **2002**, *27* (2), 79–87.
3. Renger, G. *Curr. Sci.* **2010**, *98*, 1305–1319.
4. Heathcote, P.; Jones, M. R. *Comprehensive Biophysics*, Vol. 8. E. H. Egelman, S. Ferguson (Eds.). Oxford, UK: Academic Press; **2012**. pp. 115–144.
5. Blankenship, R. E. *Molecular Mechanisms of Photosynthesis*, 2nd ed. Wiley-Blackwell; **2014**.
6. Nelson, N.; Ben-Shem, A. *Nat. Rev. Mol. Cell Biol.* **2004**, *5* (12), 971–982.
7. Fromme, P.; Yu, H.; DeRuyter, Y. S.; Jolley, C.; Chauhan, D. K.; Melkozernov, A.; Grotjohann, I. *C. R. Chim.* **2006**, *9* (2), 188–200.
8. Nelson, N.; Yocum, C. F. *Annu. Rev. Plant Biol.* **2006**, *57* (1), 521–565.
9. Caffarri, S.; Tibiletti, T.; Jennings, R.; Santabarbara, S. A. *Curr. Protein Pept. Sci.* **2014**, *15* (4), 296–331.
10. Nelson, N.; Junge, W. *Annu. Rev. Biochem.* **2015**, *84* (1), 659–683.
11. Feher, G.; Allen, J. P.; Okamura, M. Y.; Rees, D. C. *Nature* **1989**, *339* (6220), 111–116.
12. Fleming, G. R.; Van Grondelle, R. *Phys. Today* **1994**, *47* (2), 48–55.
13. Hoff, A. J.; Deisenhofer, J. *Phys. Reports* **1997**, *287* (1–2), 1–247.
14. Zinth, W.; Huppmann, P.; Arlt, T.; Wachtveitl, J. *Philos. Trans. R. Soc. A Math. Phys. Eng. Sci.* **1998**, *356* (1736), 465–476.
15. Zinth, W.; Wachtveitl, J. *ChemPhysChem* **2005**, *6* (5), 871–880.

16. Jones, M. R.; Blankenship, R. E.; Hu, X. C.; Ritz, T.; Damjanović, A.; Autenrieth, F.; Schulten, K.; Cogdell, R. J.; Gardiner, A. T.; Roszak, A. W. et al. *Biochem. Soc. Trans.* **2009**, *37* (Pt 2), 400–407.
17. Schubert, W. D.; Klukas, O.; Saenger, W.; Witt, H. T.; Fromme, P.; Krauß, N. A. *J. Mol. Biol.* **1998**, *280* (2), 297–314.
18. Ohashi, S.; Iemura, T.; Okada, N.; Itoh, S.; Furukawa, H.; Okuda, M.; Ohnishi-Kameyama, M. et al. *Photosynth. Res.* **2010**, *104* (2), 305–319.
19. Croce, R.; Van Amerongen, H. *Nat. Chem. Biol.* **2014**, *10* (7), 492–501.
20. van Grondelle, R.; Dekker, J. P.; Gillbro, T.; Sundstrom, V. *BBA - Bioenerg.* **1994**, *1187* (1), 1–65.
21. Yang, M.; Agarwal, R.; Fleming, G. R. *J. Photochem. Photobiol. A Chem.* **2001**, *142* (2–3), 107–119.
22. Cheng, Y.-C.; Fleming, G. R. *Annu. Rev. Phys. Chem.* **2009**, *60* (1), 241–262.
23. Scholes, G. D.; Fleming, G. R.; Olaya-Castro, A.; Van Grondelle, R. *Nat. Chem.* **2011**, *3* (10), 763–774.
24. Croce, R.; Van Amerongen, H. *Photosynth. Res.* **2013**, *116* (2–3), 153–166.
25. Chenu, A.; Scholes, G. D. *Annu. Rev. Phys. Chem.* **2015**, *66* (1), 69–96.
26. Mirkovic, T.; Ostroumov, E. E.; Anna, J. M.; Van Grondelle, R.; Govindjee; Scholes, G. D. *Chem. Rev.* **2017**, *117* (2), 249–293.
27. Saer, R. G.; Blankenship, R. E. *Biochem. J.* **2017**, *474* (13), 2107–2131.
28. Van Brederode, M. E.; Van Grondelle, R. *FEBS Lett.* **1999**, *455* (1–2), 1–7.
29. Bolton, J. R.; Hall, O. *Photochem. Photobiol.* **1991**, *53* (4), 545–548.
30. Zhu, X. G.; Long, S. P.; Ort, D. R. *Curr. Opin. Biotechnol.* **2008**, *19* (2), 153–159.
31. Blankenship, R. E.; Tiede, D. M.; Barber, J.; Brudvig, G. W.; Fleming, G.; Ghirardi, M.; Gunner, M. R. et al. *Science* **2011**, *332* (6031), 805–809.
32. Chitnis, P. R. *Annu. Rev. Plant Physiol. Plant Mol. Biol.* **2001**, *52*, 593–626.
33. Grotjohann, I.; Fromme, P. *Photosynth. Res.* **2005**, *85* (1), 51–72.
34. Jensen, P. E.; Bassi, R.; Boekema, E. J.; Dekker, J. P.; Jansson, S.; Leister, D.; Robinson, C.; Scheller, H. V. *Biochim. Biophys. Acta - Bioenerg.* **2007**, *1767* (5), 335–352.
35. Amunts, A.; Nelson, N. *Plant Physiol. Biochem.* **2008**, *46* (3), 228–237.
36. Amunts, A.; Nelson, N. *Structure* **2009**, *17* (5), 637–650.
37. Busch, A.; Hippler, M. *Biochim. Biophys. Acta - Bioenerg.* **2011**, *1807* (8), 864–877.
38. Kargul, J.; Janna Olmos, J. D.; Krupnik, T. *J. Plant Physiol.* **2012**, *169* (16), 1639–1653.
39. Blankenship, R. E. *Photosynth. Res.* **1992**, *33*, 91–111.
40. Büttner, M.; Xie, D. L.; Nelson, H.; Pinther, W.; Hauska, G.; Nelson, N. *Proc. Natl. Acad. Sci. U. S. A.* **1992**, *89* (17), 8135–8139.
41. Büttner, M.; Xie, D. L.; Nelson, H.; Pinther, W.; Hauska, G.; Nelson, N. *Biochim. Biophys. Acta - Bioenerg.* **1992**, *1101* (2), 154–156.
42. Permentier, H. P.; Schmidt, K. A.; Kobayashi, M.; Akiyama, M.; Hager-Braun, C.; Neerken, S.; Miller, M.; Amesz, J. *Photosynth. Res.* **2000**, *64*, 27–39.
43. Hauska, G.; Schoedl, T.; Remigy, H.; Tsiotis, G. *Biochim. Biophys. Acta - Bioenerg.* **2001**, *1507* (1–3), 260–277.
44. Liebl, U.; Mockensturm-Wilson, M.; Trost, J. T.; Brune, D. C.; Blankenship, R. E.; Vermaas, W. *Proc. Natl. Acad. Sci. U. S. A.* **1993**, *90* (15), 7124–7128.
45. Neerken, S.; Amesz, J. *Biochim. Biophys. Acta - Bioenerg.* **2001**, *1507* (1–3), 278–290.
46. Hohmann-Marriott, M. F.; Blankenship, R. E. *Evol. Photosynth.* **2011**, *62*, 515–548.
47. Cardona, T. *Photosynth. Res.* **2015**, *126* (1), 111–134.
48. Gisriel, C.; Sarrou, I.; Ferlez, B.; Golbeck, J. H.; Redding, K. E.; Fromme, R. *Science* **2017**, *357* (6355), 1021–1025.
49. Fromme, P.; Jordan, P.; Krauß, N. *Biochim. Biophys. Acta - Bioenerg.* **2001**, *1507* (1–3), 5–31.
50. Jordan, P.; Fromme, P.; Witt, H. T.; Klukas, O.; Saenger, W.; Krauss, N. *Nature* **2001**, *411* (6840), 909–917.

51. Ben-Shem, A.; Frolow, F.; Nelson, N. *Nature* **2003**, *426* (December), 630–635.
52. Amunts, A.; Drory, O.; Nelson, N. *Nature* **2007**, *447* (7140), 58–63.
53. Amunts, A.; Toporik, H.; Borovikova, A.; Nelson, N. *J. Biol. Chem.* **2010**, *285* (5), 3478–3486.
54. Qin, X.; Suga, M.; Kuang, T.; Shen, J. R. *Science* **2015**, *348* (6238), 989–995.
55. Mazor, Y.; Borovikova, A.; Nelson, N. *Elife* **2015**, *4* (June), 1–18.
56. Mazor, Y.; Borovikova, A.; Caspy, I.; Nelson, N. *Nat. Plants* **2017**, *3* (March), 1–9.
57. Webber, A. N.; Lubitz, W. *Biochim. Biophys. Acta - Bioenerg.* **2001**, *1507* (1–3), 61–79.
58. Kass, H.; Fromme, P.; Witt, H. T.; Lubitz, W. *J. Phys. Chem. B* **2001**, *105* (6), 1225–1239.
59. Poluektov, O. G.; Utschig, L. M.; Schlesselman, S. L.; Lakshmi, K. V; Brudvig, G. W.; Kothe, G.; Thurnauer, M. C. *J. Phys. Chem. B* **2002**, *106* (35), 8911–8916.
60. Brettel, K.; Leibl, W. *Biochim. Biophys. Acta - Bioenerg.* **2001**, *1507* (1–3), 100–114.
61. Semenov, A. Y.; Kurashov, V. N.; Mamedov, M. D. *J. Photochem. Photobiol. B Biol.* **2011**, *104* (1–2), 326–332.
62. Mamedov, M.; Govindjee; Nadtochenko, V.; Semenov, A. *Photosynth. Res.* **2015**, *125* (1–2), 51–63.
63. Joliot, P.; Joliot, A. *Biochemistry* **1999**, *38* (34), 11130–11136.
64. Guergova-Kuras, M.; Boudreaux, B.; Joliot, A.; Joliot, P.; Redding, K. *Proc. Natl. Acad. Sci. U. S. A.* **2001**, *98* (8), 4437–4442.
65. Muhiuddin, I. P.; Heathcote, P.; Carter, S.; Purton, S.; Rigby, S. E. J.; Evans, M. C. W. *FEBS Lett.* **2001**, *503* (1), 56–60.
66. Fairclough, W. V.; Forsyth, A.; Evans, M. C. W.; Rigby, S. E. J.; Purton, S.; Heathcote, P. *Biochim. Biophys. Acta - Bioenerg.* **2003**, *1606* (1–3), 43–55.
67. Ramesh, V. M.; Gibasiewicz, K.; Lin, S.; Bingham, S. E.; Webber, A. N. *Biochemistry* **2004**, *43* (5), 1369–1375.
68. Bautista, J. A.; Rappaport, F.; Guergova-Kuras, M.; Cohen, R. O.; Golbeck, J. H.; Wang, J. Y.; Béal, D.; Diner, B. A. *J. Biol. Chem.* **2005**, *280* (20), 20030–20041.
69. Dashdorj, N.; Xu, W.; Cohen, R. O.; Golbeck, J. H.; Savikhin, S. *Biophys. J.* **2005**, *88* (2), 1238–1249.
70. Poluektov, O. G.; Paschenko, S. V; Utschig, L. M.; Lakshmi, K. V; Thurnauer, M. C. *J. Am. Chem. Soc.* **2005**, *127* (34), 11910–11911.
71. Santabarbara, S.; Kuprov, I.; Fairclough, W. V; Purton, S.; Hore, P. J.; Heathcote, P.; Evans, M. C. W. *Biochemistry* **2005**, *44* (6), 2119–2128.
72. Santabarbara, S.; Kuprov, I.; Hore, P. J.; Casal, A.; Heathcote, P.; Evans, M. C. W. *Biochemistry* **2006**, *45* (23), 7389–7403.
73. Ali, K.; Santabarbara, S.; Heathcote, P.; Evans, M. C. W.; Purton, S. *Biochim. Biophys. Acta - Bioenerg.* **2006**, *1757* (12), 1623–1633.
74. Li, Y.; van der Est, A.; Lucas, M. G.; Ramesh, V. M.; Gu, F.; Petrenko, A.; Lin, S.; Webber, A. N.; Rappaport, F.; Redding, K. *Proc. Natl. Acad. Sci. U. S. A.* **2006**, *103* (7), 2144–2149.
75. Giera, W.; Gibasiewicz, K.; Ramesh, V. M.; Lin, S.; Webber, A. *Phys. Chem. Chem. Phys.* **2009**, *11* (25), 5186–5191.
76. Muller, M. G.; Slavov, C.; Luthra, R.; Redding, K. E.; Holzwarth, A. R. *Proc. Natl. Acad. Sci.* **2010**, *107* (9), 4123–4128.
77. Mathis, P.; Sétif, P. *FEBS Lett.* **1988**, *237* (1–2), 65–68.
78. Sétif, P.; Brettel, K. *Biochemistry* **1993**, *32* (31), 7846–7854.
79. Badura, A.; Kothe, T.; Schuhmann, W.; Rögner, M. *Energy Environ. Sci.* **2011**, *4* (9), 3263–3274.
80. Wang, F.; Liu, X.; Willner, I. *Adv. Mater.* **2013**, *25* (3), 349–377.
81. Nguyen, K.; Bruce, B. D. *Biochim. Biophys. Acta - Bioenerg.* **2014**, *1837* (9), 1553–1566.
82. Yehezkeli, O.; Tel-Vered, R.; Michaeli, D.; Willner, I.; Nechushtai, R. *Photosynth. Res.* **2014**, *120* (1–2), 71–85.

83. Ravi, S. K.; Tan, S. C. *Energy Environ. Sci.* **2015**, *8* (9), 2551–2573.
84. Iwuchukwu, I. J.; Vaughn, M.; Myers, N.; O'Neill, H.; Frymier, P.; Bruce, B. D. *Nat. Nanotechnol.* **2010**, *5* (1), 73–79.
85. Leblanc, G.; Chen, G.; Jennings, G. K.; Cliffel, D. E. *Langmuir* **2012**, *28* (21), 7952–7956.
86. Zhao, F.; Conzuelo, F.; Hartmann, V.; Li, H.; Nowaczyk, M. M.; Plumeré, N.; Rögner, M.; Schuhmann, W. *J. Phys. Chem. B* **2015**, *119* (43), 13726–13731.
87. Kim, Y.; Shin, D.; Chang, W. J.; Jang, H. L.; Lee, C. W.; Lee, H. E.; Nam, K. T. *Adv. Funct. Mater.* **2015**, *25* (16), 2369–2377.
88. Ihara, M.; Nakamoto, H.; Kamachi, T.; Okura, I.; Maeda, M. *Photochem. Photobiol.* **2006**, *82* (6), 1677–1685.
89. Ihara, M.; Nishihara, H.; Yoon, K.; Lenz, O.; Friedrich, B.; Nakamoto, H.; Kojima, K.; Honma, D.; Kamachi, T.; Okura, I. *Photochem. Photobiol.* **2006**, *82* (3), 676–682.
90. Krassen, H.; Schwarze, A.; Friedrich, B.; Ataka, K.; Lenz, O.; Heberle, J. *ACS Nano* **2009**, *3* (12), 4055–4061.
91. Schwarze, A.; Kopczak, M. J.; Rogner, M.; Lenz, O. *Appl. Environ. Microbiol.* **2010**, *76* (8), 2641–2651.
92. Lubner, C. E.; Grimme, R.; Bryant, D. A.; Golbeck, J. H. *Biochemistry* **2010**, *49* (3), 404–414.
93. Lubner, C. E.; Knörzer, P.; Silva, P. J. N.; Vincent, K. A.; Happe, T.; Bryant, D. A.; Golbeck, J. H. *Biochemistry* **2010**, *49* (48), 10264–10266.
94. Lubner, C. E.; Applegate, A. M.; Knorzer, P.; Ganago, A.; Bryant, D. A.; Happe, T.; Golbeck, J. H. *Proc. Natl. Acad. Sci.* **2011**, *108* (52), 20988–20991.
95. Ducat, D. C.; Sachdeva, G.; Silver, P. A. *Proc. Natl. Acad. Sci. U. S. A.* **2011**, *108* (10), 3941–3946.
96. Yacoby, I.; Pochekailov, S.; Toporik, H.; Ghirardi, M. L.; King, P. W.; Zhang, S. *Proc. Natl. Acad. Sci.* **2011**, *108* (23), 9396–9401.
97. Utschig, L. M.; Soltau, S. R.; Tiede, D. M. *Curr. Opin. Chem. Biol.* **2015**, *25*, 1–8.
98. Ciornii, D.; Feifel, S. C.; Hejazi, M.; Kölsch, A.; Lokstein, H.; Zouni, A.; Lisdat, F. *Phys. Status Solidi Appl. Mater. Sci.* **2017**, *214* (9), 1700017.
99. Simmerman, R. F.; Zhu, T.; Baker, D. R.; Wang, L.; Mishra, S. R.; Lundgren, C. A.; Bruce, B. D. *Bioconjug. Chem.* **2015**, *26* (10), 2097–2105.
100. Zhao, F.; Plumeré, N.; Nowaczyk, M. M.; Ruff, A.; Schuhmann, W.; Conzuelo, F. *Small* **2017**, *13* (26), 1–8.
101. Kato, Y.; Tsujii, M.; Watanabe, T. *Electrochemistry* **2011**, *79*, 845–847.
102. Terasaki, N.; Yamamoto, N.; Hiraga, T.; Yamanoi, Y.; Yonezawa, T.; Nishihara, H.; Ohmori, T. et al. *Angew. Chemie - Int. Ed.* **2009**, *48* (9), 1585–1587.
103. Yehezkeli, O.; Tel-Vered, R.; Michaeli, D.; Nechushtai, R.; Willner, I. *Small* **2013**, *9* (17), 2970–2978.
104. Efrati, A.; Yehezkeli, O.; Tel-Vered, R.; Michaeli, D.; Nechushtai, R.; Willner, I. *ACS Nano* **2012**, *6* (10), 9258–9266.
105. Le, R. K.; Raeeszadeh-Sarmazdeh, M.; Boder, E. T.; Frymier, P. D. *Langmuir* **2015**, *31* (3), 1180–1188.
106. Saboe, P. O.; Lubner, C. E.; McCool, N. S.; Vargas-Barbosa, N. M.; Yan, H.; Chan, S.; Ferlez, B.; Bazan, G. C.; Golbeck, J. H.; Kumar, M. *Adv. Mater.* **2014**, *26* (41), 7064–7069.
107. Shah, V. B.; Henson, W. R.; Chadha, T. S.; Lakin, G.; Liu, H.; Blankenship, R. E.; Biswas, P. *Langmuir* **2015**, *31* (5), 1675–1682.
108. Yu, D.; Wang, M.; Zhu, G.; Ge, B.; Liu, S.; Huang, F. *Sci. Rep.* **2015**, *5*, 1–9.
109. Carter, J. R.; Baker, D. R.; Witt, T. A.; Bruce, B. D. *Photosynth. Res.* **2016**, *127* (2), 161–170.
110. Beam, J. C.; LeBlanc, G.; Gizzie, E. A.; Ivanov, B. L.; Needell, D. R.; Shearer, M. J.; Jennings, G. K.; Lukehart, C. M.; Cliffel, D. E. *Langmuir* **2015**, *31* (36), 10002–10007.

111. LeBlanc, G.; Gizzie, E.; Yang, S.; Cliffel, D. E.; Jennings, G. K. *Langmuir* **2014**, *30* (37), 10990–11001.

112. Gizzie, E. A.; Scott Niezgoda, J.; Robinson, M. T.; Harris, A. G.; Kane Jennings, G.; Rosenthal, S. J.; Cliffel, D. E. *Energy Environ. Sci.* **2015**, *8* (12), 3572–3576.

113. Toporik, H.; Carmeli, I.; Volotsenko, I.; Molotskii, M.; Rosenwaks, Y.; Carmeli, C.; Nelson, N. *Adv. Mater.* **2012**, *24* (22), 2988–2991.

114. Peters, K.; Lokupitiya, H. N.; Sarauli, D.; Labs, M.; Pribil, M.; Rathouský, J.; Kuhn, A.; Leister, D.; Stefik, M.; Fattakhova-Rohlfing, D. *Adv. Funct. Mater.* **2016**, *26* (37), 6682–6692.

115. Janna Olmos, J. D.; Becquet, P.; Gront, D.; Sar, J.; Dąbrowski, A.; Gawlik, G.; Teodorczyk, M.; Pawlak, D.; Kargul, J. *RSC Adv.* **2017**, *7* (75), 47854–47866.

116. Szalkowski, M.; Janna Olmos, J. D.; Buczyńska, D.; Maćkowski, S.; Kowalska, D.; Kargul, J. *Nanoscale* **2017**, *9* (29), 10475–10486.

117. Kirchhofer, N. D.; Rasmussen, M. A.; Dahlquist, F. W.; Minteer, S. D.; Bazan, G. C. *Energy Environ. Sci.* **2015**, *8* (9), 2698–2706.

118. Frolov, L.; Rosenwaks, Y.; Carmeli, C.; Carmeli, I. *Adv. Mater.* **2005**, *17* (20), 2434–2437.

119. Frolov, L.; Rosenwaks, Y.; Richter, S.; Carmeli, C.; Carmeli, I. *J. Phys. Chem. C* **2008**, *112* (35), 13426–13430.

120. Carmeli, I.; Mangold, M.; Frolov, L.; Zebli, B.; Carmeli, C.; Richter, S.; Holleitner, A. W. *Adv. Mater.* **2007**, *19* (22), 3901–3905.

121. Mershin, A.; Matsumoto, K.; Kaiser, L.; Yu, D.; Vaughn, M.; Nazeeruddin, M. K.; Bruce, B. D.; Graetzel, M.; Zhang, S. *Sci. Rep.* **2012**, *2*, 1–7.

122. Deisenhofer, J.; Epp, O.; Miki, K.; Huber, R.; Michel, H. *J. Mol. Biol.* **1984**, *180* (2), 385–398.

123. Deisenhofer, J.; Epp, O.; Miki, K.; Huber, R.; Michel, H. *Nature* **1985**, *318* (6047), 618–624.

124. Deisenhofer, J.; Epp, O.; Sinning, I.; Michel, H. *J. Mol. Biol.* **1995**, *246* (3), 429–457.

125. Allen, J. P.; Feher, G.; Yeates, T. O.; Rees, D. C.; Deisenhofer, J.; Michel, H.; Huber, R. *Proc. Natl. Acad. Sci. U. S. A.* **1986**, *83* (22), 8589–8593.

126. Allen, J. P.; Feher, G.; Yeates, T. O.; Komiya, H.; Rees, D. C. *Proc. Natl. Acad. Sci. U. S. A.* **1987**, *84* (17), 6162–6166.

127. Allen, J. P.; Feher, G.; Yeates, T. O.; Komiya, H.; Rees, D. C. *Proc. Natl. Acad. Sci. U. S. A.* **1987**, *84* (August), 5730–5734.

128. Allen, J. P.; Feher, G.; Yeates, T. O.; Komiya, H.; Rees, D. C. *Proc. Natl. Acad. Sci. U. S. A.* **1988**, *85* (5), 8487–8491.

129. Yeates, T. O.; Komiya, H.; Chirino, A.; Rees, D. C.; Allen, J. P.; Feher, G. *Proc. Natl. Acad. Sci. U. S. A.* **1988**, *85*, 7993–7997.

130. Chang, C. H.; El-Kabbani, O.; Tiede, D.; Norris, J.; Schiffer, M. *Biochemistry* **1991**, *30* (22), 5352–5360.

131. Ermler, U.; Fritzsch, G.; Buchanan, S. K.; Michel, H. *Structure* **1994**, *2* (10), 925–936.

132. Ermler, U.; Michel, H.; Schiffer, M. *J. Bioenerg. Biomembr.* **1994**, *26* (1), 5–15.

133. Woodbury, N. W.; Allen, J. P., Ed. R. E. Blankenship, M. T. Madigan and C. E. Bauer, *Advances in Photosynthesis* **1995**, *2*, 527–557.

134. Kellog, E. C.; Kolaczkowski; Wasielewski, M. R.; Tiede, D. M. *Photosynth. Res.* **1989**, *22*, 47–59.

135. Heller, B. A.; Holten, D.; Kirmaier, C. *Science* **1995**, *269*, 940–945.

136. Axelrod, H. L.; Okamura, M. Y. *Photosynth. Res.* **2005**, *85*, 101–114.

137. Pogorelov, T. V; Autenrieth, F.; Roberts, E.; Luthey-Schulten, Z. A. *J. Phys. Chem. B* **2007**, *111* (3), 618–634.

138. Okamura, M. Y.; Paddock, M. L.; Graige, M. S.; Feher, G. *Biochim. Biophys. Acta - Bioenerg.* **2000**, *1458* (1), 148–163.

139. Wraight, C. A. *Biophysics (Oxf)* **2004**, *9*, 309–337.

140. Wraight, C. A.; Gunner, M. R., Ed. C.N. Hunter, F. Daldal, M. C. Thurnauer, J. T. Beatty. **2009**, *28*, 379–405.

141. Wakeham, M. C.; Jones, M. R. *Biochem. Soc. Trans.* **2005**, *33* (Pt 4), 851–857.

142. Kressel, L.; Faries, K. M.; Wander, M. J.; Zogzas, C. E.; Mejdrich, R. J.; Hanson, D. K.; Holten, D.; Laible, P. D.; Kirmaier, C. *Biochim. Biophys. Acta - Bioenerg.* **2014**, *1837* (11), 1892–1903.

143. Faries, K. M.; Kressel, L. L.; Dylla, N. P.; Wander, M. J.; Hanson, D. K.; Holten, D.; Laible, P. D.; Kirmaier, C. *Biochim. Biophys. Acta - Bioenerg.* **2016**, *1857* (2), 150–159.

144. Hunte, C.; Palsdottir, H.; Trumpower, B. L. *FEBS Lett.* **2003**, *545* (1), 39–46.

145. Crofts, A. R. *Annu. Rev. Physiol.* **2004**, *66* (1), 689–733.

146. Xia, D.; Esser, L.; Tang, W.-K.; Zhou, F.; Zhou, Y.; Yu, L.; Yu, C. *Biochim Biophys Acta.* **2013**, *1827*, 1278–1294.

147. Mitchell, P. *FEBS Lett.* **1975**, *56* (1), 1–6.

148. Crofts, A. R.; Meinhardt, S. W.; Jones, K. R.; Snozzi, M. *BBA - Bioenerg.* **1983**, *723* (2), 202–218.

149. Trumpower, B. L. *J. Biol. Chem.* **1990**, *265* (20), 11409–11412.

150. Ortega, J. M.; Mathis, P. *Biochemistry* **1993**, *32* (4), 1141–1151.

151. Verméglio, A.; Nagashima, S.; Alric, J.; Arnoux, P.; Nagashima, K. V. P. *Biochim. Biophys. Acta - Bioenerg.* **2012**, *1817* (5), 689–696.

152. Den Hollander, M. J.; Magis, J. G.; Fuchsenberger, P.; Aartsma, T. J.; Jones, M. R.; Frese, R. N. *Langmuir* **2011**, *27* (16), 10282–10294.

153. Stanley, R. J.; King, B.; Boxer, S. G. *J. Phys. Chem.* **1996**, *100* (29), 12052–12059.

154. Arnett, D. C.; Moser, C. C.; Dutton, P. L.; Scherer, N. F. *J. Phys. Chem. B* **1999**, *103* (11), 2014–2032.

155. King, B. A.; McAnaney, T. B.; DeWinter, A.; Boxer, S. G. *J. Phys. Chem. B* **2000**, *104* (37), 8895–8902.

156. Hu, X.; Damjanovi, A.; Ritz, T.; Schulten, K. *Comput. Biomol. Sci.* **1998**, *95* (May), 5935–5941.

157. Hu, X.; Ritz, T.; Damjanović, A.; Autenrieth, F.; Schulten, K. *Q. Rev. Biophys.* **2002**, *35* (1), 1–62.

158. Verméglio, A.; Joliot, P. *Trends Microbiol.* **1999**, *7* (11), 435–440.

159. Law, C. J.; Roszak, A. W.; Southall, J.; Gardiner, A. T.; Isaacs, N. W.; Cogdell, R. J. *Mol. Membr. Biol.* **2004**, *21* (3), 183–191.

160. Scheuring, S.; Lévy, D.; Rigaud, J. L. *Biochim. Biophys. Acta - Biomembr.* **2005**, *1712* (2), 109–127.

161. Cogdell, R. J.; Gall, A.; Köhler, J. *Q. Rev. Biophys.* **2006**, *39* (3), 227–324.

162. Scheuring, S. *Curr. Opin. Chem. Biol.* **2006**, *10* (5), 387–393.

163. Sener, M. K.; Olsen, J. D.; Hunter, C. N.; Schulten, K. *Proc. Natl. Acad. Sci. U. S. A.* **2007**, *104* (40), 15723–15728.

164. Sturgis, J. N.; Niederman, R. A. *Photosynth. Res.* **2008**, *95* (2–3), 269–278.

165. Scheuring, S.; Sturgis, J. N. *Photosynth. Res.* **2009**, *102* (2), 197–211.

166. Fleming, G. R.; van Grondellet, R. *Curr. Opin. Struct. Biol.* **1997**, *7* (5), 738–748.

167. Roszak, A. W.; Howard, T. D.; Southall, J.; Gardiner, A. T.; Law, C. J.; Isaacs, N. W.; Cogdell, R. J. *Science* **2003**, *302* (December), 1969–1972.

168. Qian, P.; Hunter, C. N.; Bullough, P. A. *J. Mol. Biol.* **2005**, *349* (5), 948–960.

169. Qian, P.; Bullough, P. A.; Hunter, C. N. *J. Biol. Chem.* **2008**, *283* (20), 14002–14011.

170. Qian, P.; Papiz, M. Z.; Jackson, P. J.; Brindley, A. A.; Ng, I. W.; Olsen, J. D.; Dickman, M. J.; Bullough, P. A.; Hunter, C. N. *Biochemistry* **2013**, *52* (43), 7575–7585.

171. Niwa, S.; Yu, L. J.; Takeda, K.; Hirano, Y.; Kawakami, T.; Wang-Otomo, Z. Y.; Miki, K. *Nature* **2014**, *508* (7495), 228–232.

172. Francia, F.; Wang, J.; Venturoli, G.; Melandri, B. A.; Barz, W. P.; Oesterhelt, D. *Biochemistry* **1999**, *38* (21), 6834–6845.

173. Jungas, C.; Ranck, J.; Rigaud, J.; Joliot, P.; Vermé Glio, A. *EMBO J.* **1999**, *18* (3), 534–542.

174. Siebert, C. A.; Qian, P.; Fotiadis, D.; Engel, A.; Hunter, C. N.; Bullough, P. A. *EMBO J.* **2004**, *23* (4), 690–700.

175. Scheuring, S.; Francia, F.; Busselez, J.; Melandri, B. A.; Rigaud, J. L.; Lévy, D. *J. Biol. Chem.* **2004**, *279* (5), 3620–3626.

176. Bahatyrova, S.; Frese, R. N.; Siebert, C. A.; Olsen, J. D.; Van Der Werf, K. O.; Van Grondelle, R.; Niederman, R. A.; Bullough, P. A.; Otto, C.; Hunter, C. N. *Nature* **2004**, *430* (7003), 1058–1062.

177. Holden-Dye, K.; Crouch, L. I.; Jones, M. R. *Biochim. Biophys. Acta - Bioenerg.* **2008**, *1777* (7–8), 613–630.

178. D'Haene, S. E.; Crouch, L. I.; Jones, M. R.; Frese, R. N. *Biochim. Biophys. Acta - Bioenerg.* **2014**, *1837* (10), 1665–1673.

179. Kropacheva, T. N.; Hoff, A. J. *J. Phys. Chem. B* **2001**, *105* (23), 5536–5545.

180. Noy, D.; Moser, C. C.; Dutton, P. L. *Biochim. Biophys. Acta - Bioenerg.* **2006**, *1757* (2), 90–105.

181. Lu, Y.; Yuan, M.; Liu, Y.; Tu, B.; Xu, C.; Liu, B.; Zhao, D.; Kong, J. *Langmuir* **2005**, *21* (9), 4071–4076.

182. Ham, M. H.; Choi, J. H.; Boghossian, A. A.; Jeng, E. S.; Graff, R. A.; Heller, D. A.; Chang, A. C. et al. *Nat. Chem.* **2010**, *2* (11), 929–936.

183. Swainsbury, D. J. K.; Friebe, V. M.; Frese, R. N.; Jones, M. R. *Biosens. Bioelectron.* **2014**, *58*, 172–178.

184. Caterino, R.; Csiki, R.; Lyuleeva, A.; Pfisterer, J.; Wiesinger, M.; Janssens, S. D.; Haenen, K.; Cattani-Scholz, A.; Stutzmann, M.; Garrido, J. A. *ACS Appl. Mater. Interfaces* **2015**, *7* (15), 8099–8107.

185. Gebert, J.; Reiner-Rozman, C.; Steininger, C.; Nedelkovski, V.; Nowak, C.; Wraight, C. A.; Naumann, R. L. C. *J. Phys. Chem. C* **2015**, *119* (2), 890–895.

186. Szabó, T.; Nyerki, E.; Tóth, T.; Cseko, R.; Magyar, M.; Horváth, E.; Hernádi, K. et al. *Phys. Status Solidi Basic Res.* **2015**, *252* (11), 2614–2619.

187. Friebe, V. M.; Millo, D.; Swainsbury, D. J. K.; Jones, M. R.; Frese, R. N. *ACS Appl. Mater. Interfaces* **2017**, *9* (28), 23379–23388.

188. Takshi, A.; Yaghoubi, H.; Wang, J.; Jun, D.; Beatty, J. T. *Biosensors* **2017**, *7* (2), 1–7.

189. Yaghoubi, H.; Schaefer, M.; Yaghoubi, S.; Jun, D.; Schlaf, R.; Beatty, J. T.; Takshi, A. A. *Nanotechnology* **2017**, *28* (5).

190. Yaghoubi, H.; Lafalce, E.; Jun, D.; Jiang, X.; Beatty, J. T.; Takshi, A. *Biomacromolecules* **2015**, *16* (4), 1112–1118.

191. Friebe, V. M.; Delgado, J. D.; Swainsbury, D. J. K.; Gruber, J. M.; Chanaewa, A.; Grondelle, R. Van; Hauff, E. Von; Millo, D.; Jones, M. R.; Frese, R. N. *Adv. Funct. Mater.* **2016**, *26* (2), 285–292.

192. Tan, S. C.; Crouch, L. I.; Mahajan, S.; Jones, M. R.; Welland, M. E. *ACS Nano* **2012**, *6* (10), 9103–9109.

193. Tan, S. C.; Crouch, L. I.; Jones, M. R.; Welland, M. *Angew. Chemie - Int. Ed.* **2012**, *51* (27), 6667–6671.

194. Tan, S. C.; Yan, F.; Crouch, L. I.; Robertson, J.; Jones, M. R.; Welland, M. E. *Adv. Funct. Mater.* **2013**, *23* (44), 5556–5563.

195. Singh, V. K.; Ravi, S. K.; Ho, J. W.; Wong, J. K. C.; Jones, M. R.; Tan, S. C. *Adv. Funct. Mater.* **2017**, *1703689*, 1–8.

196. Ravi, S. K.; Swainsbury, D. J. K.; Singh, V. K.; Ngeow, Y. K.; Jones, M. R.; Tan, S. C. A. *Adv. Mater.* **2018**, *30* (5), 1–8.

197. Ravi, S. K.; Yu, Z.; Swainsbury, D. J. K.; Ouyang, J.; Jones, M. R.; Tan, S. C. *Adv. Energy Mater.* **2017**, *7* (7), 1–7.

198. Das, R.; Kiley, P. J.; Segal, M.; Norville, J.; Yu, A. A.; Wang, L.; Trammell, S. A. et al. *Nano Lett.* **2004**, *4* (6), 1079–1083.

199. Trammell, S. A.; Griva, I.; Spano, A.; Tsoi, S.; Tender, L. M.; Schnur, J.; Lebedev, N. *J. Phys. Chem. C* **2007**, *111* (45), 17122–17130.

200. Lebedev, N.; Trammell, S. A.; Tsoi, S.; Spano, A.; Kim, J. H.; Xu, J.; Twigg, M. E.; Schnur, J. M. *Langmuir* **2008**, *24* (16), 8871–8876.

201. Kondo, M.; Iida, K.; Dewa, T.; Tanaka, H.; Ogawa, T.; Nagashima, S.; Nagashima, K. V. P. et al. *Biomacromolecules* **2012**, *13* (2), 432–438.

202. Kamran, M.; Delgado, J. D.; Friebe, V.; Aartsma, T. J.; Frese, R. N. *Biomacromolecules* **2014**, *15* (8), 2833–2838.

203. Suemori, Y.; Nagata, M.; Nakamura, Y.; Nakagawa, K.; Okuda, A.; Inagaki, J. I.; Shinohara, K. et al. *Photosynth. Res.* **2006**, *90* (1), 17–21.

204. Kondo, M.; Nakamura, Y.; Fujii, K.; Nagata, M.; Suemori, Y.; Dewa, T.; Iida, K.; Gardiner, A. T.; Cogdell, R. J.; Nango, M. *Biomacromolecules* **2007**, *8* (8), 2457–2463.

205. Sumino, A.; Dewa, T.; Sasaki, N.; Kondo, M.; Nango, M. *J. Phys. Chem. Lett.* **2013**, *4* (7), 1087–1092.

206. Ogawa, M.; Shinohara, K.; Nakamura, Y.; Suemori, Y.; Nagata, M.; Iida, K.; Gardiner, A. T.; Cogdell, R. J.; Nango, M. *Chem. Lett.* **2004**, *33*, 772–773.

207. Suemori, Y.; Fujii, K.; Ogawa, M.; Nakamura, Y.; Shinohara, K.; Nakagawa, K.; Nagata, M. et al. *Colloids Surf. B Biointerfaces* **2007**, *56* (1–2), 182–187.

208. Magis, G. J.; den Hollander, M. J.; Onderwaater, W. G.; Olsen, J. D.; Hunter, C. N.; Aartsma, T. J.; Frese, R. N. *Biochim. Biophys. Acta - Biomembr.* **2010**, *1798* (3), 637–645.

209. Harrold, J. W.; Woronowicz, K.; Lamptey, J. L.; Awong, J.; Baird, J.; Moshar, A.; Vittadello, M.; Falkowski, P. G.; Niederman, R. A. *J. Phys. Chem. B* **2013**, *117* (38), 11249–11259.

210. Mahmoudzadeh, A.; Saer, R.; Jun, D.; Mirvakili, S. M.; Takshi, A.; Iranpour, B.; Ouellet, E.; Lagally, E. T.; Madden, J. D. W.; Beatty, J. T. *Smart Mater. Struct.* **2011**, *20* (9), 94019.

211. Friebe, V. M.; Swainsbury, D. J. K.; Fyfe, P. K.; van der Heijden, W.; Jones, M. R.; Frese, R. N. *Biochim. Biophys. Acta - Bioenerg.* **2016**, *1857* (12), 1925–1934.

212. Kamran, M.; Friebe, V. M.; Delgado, J. D.; Aartsma, T. J.; Frese, R. N.; Jones, M. R. *Nat. Commun.* **2015**, *6*, 1–9.

213. Lu, Y.; Xu, J.; Liu, Y.; Liu, B.; Xu, C.; Zhao, D.; Kong, J. *Chem. Commun.* **2006**, No. 7, 785.

214. Xu, J.; Lu, Y.; Liu, B.; Xu, C.; Kong, J. *J. Solid State Electrochem.* **2007**, *11* (12), 1689–1695.

215. Kern, J. Renger, G. *Photosynth. Res.* **2007**, *94* (2–3), 183–202.

216. Rappaport, F.; Diner, B. A. *Coord. Chem. Rev.* **2008**, *252* (3–4), 259–272.

217. Renger, G.; Renger, T. *Photosynth. Res.* **2008**, *98* (1–3), 53–80.

218. Renger, T.; Schlodder, E. *ChemPhysChem* **2010**, *11* (6), 1141–1153.

219. Renger, T.; Schlodder, E. *J. Photochem. Photobiol. B Biol.* **2011**, *104* (1–2), 126–141.

220. Cardona, T.; Sedoud, A.; Cox, N.; Rutherford, A. W. *Biochim. Biophys. Acta - Bioenerg.* **2012**, *1817* (1), 26–43.

221. Müh, F.; Glöckner, C.; Hellmich, J.; Zouni, A. *Biochim. Biophys. Acta - Bioenerg.* **2012**, *1817* (1), 44–65.

222. Barber, J. *Q. Rev. Biophys.* **2016**, *49*, e14.

223. Zouni, A.; Witt, H. T.; Kern, J.; Fromme, P.; Krauss, N.; Saenger, W.; Orth, P. *Cryst. Nature* **2001**, *409* (1988), 739–743.

224. Kamiya, N.; Shen, J.-R. *Proc. Natl. Acad. Sci.* **2003**, *100* (1), 98–103.

225. Ferreira, K. N.; Iverson, T. M.; Maghlaoui, K.; Barber, J.; Iwata, S. *Science* **2004**, *303* (5665), 1831–1838.

226. Biesiadka, J.; Loll, B.; Kern, J.; Irrgang, K.-D.; Zouni, A. *Phys. Chem. Chem. Phys.* **2004**, *6* (20), 4733–4736.

227. Loll, B.; Kern, J.; Saenger, W.; Zouni, A.; Biesiadka, J. *Nature* **2005**, *438* (7070), 1040–1044.

228. Umena, Y.; Kawakami, K.; Shen, J. R.; Kamiya, N. *Nature* **2011**, *473* (7345), 55–60.

229. Suga, M.; Akita, F.; Hirata, K.; Ueno, G.; Murakami, H.; Nakajima, Y.; Shimizu, T. et al. *Nature* **2014**, *517* (7532), 99–103.

230. Guskov, A.; Kern, J.; Gabdulkhakov, A.; Broser, M.; Zouni, A.; Saenger, W. *Nat. Struct. Mol. Biol.* **2009**, *16* (3), 334–342.

231. Broser, M.; Gabdulkhakov, A.; Kern, J.; Guskov, A.; Müh, F.; Saenger, W.; Zouni, A. *J. Biol. Chem.* **2010**, *285* (34), 26255–26262.

232. Broser, M.; Glöckner, C.; Gabdulkhakov, A.; Guskov, A.; Buchta, J.; Kern, J.; Müh, F.; Dau, H.; Saenger, W.; Zouni, A. *J. Biol. Chem.* **2011**, *286* (18), 15964–15972.

233. Hellmich, J.; Bommer, M.; Burkhardt, A.; Ibrahim, M.; Kern, J.; Meents, A.; Müh, F.; Dobbek, H.; Zouni, A. *Structure* **2014**, *22*, 1607–1615.

234. Ayyer, K.; Yefanov, O. M.; Oberthür, D.; Roy-Chowdhury, S.; Galli, L.; Mariani, V.; Basu, S. et al. *Nature* **2016**, *530* (7589), 202–206.

235. Young, I. D.; Ibrahim, M.; Chatterjee, R.; Gul, S.; Fuller, F. D.; Koroidov, S.; Brewster, A. S. et al. *Nature* **2016**, *540* (7633), 453–457.

236. Kawakami, K.; Umena, Y.; Kamiya, N.; Shen, J.-R. *Proc. Natl. Acad. Sci.* **2009**, *106* (21), 8567–8572.

237. Koua, F. H. M.; Umena, Y.; Kawakami, K.; Shen, J.-R. *Proc. Natl. Acad. Sci.* **2013**, *110* (10), 3889–3894.

238. Tanaka, A.; Fukushima, Y.; Kamiya, N. *J. Am. Chem. Soc.* **2017**, *139* (5), 1718–1721.

239. Suga, M.; Akita, F.; Sugahara, M.; Kubo, M.; Nakajima, Y.; Nakane, T.; Yamashita, K. et al. *Nature* **2017**, *543* (7643), 131–135.

240. Ago, H.; Adachi, H.; Umena, Y.; Tashiro, T.; Kawakami, K.; Tian, N. K. L.; Han, G. et al. *J. Biol. Chem.* **2016**, *291* (11), 5676–5687.

241. Olson, J. M.; Blankenship, R. E. *Photosynth. Res.* **2004**, *80* (1–3), 373–386.

242. Van Amerongen, H.; Croce, R. *Photosynth. Res.* **2013**, *116* (2–3), 251–263.

243. Barber, J.; Archer, M. D. *J. Photochem. Photobiol. A Chem.* **2001**, *142* (2), 97–106.

244. Durrant, J. R.; Klug, D. R.; Kwa, S. L.; van Grondelle, R.; Porter, G.; Dekker, J. P. A. *Proc. Natl. Acad. Sci. U. S. A.* **1995**, *92* (May), 4798–4802.

245. Dekker, J. P.; van Grondelle, R. *Photosynth. Res.* **2000**, *63* (3), 195–208.

246. Barber, J.; Anderson, B. *Trends Biochem. Sci.* **1992**, *17* (2), 61–66.

247. Niyogi, K. K. *Annu. Rev. Plant Physiol. Plant Mol. Biol.* **1999**, *50* (1), 333–359.

248. Nixon, P. J.; Michoux, F.; Yu, J.; Boehm, M.; Komenda, J. *Ann. Bot.* **2010**, *106* (1), 1–16.

249. Komenda, J.; Sobotka, R.; Nixon, P. J. *Curr. Opin. Plant Biol.* **2012**, *15* (3), 245–251.

250. Nath, K.; Jajoo, A.; Poudyal, R. S.; Timilsina, R.; Park, Y. S.; Aro, E. M.; Nam, H. G.; Lee, C. H. *FEBS Lett.* **2013**, *587* (21), 3372–3381.

251. Järvi, S.; Suorsa, M.; Aro, E. M. *Biochim. Biophys. Acta - Bioenerg.* **2015**, *1847* (9), 900–909.

252. Aro, E. M.; Virgin, I.; Andersson, B. Photoinhibition of Photosystem II. Inactivation, Protein Damage and Turnover. *BBA - Bioenerg.* **1993**, *1143* (2), 113–134.

253. Badura, A.; Esper, B.; Ataka, K.; Grunwald, C.; Wöll, C.; Kuhlmann, J.; Heberle, J.; Rögner, M. *Photochem. Photobiol.* **2006**, *82* (5), 1385–1390.

254. Badura, A.; Guschin, D.; Esper, B.; Kothe, T.; Neugebauer, S.; Schuhmann, W.; Rögner, M. *Electroanalysis* **2008**, *20* (10), 1043–1047.

255. Hartmann, V.; Kothe, T.; Pöller, S.; El-Mohsnawy, E.; Nowaczyk, M. M.; Plumeré, N.; Schuhmann, W.; Rögner, M. *Phys. Chem. Chem. Phys.* **2014**, *16* (24), 11936–11941.

256. Kato, M.; Cardona, T.; Rutherford, A. W.; Reisner, E. *J. Am. Chem. Soc.* **2012**, *134* (20), 8332–8335.

257. Kato, M.; Cardona, T.; Rutherford, A. W.; Reisner, E. *J. Am. Chem. Soc.* **2013**, *135* (29), 10610–10613.

258. Kothe, T.; Plumeré, N.; Badura, A.; Nowaczyk, M. M.; Guschin, D. A.; Rögner, M.; Schuhmann, W. *Angew. Chemie - Int. Ed.* **2013**, *52* (52), 14233–14236.

259. Maly, J.; Krejci, J.; Ilie, M.; Jakubka, L.; Masojídek, J.; Pilloton, R.; Sameh, K.; Steffan, P.; Stryhal, Z.; Sugiura, M. *Anal. Bioanal. Chem.* **2005**, *381* (8), 1558–1567.

260. Mersch, D.; Lee, C. Y.; Zhang, J. Z.; Brinkert, K.; Fontecilla-Camps, J. C.; Rutherford, A. W.; Reisner, E. *J. Am. Chem. Soc.* **2015**, *137* (26), 8541–8549.

261. Sokol, K. P.; Mersch, D.; Hartmann, V.; Zhang, J. Z.; Nowaczyk, M. M.; Rögner, M.; Ruff, A.; Schuhmann, W.; Plumeré, N.; Reisner, E. *Energy Environ. Sci.* **2016**, *9* (12), 3698–3709.

262. Terasaki, N.; Iwai, M.; Yamamoto, N.; Hiraga, T.; Yamada, S.; Inoue, Y. *Thin Solid Films* **2008**, *516* (9), 2553–2557.

263. Vöpel, T.; Ning Saw, E.; Hartmann, V.; Williams, R.; Müller, F.; Schuhmann, W.; Plumeré, N.; Nowaczyk, M.; Ebbinghaus, S.; Rögner, M. *Biointerphases* **2016**, *11* (1), 19001.

264. Yehezkeli, O.; Tel-Vered, R.; Wasserman, J.; Trifonov, A.; Michaeli, D.; Nechushtai, R.; Willner, I. *Nat. Commun.* **2012**, *3*, 742–747.

265. Zhang, J. Z.; Sokol, K. P.; Paul, N.; Romero, E.; Van Grondelle, R.; Reisner, E. *Nat. Chem. Biol.* **2016**, *12* (12), 1046–1052.

266. Cai, P.; Feng, X.; Fei, J.; Li, G.; Li, J.; Huang, J.; Li, J. *Nanoscale* **2015**, *7* (25), 10908–10911.

267. Li, Z.; Wang, W.; Ding, C.; Wang, Z.; Liao, S.; Li, C. *Energy Environ. Sci.* **2017**, *10* (3), 765–771.

268. Li, G.; Feng, X.; Fei, J.; Cai, P.; Li, J.; Huang, J.; Li, J. *Adv. Mater. Interfaces* **2017**, *4* (1), 1600619.

269. Larom, S.; Kallmann, D.; Saper, G.; Pinhassi, R.; Rothschild, A.; Dotan, H.; Ankonina, G.; Schuster, G.; Adir, N. *Photosynth. Res.* **2015**, *126* (1), 161–169.

270. McEvoy, J. P.; Brudvig, G. W. *Chem. Rev.* **2006**, *106* (11), 4455–4483.

271. Barber, J. *Chem. Soc. Rev.* **2009**, *38* (1), 185–196.

272. Dau, H.; Limberg, C.; Reier, T.; Risch, M.; Roggan, S.; Strasser, P. *ChemCatChem* **2010**, *2* (7), 724–761.

273. Najafpour, M. M.; Renger, G.; Hołyńska, M.; Moghaddam, A. N.; Aro, E. M.; Carpentier, R.; Nishihara, H.; Eaton-Rye, J. J.; Shen, J. R.; Allakhverdiev, S. I. *Chem. Rev.* **2016**, *116* (5), 2886–2936.

274. Askerka, M.; Brudvig, G. W.; Batista, V. S. *Acc. Chem. Res.* **2017**, *50* (1), 41–48.

275. Nocera, D. G. The Artificial Leaf. *Acc. Chem. Res.* **2012**, *45* (5), 767–776.

276. Okamura, M.; Kondo, M.; Kuga, R.; Kurashige, Y.; Yanai, T.; Hayami, S.; Praneeth, V. K. K. et al. *Nature* **2016**, *530* (7591), 465–468.

277. Efrati, A.; Tel-Vered, R.; Michaeli, D.; Nechushtai, R.; Willner, I. *Energy Environ. Sci.* **2013**, *6* (10), 2950–2956.

278. Raszewski, G.; Diner, B. A.; Schlodder, E.; Renger, T. *Biophys. J.* **2008**, *95* (1), 105–119.

279. Groot, M. L.; Pawlowicz, N. P.; van Wilderen, L. J. G. W.; Breton, J.; van Stokkum, I. H. M.; van Grondelle, R. *Proc. Natl. Acad. Sci. U. S. A.* **2005**, *102* (37), 13087–13092.

280. Holzwarth, A. R.; Muller, M. G.; Reus, M.; Nowaczyk, M.; Sander, J.; Rogner, M. *Proc. Natl. Acad. Sci.* **2006**, *103* (18), 6895–6900.

281. Di Donato, M.; Cohen, R. O.; Diner, B. A.; Breton, J.; Van Grondelle, R.; Groot, M. L. *Biophys. J.* **2008**, *94* (12), 4783–4795.

282. Novoderezhkin, V. I.; Dekker, J. P.; Van Grondelley, R. *Biophys. J.* **2007**, *93* (4), 1293–1311.

283. Romero, E.; Van Stokkum, I. H. M.; Novoderezhkin, V. I.; Dekker, J. P.; Van Grondelle, R. *Biochemistry* **2010**, *49* (20), 4300–4307.

284. Diner, B. A.; Schlodder, E.; Nixon, P. J.; Coleman, W. J.; Rappaport, F.; Lavergne, J.; Vermaas, W. F. J.; Chisholm, D. A. *Biochemistry* **2001**, *40* (31), 9265–9281.

285. Shelaev, I. V.; Gostev, F. E.; Nadtochenko, V. A.; Shkuropatov, A. Y.; Zabelin, A. A.; Mamedov, M. D.; Semenov, A. Y.; Sarkisov, O. M.; Shuvalov, V. A. *Photosynth. Res.* **2008**, *98* (1–3), 95–103.
286. Shelaev, I. V; Gostev, F. E.; Vishnev, M. I.; Shkuropatov, A. Y.; Ptushenko, V. V; Mamedov, M. D.; Sarkisov, O. M.; Nadtochenko, V. A.; Semenov, A. Y.; Shuvalov, V. A. *J. Photochem. Photobiol. B* **2011**, *104* (1–2), 44–50.
287. Nadtochenko, V. A.; Semenov, A. Y.; Shuvalov, V. A. *Biochim. Biophys. Acta - Bioenerg.* **2014**, *1837* (9), 1384–1388.
288. Müller, M. G.; Niklas, J.; Lubitz, W.; Holzwarth, A. R. *Biophys. J.* **2003**, *85* (6), 3899–3922.
289. Di Donato, M.; Stahl, A. D.; Van Stokkum, I. H. M.; Grondelle, R. Van; Groot, M. L. *Biochemistry* **2011**, *50* (4), 480–490.
290. Holzwarth, A. R.; Müller, M. G.; Niklas, J.; Lubitz, W. *Biophys. J.* **2006**, *90* (2), 552–565.
291. Shelaev, I. V; Gostev, F. E.; Mamedov, M. D.; Sarkisov, O. M.; Nadtochenko, V. A.; Shuvalov, V. A.; Semenov, A. Y. *Biochim. Biophys. Acta - Bioenerg.* **2010**, *1797* (8), 1410–1420.
292. Semenov, A. Y.; Shelaev, I. V; Gostev, F. E.; Mamedov, M. D.; Shuvalov, V. A.; Sarkisov, O. M.; Nadtochenko, V. A. *Biochem.* **2012**, *77* (9), 1011–1020.
293. Engel, G. S.; Calhoun, T. R.; Read, E. L.; Ahn, T. K.; Mančal, T.; Cheng, Y. C.; Blankenship, R. E.; Fleming, G. R. *Nature* **2007**, *446* (7137), 782–786.
294. Lewis, K. L. M.; Ogilvie, J. P. *J. Phys. Chem. Lett.* **2012**, *3* (4), 503–510.
295. Anna, J. M.; Scholes, G. D.; Van Grondelle, R. *Bioscience* **2014**, *64* (1), 14–25.
296. Fassioli, F.; Dinshaw, R.; Arpin, P. C.; Scholes, G. D. *J. R. Soc. Interface* **2013**, *11* (92), 20130901–20130901.
297. Fuller, F. D.; Pan, J.; Gelzinis, A.; Butkus, V.; Senlik, S. S.; Wilcox, D. E.; Yocum, C. F.; Valkunas, L.; Abramavicius, D.; Ogilvie, J. P. *Nat. Chem.* **2014**, *6* (8), 706–711.
298. Romero, E.; Augulis, R.; Novoderezhkin, V. I.; Ferretti, M.; Thieme, J.; Zigmantas, D.; Van Grondelle, R. *Nat. Phys.* **2014**, *10* (9), 676–682.
299. Scholes, G. D.; Fleming, G. R.; Chen, L. X.; Aspuru-Guzik, A.; Buchleitner, A.; Coker, D. F.; Engel, G. S. et al. *Nature* **2017**, *543* (7647), 647–656.
300. Brédas, J. L.; Sargent, E. H.; Scholes, G. D. *Nat. Mater.* **2016**, *16* (1), 35–44.
301. Romero, E.; Novoderezhkin, V. I.; Van Grondelle, R. *Nature* **2017**, *543* (7645), 355–365.

5 Bio-photoelectrochemical Cells

Protein Immobilization Routes and Electron Transfer Modes

Sai Kishore Ravi, Vishnu Saran Udayagiri,
Anuraj Singh Rawat, and Swee Ching Tan

CONTENTS

5.1 INTRODUCTION

Effectively fixating the proteins onto electrodes is always considered to be vital for optimal performance of any photo-bioelectrochemical cell.[1] Immobilization of the protein complexes also ensures they retain their functions[2] and effectively transfer the electrons from the complexes to the electrodes. One of the biggest problems with protein immobilization in a device environment is the loss/reduction in biological activity.[3] In order to prevent this loss, an artificial environment has to be re-created[3] to match as much as possible the natural setting in which the protein is extracted from. Proteins can be immobilized using physical or chemical methods.[3] Physical methods include adherence to electrode by electrostatic and van der Waals forces. These methods are economic and facile but with one major limitation. Physical means to immobilize proteins create a heterogeneous distribution of proteins that affects the device performance to a great deal.[4] Chemical methods include functionalization on electrode forming strong covalent bonds between the electrode surface and the protein or even coordination bonds. A major concern in these methods is the possibility of chemical conformation changes in the proteins, which affects the performance.[1,5,6] This chapter outlines the different approaches that are in use to integrate/immobilize photosynthetic reaction center (RC) proteins in bio-photoelectrochemical cells.

5.2 IMMOBILIZATION OF RCS: BARE ELECTRODES VS CHEMICAL LINKERS

Starting off with bare electrodes, more complex methods of immobilization such as chemical linking and the usage of nanomaterials emerged. For instance, the Langmuir-Blodgett (LB)[7-9] method was utilized to coat the RCs onto the electrodes as well as control their orientation. The LB technique uses film-forming materials that are insoluble in water.[10] Multiple films are deposited on top of each other in the same arrangement and by repeating the process used to make these films. An artificial lipid bilayer film is then used to coat onto the RCs, immobilizing them; this also provides them with a suitable setting, similar to their initial environment and thus possibly improving their performance.[10,11] Another common method that was used to immobilize the RCs onto the electrode was through the usage of cross linkers that allow the RC to bond with the electrode. These cross linkers allow better covalent bonding between the electrode and the RCs, which makes it possible to functionalize the RC just via physical adsorption.[12] Various physical and chemical methods are being used to attach the RCs onto the electrode surfaces, and each method has its advantages and disadvantages. In order to further enhance the adhesiveness of the RCs onto electrodes, the electrodes were pre-coated with a Self-Assembled Monolayer (SAM)[11,12] that serves as a means to control the orientation and bonding between the RCs and electrode surface. The SAM is prepared using bifunctional reagents that enable the modification and control of the arrangement and orientation of the RCs onto the electrode.[13] In addition to these methods, there were also attempts to immobilize the proteins in a sol-gel or a polymer gel matrix.[14] Another unique method is the usage of electrodes that are fabricated on the nanoscale, which provides greater control and better bonding between the RCs and the surface. This chapter presents the various ways of immobilization of RCs onto the electrodes and recounts the progress made in different systems.

The easiest and most effective form of immobilization was to simply coat the protein onto the bare electrodes, making use of physical adsorption to attach the RCs onto the surface of the electrodes. This method was one of the earliest methods employed to integrate the protein into biohybrid solar cells. In 1980, Janzen and Seibert demonstrated this principle by fabricating a photoelectrochemical cell that consisted of RCs coated onto an SnO_2 sputtered glass electrode.[15] The system consisted of another electrode that was either Pt or SnO_2. The electrolyte that allowed charge transfer to be made possible was 0.1 M Na_2SO_4, and this also contained sufficient amounts of buffer solution.[15] The RCs were immobilized on the electrode via a very simple method of submerging the electrode into an RCs concentrate, and then they were removed and left to be air dried.[15,16] Initially, a platinized platinum-coated glass electrode was used, but this resulted in the backflow of electrons from the electrode to the oxidized RCs. Therefore, to overcome this problem, a SnO_2 semiconductor electrode was used.[15,16] This resulted in a functional setup, giving a photocurrent of about 0.3 µA cm^{-2}, which was achieved when light of wavelengths greater than 600 nm was used.[15] Following this, a secondary experiment was conducted by using antimony-doped SnO_2 as the electrode, and a secondary quinone was also added to the RCs before the electrode was submerged into the solution. This resulted in an output photocurrent of 0.46 µA cm^{-2}. The secondary quinone was added to optimize the kinetics of the electrolytic solution, allowing electron transfer to be more efficient.[16] It also stabilized the charge separation, thus giving more time for the electrons to tunnel through the electrolyte to eventually reach the other electrode.

Physical adsorption of proteins onto the electrodes, though simple and economic, does not provide an effective binding between the electrodes with the proteins, especially when there are multiple layers. Hence, it became important to develop functionalization routes through the usage of chemical linkers, which not only effectively bind the proteins to the electrode but also control their orientation and the charge transfer in the device. One of the most widely known ways to chemically bind proteins to electrodes is by using SAMs. SAMs are similar to conventional surfactant monolayers, apart from the fact that one end of the SAM[13] is engineered to have a favorable contact with the area of interest. This creates a stable, thin monolayer film that remains in the same orientation throughout substrate. Studies have been conducted on biohybrid cells with immobilized RC monolayers on a platinum electrode[17] and pyrolytic graphite[18] electrodes. Further modifications were also done by utilizing organic functional groups. Bifunctional reagent groups with condensed aromatic groups and cysteine thiol groups were used, which showed a large increase in photocurrent produced, due to the optimal orientation of the RCs with the usage of these chemical linkers. Furthermore, there were also attempts on varying bifunctional reagent groups that allowed the RCs to bind to specific sites only.[19,20]

For instance, when aminothiophenol (ATP) was utilized as a linker (Figure 5.1a), the binding site was observed to be the non-heme iron, and electron transfer was observed to be between the non-heme iron and the primary quinone.[21] When the linker was changed to mercaphtoethylamine (MEA), the electron transfer was observed between the primary donor (P) and the bacteriopheophytin (Bphe), and a greater current was observed as compared to using ATP as a linker.[21] The RC-MEA system (Figure 5.1b) generated a photocurrent of 40 nA cm^{-2} while the RC – ATP system generated a photocurrent of 30 nA cm^{-2}.[21] This highlights the fact that the right type of chemical linker is necessary for high photocurrent generation, as the orientation of the RCs will also be more favorable, providing improved electron transfer. Furthermore, the usage of the correct chemical linker will result in better adsorption of the RCs onto the electrode.[22] The RCs exhibited a higher stability when the chemical linker was an amino group-terminated SAM.[22] When the chemical linker utilized carbonyl-terminating SAMs in the same type of setup, the RCs were only partially stable. On the other hand, when the chemical linker had methyl groups as the terminal points, the RCs tended to denature. This further emphasizes the need for the right type of chemical linker, as it greatly affects the orientation of the RCs and thereby the device performance.[22] In addition to the right type of SAMs, the selection of electrolyte and its constituents is also critical. The addition of electron transfer mediators serves to enhance electron transfer in most cases,[17,18]

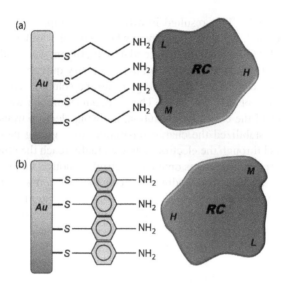

FIGURE 5.1 (a) RC bound to gold electrode by Aminothiophenol (ATP) linker. (b) RC bound to gold electrode by Mercaphtoethylamine (MEA) linker. (The illustration is created, inspired from Zhao, J.Q. et al., *Biosens. Bioelectron.*, 17, 711–718, 2002.)

generating higher levels of photocurrent. Common mediators such as ubiquinone-10, cytochrome *c*, and ferrocene are used for this purpose. The most common approach has been to add two types of transfer mediators, one serving as an electron donor and the other as an acceptor. An example of this is to use ubiquinone-10 and cytochrome *c* in the electrode where the former serves as the electron acceptor and the latter as the electron donor.[23–26]

5.3 IMMOBILIZATION BY ELECTROSTATIC ADSORPTION

Electrostatic adsorption utilizes electrostatic charges to attach the RCs to the electrodes. The RCs are mostly negatively charged and therefore adsorbed onto the electrode after inducing a positive charge on the electrode's surface.[27] Another form of electrostatic adsorption is by linking multiple RC layers by electrostatic forces, but the initial RC layer that is on the electrode surface can be chemically linked.[20] There are two major approaches in improving the performance of the biohybrid cells that utilize electrostatic adsorption. Firstly, increasing the number of RC layers increases the photocurrent. A higher photocurrent is generated when multiple RC layers are used. This stacking of multiple RC layers was achieved by manipulating the pH of the environment to enable the negatively charged RCs to electrostatically adsorb to the positively charged electrolyte, commonly poly(diallyldimethylammoniumchlor ide) (PDDA),[27] and this RC multilayer is then chemically linked to an Au electrode by using a bifunctional reagent, such as 2-mercaptoacetic acid (MAA).[20] A biohybrid cell with 24 layers of RCs generated a photocurrent of 77 nA cm^{-2} as opposed to that with a mono-layered RC electrode, which only generated a photocurrent of 8.5 nA cm^{-2}. This points to the fact that having multiple RC layers increases the photocurrent.

Electrostatic linkage is also possible without the usage of a chemical linker simply by using a charged electrode surface. For instance, a clean quartz electrode whose surface is negatively charged can adsorb a negatively charged RC layer by using the positively charged PDDA like a glue in between. The second approach is to increase the protein loading by integrating the proteins in a sol-gel. The sol is a colloidal or molecular suspension of solid particles of ions in a solvent. The gel is a viscous mass that forms when the solvent from the sol begins to evaporate, and the particles and ions that were initially in that solvent begin to form a continuous network between themselves.[14] Utilizing a sol-gel has been observed to enhance the photocurrent performance of the cell. The RCs were immobilized onto a glassy carbon electrode using an Al_2O_3 sol-gel matrix.[28] This matrix electrostatically adsorbs the negatively charged RCs. Under optimal conditions, photocurrents in the order of a few microamperes were observed.

5.4   EFFECT OF RC ORIENTATION ON CELL PERFORMANCE

Achieving a favorable protein orientation on a bio-photoelectrode has been a prime motive in a number of different reports on biohybrid photoelectrochemical cells. Comparison between two opposite protein orientations has been studied in a device; one device configuration was with a protein's primary donor (P-side) facing the electrode, and the other with the acceptor (H subunit side) facing the electrode (Figure 5.2).[25] The reaction center proteins were immobilized on a carbon-coated gold electrode. In the first configuration, the RC is attached onto the electrode using a

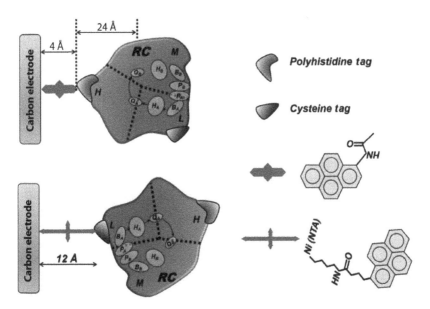

FIGURE 5.2   Two possible orientations of RCs and the respective electron transfer paths between the electrodes and the RCs. (The illustration is created, inspired from Trammell, S.A. et al., *Biosens. Bioelectron.*, 21, 1023–1028, 2006.)

bifunctional agent with one end having an NTA (Nitrilotriacetic acid) group with the Ni^{2+} cation, which enables binding with the His-tag in the RC. The other end of the agent is a pyrene group that is suitable to bind with the carbon-layered gold electrode. In the second configuration, N-(1-pyrene) iodoacetamide was used as the binding agent that forms a link with a cysteine group in the RC.[25] In these two configurations, the mediators Ubiquinone-10 and cytochrome c were used. From this study, two crucial conclusions were drawn. First, the photosynthetic RCs acted like rectifiers, which implies that the photocurrent always flows in the same direction, which is from the primary donor to the primary acceptor. This direction of current flow remains fixed, no matter what orientation is used. This implies that the current will be cathodic if the P side faces the electrode and anodic if the H subunit is oriented onto the electrode.[25] The second conclusion is that the orientation in which the P side is facing the electrode yielded a much higher photocurrent with better current stability compared to the other orientation with the H subunit facing the electrode.[25] A few explanations to this observation were put forth. Any difference in surface area between the two configurations might not be a factor as almost an equal surface coverage was ensured in the experimental conditions.[25] The length of the bifunctional agent used to link H-side to the electrode (4 Å) is shorter than the agent used to link the P-side (12 Å) to the electrode, but the electron transfer rate in the "H-side on electrode" orientation is much lower[25] than that of the "P-side on electrode" configuration. X-ray crystallography studies conducted to understand the protein structure indicate that the total distance between the electrode at the H subunit and the electron acceptor is 28 Å, which includes the length of the H subunit 24 Å and the length of the bifunctional linker 4 Å.[25] There is an estimation that for a change of 20 Å in the distance between the electron donor and electron acceptor there will be a 10^{12} fold change in the electron transfer rate.[29] Therefore, the reason the configuration with the "H-side on electrode" orientation had a lower photocurrent was due to the longer electron tunneling distance from the electrode to the electron acceptors because of the thicker H subunit.[25] Another study by Kondo et al.[30] shows the importance of reducing the distance between the electron acceptor and electrode in which the photoelectrodes were modified with RC-LH1 (extracted from *Rhodopseudomonas palustris*). It was observed that when the proteins were oriented with the H subunit facing the electrode, there was a higher photocurrent compared to the opposite orientation.[30] To further demonstrate the dependence of the electron transfer rate on the distance between the electrode and the electron acceptor,[24] a series of experiments were conducted, using a range of MHisRCs/Ni-NTA SAM/Au photoelectrodes (Figure 5.3), with differing thicknesses of the SAM, where MHisRCs are genetically engineered RCs having a polyhistide tag at the M subunit.

The differing thicknesses were reached by the different number of methylene units (n) in the linking reagent, where n took the value of 3, 6, 10, and 15 in different configurations. To facilitate the electron transfer, the electron acceptor ubiquinone (Q2) and the electron donor cytochrome c were used. The cytochrome c also acted as the conductive wire between the working electrode and the RC's special pair.[24] From photocurrent measurements, it was deduced that the photocurrent is independent of the linker length at short distances of separation between the protein and the electrode, and it reduces by a large deal at larger distances of separation.

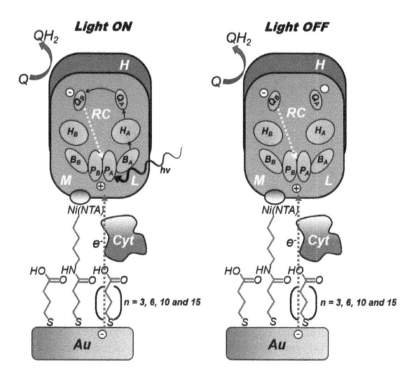

FIGURE 5.3 Electron transfer reactions in RC-Cyt-SAM-Au electrode. (The illustration is created, inspired from Trammell, S.A. et al., *J. Phys. Chem. C*, 111, 17122–17130, 2007.)

A maximum photocurrent of 167 nA cm^{-2} was measured when 7-carboxyheptyl disulphide acid was used as the linking reagent with 6 methylene units. The photocurrent, when a linker with 3 methylene units was used, was 161 nA cm^{-2}, and it was 158 nA cm^{-2} when a linker with 10 methylene units was used. While these were still close to the maximum generated photocurrent, there was a drastic drop in the measured photocurrent (25 nA cm^{-2}) when a linker with 15 methylene units was used. This study emphasizes the importance of the optimizing distance of separation between the RCs and the electrode in order to achieve high photocurrent.[24] These observations are also in good agreement with those reported by Kondo et al.,[30] where the photoelectric current produced by RC-LH1/alkanethiol-SAM/Au photoelectrode varied with the SAM thickness. SAMs of varying linker lengths of alkanethiols $NH_2(CH_2)_nSH$ ($n = 2, 6, 8, 11$) were employed.[30] The maximum photocurrent measured was when a linker of length $n = 6$ was used, and similar to the former study, the photocurrent decreased with increasing linker lengths. In other words, photocurrent decreased with increasing distance of separation between the protein and the electrode. The linker with $n = 6$ had a separation of 1 nm, and when the liker length with $n = 11$ was used, the separation was 2.1 nm.[22] An interesting point to note is that the shortest distance of separation did not necessarily yield the highest photocurrent. The maximum photocurrent measured was not at $n = 2$, as the adsorption of the RCs onto the electrode was poor. The adsorption betters with increasing distance from the electrode but at the same time lowers electron transfer

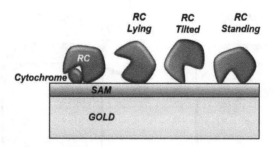

FIGURE 5.4 Different RC orientations with cytochrome c on NTA SAM modified electrode. (The illustration is created, inspired from Lebedev, N. et al., *J. Am. Chem. Soc.*, 128, 12044–12045, 2006.)

rates. Therefore, there is a competition between increasing photocurrents due to stronger adsorption and decreasing photocurrents due to poorer electron transfer rate, as the distance from the electrode is increased. As a trade-off between the two conditions, the maximum current was obtained for the linker length with $n = 6$.

Furthermore, the importance of the cytochrome c in providing a better charge transfer between the RCs and electrodes was also studied. A Ni-NTA SAM-coated gold electrode was used, and the RCs were immobilized onto the electrode with His tagged M subunits[31] (Figure 5.4). When cytochrome c was used, the photocurrent displayed a time-dependent improvement in the photocurrent measured, eventually reaching to a value that was about 20 to 40 fold higher than the initial photocurrent measured with no cytochrome c.[31] When cytochrome c was not added into the system, the RCs were thought to be in one of the three possible orientations (Figure 5.4). In the first, the RC was assumed to lie on the SAM surface.[31] The second orientation was when the RC was oriented in the same way as if cytochrome c was present ("RC tilted" in Figure 5.4). In the last case, the RC was thought to stand on the surface of SAMs and the primary donor attached to the SAM surface.[31] Assuming that all the three cases had the RCs surrounded with water, in the absence of cytochrome c it was found that electron transfer only could occur with the RCs oriented to be close to the standing position.[31] Upon the addition of cytochrome c, a shorter electron tunneling path was provided, along with a more effective electron transfer mechanism, which resulted in an improvement in the photocurrent generated. Therefore, cytochrome c acts as a conductive agent/wire between the RCs and the working electrode. In addition to this study conducted, Mahmoudzadeh et al.,[26] also reported how varying the distances between the RCs and electrodes caused a difference in the measured photocurrent, due to differing electron-transfer mechanism and kinetics.

Besides optimizing photocurrents by chemically tweaking the protein orientations by different SAMs and linkers, the prospects of photocurrent enhancements by specialized protein immobilization by means of genetic modifications in the proteins were also explored. Poly-histidine tags were genetically engineered and attached to different parts of the RCs to preferentially orientate them. To demonstrate the role of genetically modified immobilization route, two different systems were analysed. The first is a "Ni-NTA modified dextran"-coated gold electrode (Figure 5.5) onto which RCs with a hexameric histide tag (His$_6$) bound to the H subunit of the RC

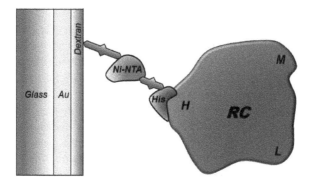

FIGURE 5.5 HHisRC linked to Ni-NTA modified gold electrode. (The illustration is created, inspired from Nakamura, C. et al., Self-assembling photosynthetic reaction centers on electrodes for current generation, *Twenty-First Symposium on Biotechnology for Fuels and Chemicals,* 2000, Springer, pp. 401–408.)

(HHisRC) are attached. The other system had the same His_6 tag attached but to the M subunit of the RC (MHisRC)[32] (Figure 5.6). When light was irradiated on these two systems, the system with HHisRC generated a much larger photocurrent than that with the MHisRC.[32] This proved that the H subunit is more hydrophilic than M, thereby reacting stronger with the hydrophilic dextran-coated gold electrode.[33] This allowed the creation of a more uniform, homogeneous, unidirectional orientation of the HHisRC as compared to the MHisRC. Despite this, even the MHisRC system also generated a modest value of cathodic photocurrent (30 nA cm^{-2}). These early studies proved that genetic modifications in the RCs could indeed affect the efficacy of immobilization and hence the device efficiency.[34,35]

Besides the developments on the various means to attach/immobilize the proteins onto conventional electrode surfaces, there has also been considerable interest in engineering the electrode material itself, rather than just its surface chemistry. RCs have been immobilized onto a nanocrystalline TiO_2 film coated on an ITO-glass (Indium Tin Oxide coated glass) photo electrode, which proved more effective than immobilizing onto a planar electrode.[37] There was a high photocurrent mainly due to

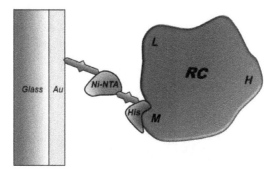

FIGURE 5.6 MHisRC linked to Ni-NTA modified gold electrode. (The illustration is created, inspired from Trammell, S.A. et al., *Biosens. Bioelectron.,* 19, 1649–1655, 2004.)

the increased adsorption of the RCs on the electrode because of the larger surface area available in the nanocrystalline matrix. The immobilization was essentially without the use of any chemical linkers in this case. A photocurrent of 8 μA cm^{-2} was observed in the photoelectrochemical cell with RC-modified nanoporous TiO$_2$ photoelectrode, Pt counter electrode, and a sodium dithionite electrolyte.[36] Further engineering of the electrode was done by introducing WO$_3$ in the electrode. WO$_3$-TiO$_2$ nanoclusters in the photoelectrode yielded a remarkably higher photocurrent compared to that obtained with the individual WO$_3$ and TiO$_2$ photoelectrodes. Immobilization of RCs in the specially designed three-dimensional, wormlike mesoporous WO$_3$-TiO$_2$ photoelectrode enhanced the photocurrent generation (Figure 5.7). The large photocurrent was due to a number of factors, most notably, the good match in the energy levels between WO$_3$-TiO$_2$ and the RCs[36] (Also refer to Section 6.3). The structure of the WO$_3$-TiO$_2$ electrode in a way provided a more compatible environment, preserving the natural function and activity of the RCs akin to their native.

The protein compatibility in the electrode was also favored by the presence of open pores of size ~7 nm, which is equivalent to the dimensions of the RCs and by an ideal hydrophilic surface with the appropriate charge.[11] The photocurrent generated had high stability, showing signs of a decrease in performance by 15% only after a continuous illumination for 1 hour.[11] A similar performance was observed when a thick film (4 μm) of the nanocrystalline porous TiO$_2$ electrode was immobilized with the RCs.[38] The RCs were immobilized/adsorbed onto the electrode by incubating in a solution of RCs for 24 hours. Though there can be photoexcitation and charge carrier generation in an unmodified semiconductor itself, the photocurrent observed with the RC-adsorbed TiO$_2$ was much greater, indicating the additional injection of electrons from RCs into the conduction band of the TiO$_2$ electrode[38] (Also refer to Section 6.4.2). Furthermore, integrating the RCs into the porous electrode also increased the available surface energy states, thereby increasing the number of electron transfer pathways, leading to an increase in the photocurrent generated.

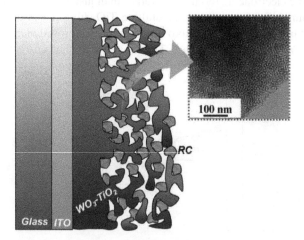

FIGURE 5.7   Immobilization of RCs in a mesoporous WO$_3$-TiO$_2$/ITO electrode. (The illustration is created, inspired from Lu, Y.D. et al., *Langmuir*, 21, 4071–4076, 2005.[36])

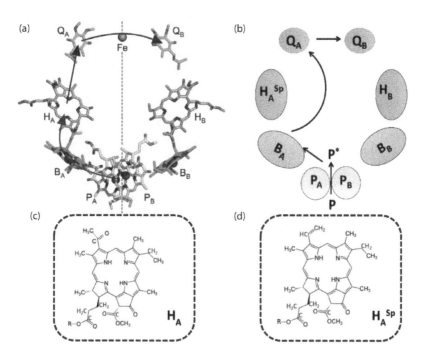

FIGURE 5.8 (a) Electron transfer in native RC (RC_{WT}). (Reproduced with permission from Jones, M.R., *Prog. Lipid Res.*, 46, 56–87, 2007.[41]); (b) Electron transfer in mutant RC (RC_{Phe}); (c) Structure of Bacteriopheophytin. (Adapted from Lu, Y.D. et al., *Chem. Commun.*, 785–787, 2006.); (d) Structure of Pheophytin from Spinach Photosystem. (Adapted from Lu, Y.D. et al., *Chem. Commun.*, 785–787, 2006.) (The illustration is created, inspired from Lu, Y.D. et al., *Chem. Commun.*, 785–787, 2006.)

This adds to the benefit of a high-protein loading capacity,[38] which is an obvious advantage of a nanoporous electrode.

For more effective immobilization in nanoelectrodes, proteins were engineered by pigment substitution. Pigment-exchanged RCs were prepared by replacing the native bacteriopheophytin in the protein with a new pheophytin found in spinach photosystems (Figure 5.8). This was aimed to manipulate the energetics and kinetics of the charge transport process at the protein/semiconductor interface and hence in the overall device. These pigment-substituted RCs are referred to as "RC_{Phe}" (Figure 5.8b). The pigment-exchanged protein exhibited a substantial decrease in the speed of excitation transfer and slower charge separation due to the higher energy level of P^+Phe^- than that of the P^+Bchl^-.[11,39] The natural electron transfer chain of "$P^* \rightarrow B_A \rightarrow H_A \rightarrow Q_A \rightarrow Q_B$" is energetically hindered to a great degree when H_A is replaced by H_A^{Sp}. As the pigment-substituted protein is integrated into a nanoporous WO_3-TiO_2 instead of the unmodified wild-type protein, upon illumination it becomes more energetically favorable for the photoexcited electrons from the special pair and bacteriochlorophyll in the protein to jump into the conduction band of the WO_3-TiO_2 semiconductor rather than tracing a hindered pathway. As the electron injection rate is greatly increased in this system, the photocurrent generated was also remarkably enhanced.[11,39]

Similar comparative studies between native RCs and pheophytin-replaced RCs[40] were also conducted in a system with SAM-coated gold electrodes.[40] The SAM layer on the gold electrode was formed by a thin layer of 2-mecraptoacetic acid (MAA) and polydimethylsiallylammonium chloride (PDDA).[40] Both the native wild-type RCs (RC_{WT}, Figure 5.8a) and mutant RCs (RC_{Phe}, Figure 5.8b) were immobilized onto the gold electrode by assembling onto the SAMs, resulting in two variants of electrodes, namely RC_{WT}-PDDA-MAA-Au and RC_{Phe}-PDDA-MAA-Au.

Upon illumination, the cell with RC_{WT}-PDDA-MAA-Au generated a photocurrent of about 30 nA cm^{-2} while that with RC_{Phe}-PDDA-MAA-Au yielded a photocurrent of about 45 nA cm^{-2}, which is a 15% enhancement in the current output. Both electrodes were completely identical with respect to the protein loading and the nature of SAM used; the only difference between the two was the type of protein used (mutant RCs or native RCs). This also implied that the main reason for the photocurrent enhancement was the relatively increased electron injection into the SAMs from the mutant RCs compared to their native counterparts.[40] This is again due to a slowed-down internal electron transfer process in the mutant RCs as opposed to the unhindered charge separation in the native RCs. The longer lifetime of the P* or P$^+$BChl$^-$ in the mutant RCs compared to the native RCs favors the electron injection into electrode. The wider energy gap between the P$^+$Q_A$^-$ and P/P$^+$ in the mutant RCs is another major contributor to the enhancement in the photoelectric performance.[40]

5.5   REACTION CENTERS IN NANOTUBES

With developments in using nanoporous and nanostructured electrodes for protein immobilization instead of simple planar electrodes, a number of different approaches emerged to expand the surface area available for electron transfer. This has been realized by engineering the electrode materials into various forms and morphologies such as nanotubes and nanopores. Nanotubes are advantageous for protein fixation in a number of ways. First, they allow a greater surface area to volume ratio, thereby providing larger inner volumes that can be occupied by the proteins.[42] Next, the inner and outer surfaces of the nanotubes have distinct properties enabling differential modification suitable for chemical or biofunctionalization. Furthermore, the open ends of the tubes make it easy for addition of biomolecules into the interiors of the tubes. The most common nanotubes for protein immobilization are of carbon, while some are based on silica[43] and boron nitride.[44] Carbon nanotubes are highly favored in the field of bioelectrochemistry mainly due to the scope of their redox potential match with that of the proteins.[45] The review by Wenrong Yang et al.[46] elaborates on the different means by which the carbon nanotubes can be modified with biomolecules. They were grouped into three main categories: the covalent attachment, non-covalent attachment, and the hybrid method. In the covalent approach, the biomolecule is chemically linked to the nanotube by means of a bifunctional spacer group or by direct reaction with a preferred site of the biomolecule or by functionalizing the nanotubes with carboxylic acid groups to facilitate chemical binding with the proteins/biomolecules.[46] In the non-covalent approach, since CNTs are hydrophobic in nature, the surface property is utilized to physically adsorb the appropriate biomolecules.[46] These hydrophobic interactions can take place either inside or outside of the CNTs, and the nanotubes are not chemically bound to any specific site in the protein/biomolecule.[46] The hybrid method puts together both covalent and non-covalent approaches. A small anchor molecule is initially non-covalently bonded to the CNT after which the biomolecules are covalently linked to the anchor molecules.[46] There have been various reports on how proteins can be functionalized onto the CNTs,[46-48] but the attempts on encapsulation of biomolecules in the CNTs were not effective. This is due to the low yield in the method and also because of the difficulty in achieving homogeneous and uniform protein distribution.[49] Therefore, effective functionalization of the proteins into the inner cavity of CNTs was challenging, also with a limitation on the size of the biomolecule to be integrated.[46] Nonetheless, successful encapsulation of reaction center proteins have been reported.[49] CNT encapsulation promises high functional density, increase in stability, as well as having a one-dimensional electron transfer.[49] Photocurrent generation by RCs immobilized onto HOPG has been compared with RCs encapsulated in densely packed multi-walled CNTs. With respect to the electron-transfer properties, the open ends of the CNTs are similar to the HOPG edge planes, and the walls of the CNTs are comparable to the basal planes of the HOPG.[45] In the device architecture put to test, the CNTs placed in an array were separated using an Al_2O_3 spacer that electrically isolated the CNTs and prevented the binding of RCs to the outer surface of CNTs. The other side of the CNT array-oxide film was coated with a submicron-thick gold layer.[49] In the case of the HOPG electrodes, the RCs were immobilized using a bifunctional reagent as the linker, which had a pyrene group on one side and Ni(NTA) group on the other. The pyrene group formed bonds with the electrode and the Ni(NTA) group served to link with the proteins, which were genetically engineered MHisRCs.[49] In the fabrication of RC-modified CNT photoelectrodes, RCs were allowed to penetrate into the CNTs by diffusion and capillary motion, by incubating the RC solution with CNTs at low temperatures (4°C, 1-2 hours).[49] The RCs were linked to the CNT by the same bifunctional reagent, the pyrene end of which non-covalently bound the electrode; and the Ni(NTA) end bound the His tagged M subunit of the RC. Comparing the two photoelectrodes, it was found that the protein loading in the CNT electrodes were several folds greater than that in the HOPG electrodes. With both types of photoelectrodes, a cathodic photocurrent was generated upon illumination, indicating that the RCs were oriented with the P-side facing the electrode. The RCs bound to the HOPG electrode without any linkers resulted in a photocurrent of about 30 nA cm^{-2} and when linkers were used, it increased to about 314 nA cm^{-2}. Similarly, the RCs linked to the CNT electrodes with a linker gave higher photocurrents with magnitudes as high as 1414 nA cm^{-2}. An implication from the study was that the electron transfer in the case of CNT electrode was much faster than that in the HOPG electrode, despite the RCs being attached to the two types of electrodes in the same way. This was attributed to the low internal resistance and high conductance along the length of the CNTs, contrary to the HOPG electrode.[49]

Engineered materials with hexagonal honeycomb-structured pores are also attractive for loading/integrating protein complexes of any size as there are defined ways to control the diameter of the tubular pores.[50,51] Studies were conducted on integrating RCs[51] and light- harvesting complexes[52] extracted from a thermophilic purple photosynthetic bacterium (*Thermochromatium tepidum*) in folded sheet silica mesoporous material (FSM), which had hexagonal pores of controllable perimeter. The binding between these RCs and the FSMs of different pore sizes have been evaluated. One of the key findings of the study was that the photocurrent generation from the proteins was optimal only when the pore size matched the proteins' dimensions.[50,52] Developing mesoporous materials of tuneable structural, electrical, and surface properties has been one of the promising approach to re-create a near-native environment for the protein complexes in the device environment.

5.6 REACTION CENTERS IN ELECTROLYTE SOLUTIONS

Besides the humongous efforts to immobilize and orientate the RCs onto the electrode materials in bio-photoelectrochemical cells, attempts to make cells with the proteins freely dispersed in the electrolyte solution with no dedicated attachment to the electrodes were also successful in photocurrent generation. In the electrolyte solution, the proteins are typically mixed with two electron transfer mediators, one serving as an electron acceptor and the other as donor[1,53–56] (Figure 5.9).

In a study by Takshi et al.,[56] the bio-photoelectrochemical cells were constructed with RCs mixed in the electrolyte solution containing two electron transfer mediators, namely ferrocene and methyl viologen. Since it was found that even in those cells where RCs are directly attached to the electrode a significant fraction of electron transfer occurs through electron transfer mediators, the study attempted to improve the performance by making the charge transfer fully diffusion controlled and without the use of any direct electron transfer between the RCs and the electrode.[55,56] Upon illumination, the protein reaches the charge-separated state ($P^+Q_B^-$), the positive and negative charges from which are migrated to the two electrodes by electrochemical reactions facilitated by the two mediators. The reactions involved (i) an electron transfer from ferrocene to P^+ (oxidation: $Cp_2Fe \rightarrow Cp_2Fe^+$) and (ii) electron transfer

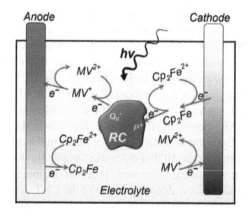

FIGURE 5.9 Illustration of electrochemical reactions in a two-mediator bio-photoelectrochemical cell with reaction centers serving as the primary photoactive species while ferrocene and methyl viologen serve as mediators in transporting the photogenerated charge carriers to the two electrodes. (The illustration is created, inspired from Takshi, A. et al., *Energies*, 3, 1721–1727, 2010.)

from Q_B^- to methyl viologen (reduction: $MV^{2+} \rightarrow MV^+$) (Figure 5.9). Ubiquinone-10 and cytochrome c had also been used for the same purpose. With proteins still dispersed in solution, attempts to induce a natural tendency in the proteins to bind to the electrode have been made without the use of any chemical linker. Genetically engineered reaction center proteins with a cysteine tag in their H subunits exhibited an increased propensity to bind to gold electrodes. On adding these proteins to the electrolyte solution in a photoelectrochemical cell, 78% of the proteins were found to be preferentially bound to the gold electrode, while a majority of the rest were in random motion in the solution.[54] A minor fraction of them were also found clinging to the counter electrode. Nevertheless, though the RCs were in direct contact with the gold electrode, the photocurrent was close to zero in the absence of the two electron transfer mediators, pointing to the least possibility of a direct electron transfer between the electrode and the protein, underscoring the importance of the mediators in achieving the electron transfer.[54]

Unlike the preferential binding of genetically engineered RCs with cysteine tags to the gold electrode, in cells using RC-LH1 proteins dispersed in the electrolyte, the proteins were still found to adhere to the electrode without the use of any tags. The cell employed FTO front electrode and Pt counter electrode with proteins dispersed in an electrolyte solution.[57] In contrast to the earlier work (Figure 5.9), the preferential adherence of RC-LH1 proteins to the FTO electrode facilitated direct electron transfer from the electrode to the protein to replenish the photooxidized special pair with electrons. As one half of the electron transfer in

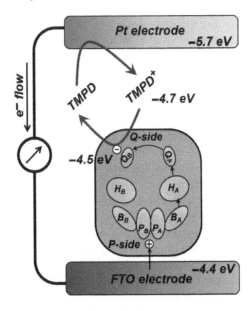

FIGURE 5.10 Illustration of a single-mediator bio-photoelectrochemical cell with RC-LH1 serving as the primary photoactive species (only the RC portion of the protein is shown). The photogenerated charges reach the two electrodes by direct electron transfer at the FTO electrode and mediated electron transfer at the Pt electrode. (The illustration is created, inspired from Tan, S.C. et al., *Angew. Chem. Int. Ed.*, 51, 6667–6671, 2012.[57])

the device is achieved by direct protein-to-electrode contact, employing a single redox mediator was sufficient for the device working, which aids in transferring the photogenerated electrons from the Q_B site in the protein to the counter electrode (Figure 5.10). This also showed that the electrolyte (N,N,N′,N′-Tetramethyl-p-phenylenediamine dihydrochloride or TMPD) used in the cell was in itself a good electron transfer mediator. A majority of RC-LH1 complexes were believed to bind to the FTO electrode with any of the two possible terminals of the complex, and the electrons were shuttled from the other terminal of the complex to the Pt counter electrode. Since RCs are hydrophilic, they attract to the hydrophilic FTO as opposed to the hydrophobic Pt electrode, thus preventing any electrical hindrance at the electrolyte/counter electrode interface. Many new device architectures in recent times employ a single type of electron transfer mediators or redox mediators, and the photoelectric performances have been on par with or superior to that in the earlier studies.[58,59]

5.7 SUMMARY

Immobilization/integration of photosynthetic proteins in devices has over the decades witnessed periodic improvements in optimizing protein orientation, protein-electrode binding, electrolyte composition, and electron transfer reactions. This chapter discussed the various methods employed to effectively attach photosynthetic reaction centers to different kinds of electrodes in a bio-photoelectrochemical cell. Starting from the use of bare methods, the diverging scope of chemically attaching proteins to electrodes was outlined, and different accounts of direct RC-to-electrode electron transfer, RC-linker-electrode electron transfer, and mediated electron transfer were discussed. The progress in photocurrent generation achieved by different bio-photoelectrochemical cells by trying different chemical linkers and by altering the protein orientation was highlighted. The photocurrent generation in different multilayer systems such as proteins electrostatically adsorbed on electrodes, proteins held by sol-gels and different protein-SAM systems was compared and evaluated. Stepping from the use of conventional planar electrodes, the need for improving the protein loading and for widening the electrode/protein contact areas led to the emergence of bio-photoelectrodes of different morphologies ranging from random nanopores to structured nanotubes.

By adopting an interdisciplinary approach, there is still plenty of room to explore newer and better ways of exploiting natural photosynthetic proteins for solar energy harnessing. Experimenting alternative electrode–electrolyte systems with new device architectures promises a great scope for developing more efficient and low-cost bio-photoelectrochemical cells. The unresolved stability concerns in photosynthetic protein-based photoelectrochemical cells point to the need for new device structures, and the recent reports on solid-state systems have been promising. Materials engineering in conjunction with biomolecular and genetic engineering has an unrestrained potential to take photosynthetic energy harvesting devices to newer dimensions with brighter commercialization prospects.

REFERENCES

1. Ravi, S. K.; Tan, S. C. *Energy & Environmental Science* **2015**, 8, (9), 2551–2573.
2. Wiseman, A. *Journal of Chemical Technology and Biotechnology* **1993**, 56, (1), 3–13.
3. Rao, S. V.; Anderson, K. W.; Bachas, L. G. *Microchimica Acta* **1998**, 128, (3), 127–143.
4. Johnson, R. D.; Todd, R. J.; Arnold, F. H. *Journal of Chromatography A* **1996**, 725, (2), 225–235.
5. Trevan, M. D. *Immobilized Enzymes: An Introduction and Applications in Biotechnology* **1980**; Wiley.
6. Mosbach, K.; Mattiasson, B. *Methods in Enzymology* **1976**, 44, 453–478.
7. Yasuda, Y.; Hirata, Y.; Sugino, H.; Kumei, M.; Hara, M.; Miyake, J.; Fujihira, M. *Thin Solid Films* **1992**, 210, (1–2), 733–735.
8. Yasuda, Y.; Sugino, H.; Toyotama, H.; Hirata, Y.; Hara, M.; Miyake, J. *Bioelectrochemistry and Bioenergetics* **1994**, 34, (2), 135–139.
9. Yasuda, Y.; Toyotama, H.; Hara, M.; Miyake, J. *Thin Solid Films* **1998**, 327, 800–803.
10. Khomutov, G. B.; Kim, V. P.; Potapenkov, K. V.; Parshintsev, A. A.; Soldatov, E. S.; Usmanov, N. N.; Saletsky, A. M.; Sybachin, A. V.; Yaroslavov, A. A.; Migulin, V. A. *Colloids and Surfaces A: Physicochemical and Engineering Aspects* **2017**.
11. Lu, Y.; Xu, J.; Liu, B.; Kong, J. *Biosensors & Bioelectronics* **2007**, 22, (7), 1173–1185.
12. Nagy, L.; Magyar, M.; Szabo, T.; Hajdu, K.; Giotta, L.; Dorogi, M.; Milano, F. *Current Protein & Peptide Science* **2014**, 15, (4), 363–373.
13. Ulman, A. *Chemical Reviews* **1996**, 96, (4), 1533–1554.
14. Brinker, C. J.; Scherer, G. W., *Sol-Gel Science: The Physics and Chemistry of Sol-Gel Processing.* Boston, MA: Academic Press, **2013**.
15. Janzen, A. F.; Seibert, M. *Nature* **1980**, 286, (5773), 584–585.
16. Seibert, M.; Janzen, A. F.; Kendalltobias, M. *Photochemistry and Photobiology* **1982**, 35, (2), 193–200.
17. Solovev, A. A.; Katz, F. Y.; Shuvalov, V. A.; Erokhin, Y. E. *Bioelectrochemistry and Bioenergetics* **1991**, 26, (1), 29–41.
18. Katz, E. *Journal of Electroanalytical Chemistry* **1994**, 365, (1–2), 157–164.
19. Zhao, J.; Feng, M.; Dougherty, D. B.; Sun, H.; Petek, H. *ACS Nano* **2014**, 8, (10), 10988–10997.
20. Zhao, J. Q.; Liu, B. H.; Zou, Y. L.; Xu, C. H.; Kong, J. L. *Electrochimica Acta* **2002**, 47, (12), 2013–2017.
21. Zhao, J. Q.; Zou, Y. L.; Liu, B. H.; Xu, C. H.; Kong, J. L. *Biosensors & Bioelectronics* **2002**, 17, (8), 711–718.
22. Kondo, M.; Nakamura, Y.; Fujii, K.; Nagata, M.; Suemori, Y.; Dewa, T.; Lida, K.; Gardiner, A. T.; Cogdell, R. J.; Nango, M. *Biomacromolecules* **2007**, 8, (8), 2457–2463.
23. Lebedev, N.; Spano, A.; Trammell, S.; Griva, I.; Tsoi, S.; Schnur, J. M. New bio-inorganic photo-electronic devices based on photosynthetic proteins. In *Organic Photovoltaics VIII*, Kafafi, Z. H.; Lane, P. A., (Eds.) **2007**; pp. 65614–65614.
24. Trammell, S. A.; Griva, I.; Spano, A.; Tsoi, S.; Tender, L. M.; Schnur, J.; Lebedev, N. *Journal of Physical Chemistry C* **2007**, 111, (45), 17122–17130.
25. Trammell, S. A.; Spano, A.; Price, R.; Lebedev, N. *Biosensors & Bioelectronics* **2006**, 21, (7), 1023–1028.
26. Mahmoudzadeh, A.; Saer, R.; Jun, D.; Mirvakili, S. M.; Takshi, A.; Iranpour, B.; Ouellet, E.; Lagally, E. T.; Madden, J. D. W.; Beatty, J. T. *Smart Materials & Structures* **2011**, 20, (9).
27. Giustini, M.; Autullo, M.; Mennuni, M.; Palazzo, G.; Mallardi, A. *Sensors and Actuators B-Chemical* **2012**, 163, (1), 69–75.

28. Zhao, J. Q.; Ma, N.; Liu, B. H.; Zhou, Y. L.; Xu, C. H.; Kong, J. L. *Journal of Photochemistry and Photobiology a-Chemistry* **2002**, 152, (1–3), 53–60.
29. Moser, C. C.; Keske, J. M.; Warncke, K.; Farid, R. S.; Dutton, P. L. *Nature* **1992**, 355, (6363), 796–802.
30. Kondo, M.; Iida, K.; Dewa, T.; Tanaka, H.; Ogawa, T.; Nagashima, S.; Nagashima, K. V. P. et al. *Biomacromolecules* **2012**, 13, (2), 432–438.
31. Lebedev, N.; Trammell, S. A.; Spano, A.; Lukashev, E.; Griva, I.; Schnur, J. *Journal of the American Chemical Society* **2006**, 128, (37), 12044–12045.
32. Nakamura, C.; Hasegawa, M.; Yasuda, Y.; Miyake, J. Self-assembling photosynthetic reaction centres on electrodes for current generation, In *Twenty-First Symposium on Biotechnology for Fuels and Chemicals*, **2000**; Springer, pp. 401–408.
33. Mikayama, T.; Miyashita, T.; Iida, K.; Suemori, Y.; Nango, M. *Molecular Crystals and Liquid Crystals* **2006**, 445, 291–296.
34. Das, R.; Kiley, P. J.; Segal, M.; Norville, J.; Yu, A. A.; Wang, L. Y.; Trammell, S. A. et al. *Nano Letters* **2004**, 4, (6), 1079–1083.
35. Trammell, S. A.; Wang, L. Y.; Zullo, J. M.; Shashidhar, R.; Lebedev, N. *Biosensors & Bioelectronics* **2004**, 19, (12), 1649–1655.
36. Lu, Y. D.; Yuan, M. J.; Liu, Y.; Tu, B.; Xu, C. H.; Liu, B. H.; Zhao, D. Y.; Kong, J. L. *Langmuir* **2005**, 21, (9), 4071–4076.
37. Lu, Y.; Liu, Y.; Xu, J.; Xu, C.; Liu, B.; Kong, J. *Sensors* **2005**, 5, (4), 258–265.
38. Lukashev, E. P.; Nadtochenko, V. A.; Permenova, E. P.; Sarkisov, O. M.; Rubin, A. B. *Doklady Biochemistry and Biophysics* **2007**, 415, (1), 211–216.
39. Lu, Y. D.; Xu, J. J.; Liu, Y.; Liu, B. H.; Xu, C. H.; Zhao, D. Y.; Kong, J. L. *Chemical Communications* **2006**, (7), 785–787.
40. Xu, J.; Lu, Y.; Liu, B.; Xu, C.; Kong, J. *Journal of Solid State Electrochemistry* **2007**, 11, (12), 1689–1695.
41. Jones, M. R. *Progress in Lipid Research* **2007**, 46, (1), 56–87.
42. Martin, C. R.; Kohli, P. *Nature Reviews Drug Discovery* **2003**, 2, (1), 29–37.
43. Kang, M. C.; Trofin, L.; Mota, M. O.; Martin, C. R. *Analytical Chemistry* **2005**, 77, (19), 6243–6249.
44. Zhi, C.; Bando, Y.; Tang, C.; Golberg, D. *Journal of the American Chemical Society* **2005**, 127, (49), 17144–17145.
45. Gooding, J. J.; Wibowo, R.; Liu, J. Q.; Yang, W. R.; Losic, D.; Orbons, S.; Mearns, F. J.; Shapter, J. G.; Hibbert, D. B. *Journal of the American Chemical Society* **2003**, 125, (30), 9006–9007.
46. Yang, W.; Thordarson, P.; Gooding, J. J.; Ringer, S. P.; Braet, F. *Nanotechnology* **2007**, 18, (41).
47. Gruner, G. *Analytical and Bioanalytical Chemistry* **2006**, 384, (2), 322–335.
48. Alvaro, M.; Atienzar, P.; la Cruz, P.; Delgado, J. L.; Troiani, V.; Garcia, H.; Langa, F.; Palkar, A.; Echegoyen, L. *Journal of the American Chemical Society* **2006**, 128, (20), 6626–6635.
49. Lebedev, N.; Trammell, S. A.; Tsoi, S.; Spano, A.; Kim, J. H.; Xu, J.; Twigg, M. E.; Schnur, J. M. *Langmuir* **2008**, 24, (16), 8871–8876.
50. Oda, I.; Iwaki, M.; Fujita, D.; Tsutsui, Y.; Ishizaka, S.; Dewa, M.; Nango, M.; Kajino, T.; Fukushima, Y.; Itoh, S. *Langmuir* **2010**, 26, (16), 13399–13406.
51. Inagaki, S.; Guan, S.; Fukushima, Y.; Ohsuna, T.; Terasaki, O. *Journal of the American Chemical Society* **1999**, 121, (41), 9611–9614.
52. Oda, I.; Hirata, K.; Watanabe, S.; Shibata, Y.; Kajino, T.; Fukushima, Y.; Iwai, S.; Itoh, S. *Journal of Physical Chemistry B* **2006**, 110, (3), 1114–1120.
53. Ravi, S. K.; Yu, Z.; Swainsbury, D. J.; Ouyang, J.; Jones, M. R.; Tan, S. C. *Advanced Energy Materials* **2017**, 7, (7).

54. Yaghoubi, H.; Li, Z.; Jun, D.; Saer, R.; Slota, J. E.; Beerbom, M.; Schlaf, R.; Madden, J. D.; Beatty, J. T.; Takshi, A. *Journal of Physical Chemistry C* **2012**, 116, (47), 24868–24877.

55. Takshi, A.; Madden, J. D.; Beatty, J. T. *Electrochimica Acta* **2009**, 54, (14), 3806–3811.

56. Takshi, A.; Madden, J. D.; Mahmoudzadeh, A.; Saer, R.; Beatty, J. T. *Energies* **2010**, 3, (11), 1721–1727.

57. Tan, S. C.; Crouch, L. I.; Jones, M. R.; Welland, M. *Angewandte Chemie-International Edition* **2012**, 51, (27), 6667–6671.

58. Ravi, S. K.; Swainsbury, D. J.; Singh, V. K.; Ngeow, Y. K.; Jones, M. R.; Tan, S. C. *Advanced Materials* **2018**, 30, (5).

59. Singh, V. K.; Ravi, S. K.; Ho, J. W.; Wong, J. K. C.; Jones, M. R.; Tan, S. C. *Advanced Functional Materials* **2017**, 1703689.

6 Electronics, Photonics, and Device Physics in Protein Biophotovoltaics

Sai Kishore Ravi and Swee Ching Tan

CONTENTS

6.1 INTRODUCTION

Supplementing the comprehensive account of structure and function of different components of the natural energy-harvesting apparatus and their roles in meeting the energy demands in any photosynthetic organism, and collating the principles of energy harvesting and device physics applied in the emerging photovoltaic technologies presented in the earlier chapters, this chapter chronicles the various possible approaches that can come in handy in designing the future "protein-integrated biophotovoltaic" devices. Photosynthesis, a process by which plants and algae turn solar energy, water, and carbon dioxide into biomass, is that one process that sustains nearly every life form on Earth, generating over 100 gigatons of biomass on an annual basis.[1–4] Evolution over billions of years has enabled photosynthesis to operate under

161

extreme environmental conditions; the structural adaptations in the photosynthetic proteins render them operative even under extreme physiological temperatures and under minimal light flux.[5,6] With the exigency of renewable and clean energy alternatives, new means to tap energy from the ambient sources are increasingly being researched to reduce our dependence on fossil fuels.[7] Solar energy has been accepted as the most "green" alternative for fossil fuel and has already found practical applications in a wide range of research fields.[8] Nature has mastered the solar energy capture through intricate photosynthetic systems equipped in most autotrophic organisms, the exact rationale in the structural adaptations and the ensuing functionalities of some of which is intriguing people in the field of biophotonics and photovoltaics. Natural photosynthetic systems facilitate the initial phases of photosynthesis including the photoinduced excitation energy transfer and charge separation processes that occur at near-unity quantum efficiencies (i.e., ideally, for every photon absorbed, there is an electron-hole pair generated).[9,10] In light of the attractive light-harvesting and energy conversion efficiencies in the natural photosystems, a wide variety of photovoltaic systems have been studied, some involving molecular systems mimicking these photosystems in a device setup to achieve artificial photosynthesis while the others employing a wide variety of actual photosynthetic complexes and biomolecules interfaced with human-made electrode/electrolyte materials for various optoelectronic applications.[9,11,12] Photosynthetic complexes at different structural levels from different species of plants, algae, and bacteria have been experimented for general application in optoelectronic and photoelectrochemical devices and some even for specialized applications such as biosensing, photodetection, solar fuel synthesis, and biocomputing.[9,11,12]

Photosynthetic complexes and subunits isolated at different dimensional levels from different species of plants and bacteria have been studied for application in optoelectronic and bioelectrochemical devices. There are also numerous reports on using the whole living cell (typically of a cyanobacteria) as the photoactive component in bioreactors and photoelectrochemical cells.[13-15] However, this chapter confines its focus to those subunits of photosynthetic machinery isolated from plant/bacteria that can be made use of in a device setup without relying on the life span of the photosynthetic organism. Photosynthetic subunits as big as chloroplasts (that are several microns in size) and thylakoid/photosynthetic membranes have been used in devices; and the use of the photosynthetic pigment molecules that are hardly a few nanometers in size have also been common (Figure 6.1). While the chloroplast is a photosynthetic organelle that has a complex arrangement of biological units including the photosynthetic reaction centers coupled with a number of different antenna complexes, capable both of light harvesting and energy conversion, the function of photosynthetic pigments is limited only to photoabsorption for practical use in a biophotovoltaic device. Among all photosynthetic complexes and organelles, photosystems from plants/cyanobacteria and the reaction center proteins from purple bacteria are the most commonly studied. Of these, purple bacterial reaction centers are simpler in structure and relatively well understood compared to the photosystems in higher plants.[3,16,17] Numerous efforts on integrating reaction centers as photoactive materials in bioelectrochemical cells for solar energy harvesting have been reported.[16] Though in the past, most bioelectrochemical cells employed only the core reaction

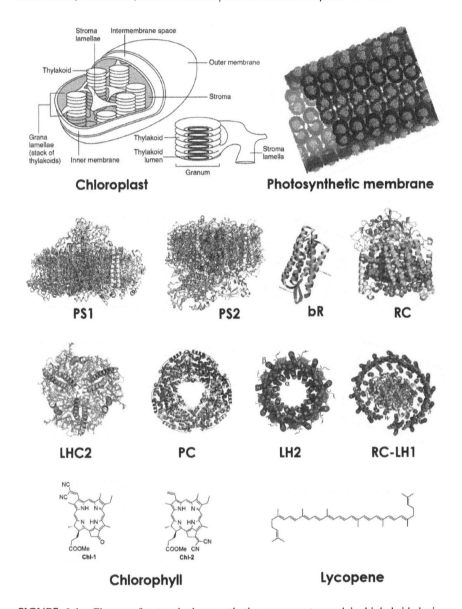

FIGURE 6.1 Classes of natural photosynthetic components used in biohybrid devices: 1. Larger Units and Organelles: *Chloroplast*: Schematic diagram of a plant chloroplast (From Blankenship, R.E.: *Molecular Mechanisms of Photosynthesis*, 11–25, 2002. Copyright Wiley-VCH Verlag GmbH & Co. KGaA. Reproduced with permission.), *Photosynthetic membrane*: A segment of the tubular photosynthetic membrane from purple bacterium (Reproduced from *Biophys. J.*, 97, Hsin, J. et al., 321–329, Copyright 2009, with permission from Elsevier.). 2. Protein complexes: *PS1*: Photosystem 1, *PS2*: Photosystem 2, *bR*: Bacteriorhodopsin, *RC*: reaction center. 3. Light-Harvesting Complexes/Proteins: *LHC2*: Light-harvesting antenna complex, which is a part of PS2 supercomplex found in plants. *PC*: Phycocyanin complex, LH2: Light-harvesting complex in purple bacterium that aids in excitation   (*Continued*)

center proteins and photosystems. In recent times, use of isolated light-harvesting
complexes such as LH1, LH2, and LHC2 in biophotovoltaic devices have also been
reported. LH1 and LH2 are the two major antenna complexes that feed into the
reaction center core with the excitation energy derived from photoabsorption of the
various antenna pigments; LHC2 is a light-harvesting complex found in the higher
plants and cyanobacteria, which does a similar function of excitation energy transfer
to the reaction center in the photosystems. The progress in photocurrent generation and device architectures in biophotovoltaic devices integrating purple bacterial
photosynthetic proteins has been discussed in a few recent reviews.[3,16,18] As opposed
to the simple structure and well-understood structure-function relations of proteins
in anoxygenic phototrophs such as purple bacteria, the photosynthetic complexes
(namely Photosystem 1 and Photosystem 2) from oxygenic phototrophs such as
plants, algae, and cyanobacteria are rather complex.[17,19–21] Photosystem 1 (PS1) and
Photosystem 2 (PS2) are the two main protein complexes crucial in the operation
of oxygenic photosynthesis, which although sharing many functional similarities
with the purple bacterial reaction centers (RCs), are not the minimal functional units
responsible for the photochemical reaction, unlike RCs.[17,19–22] RCs are the minimal
functional units capable of photochemical reaction in purple bacterial cells, which
can independently perform the photoinduced charge separation without any addi-
tional/auxiliary proteins or antenna complexes. However, it is not straightforward to
identify and isolate such a minimal unit from the photosystems.[22] The use of photosystems 1 and 2 in solar energy harvesting and other optoelectronic applications
have been summarized in a few review articles.[23–25] In addition to photosystems and
reaction centers, there are also reports on devices employing proton pump-based photosynthetic proteins such as Bacteriorhodopsin (bR)[26–28] and other light-harvesting
pigment-protein complexes such as Phycocyanin (PC).[29,30]

One of the most conventional approaches that dominated a majority of studies
in the field was to construct electrochemical cells, where either different kinds of
biophotoelectrodes were developed by coating/functionalizing a transparent electrode material with photosynthetic organelles/antenna-complexes/pigments/proteins
or different kinds of electrolyte compositions were used, dispersing different kinds
of photosynthetic components in electrolyte solutions of different redox couples or
electron transfer mediators. While this bioelectrochemistry approach is still relevant

and in use, recent developments are aimed at performance enhancement that is possible by clubbing new approaches with a bioelectrochemical design, taking insights from the other emerging photovoltaic technologies in the aspects of electronics, photonics, and device physics. This chapter presents a short overview of the bioelectrochemistry approach that is used by and large in the field and moves forward in further illustrating the other emerging approaches in biophotovoltaics, highlighting the aspects of electronics, photonics, and device physics. The photosynthetic complexes/subunits involved in the various biohybrid models described in this chapter are limited to those presented in Figure 6.1. For more detailed structural and functional descriptions of the different proteins, pigments and organelles, classic books such as ref[31] and ref[22] shall be referenced.

6.2   ELECTROCHEMICAL APPROACHES

Photocurrent generation is often the most intended purpose of integrating the photosynthetic proteins in an electrochemical cell by exploiting the highly efficient photoinduced charge separation processes in the proteins. Though both current and voltage generated are equally crucial in the mainstream photovoltaics, the importance of photovoltage has been overlooked in the field of bioelectrochemical cells as a huge number of reports do not present any photovoltage measurement.[16] Most bioelectrochemical cells are three electrode cells where the photoactive biological components (pigments/proteins/organelles) are either coated/immobilized on the working electrode or blended with the electrolyte solution that facilitates the charge transfer between the protein and the electrodes by means of electron transfer mediators or through redox couples.[39–44] For convenience and ease of miniaturization, in some cases, two electrode sealed cells are constructed without any reference electrode.[9,45,46] The photoelectrodes are typically coated with proteins by a number of immobilization techniques using different kinds of chemical linker molecules. Recent reports also adopt nonchemical means of coating proteins for ease of increasing the overall protein loading on the electrode, which directly affects the quantum of light absorbed by the device and hence the photocurrent generated. This is realized by methods such as spin coating, drop casting, and electrospraying.[47–50] One of the earliest designs of the photosynthetic protein-based photoelectrochemical cell was reported by Janzen and Seibert in the early 1980s that involved a reaction center coated working electrode, a Pt counter electrode, and a saturated calomel reference electrode with hydroquinone as a redox couple.[51,52] The design of liquid-electrolyte electrochemical cells has had a number of variations over the years, though retaining most of the common features. The major variations have only been in the method of illumination and the method of integration of the proteins in the cell (coating on electrode or blending with electrolyte) (Figure 6.2a–c). A general scheme of photoelectrochemical setup employed by most of the works on bioelectrochemical cells in the field is shown in Figure 6.2d. Most bioelectrochemical cells use liquid electrolytes to facilitate charge transfer between the protein and the counter electrode; however, in recent reports the use of gel electrolytes has been suggested to improve both the protein stability and the charge transfer.[50] Unlike conventional photovoltaics, the possible direction of charge transfer in bioelectrochemical cells is not easily controlled to be in a single direction;

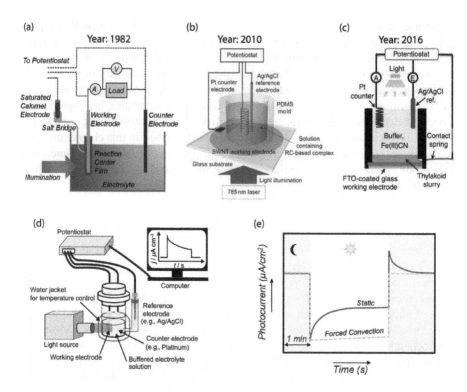

FIGURE 6.2 Designs of Bio-photoelectrochemical cells: (a) Earliest design of protein-based photoelectrochemical cell with the reaction center proteins physically adhered on the working electrode, with lateral illumination. (Inspired from Seibert, M. et al., *Photochem. Photobiol.*, 35, 193–200, 1982.) (b) Bio-photoelectrochemical cell with reaction center proteins suffused in the electrolyte, with base illumination. (Reproduced with permission from Ham, M.-H. et al., *Nat. Chem.*, 2, 929–936, 2010. Copyright 2010, Springer Nature.) (c) Thylakoid-integrated Photoelectrochemical cell with top illumination. (Reproduced from Pinhassi, R.I. et al., *Nat. Commun.*, 7, 12552, 2016.) (d) Basic three-electrode electrochemical measurement set up. (Adapted from Kato, M. et al., *Chem. Soc. Rev.*, 43, 6485–6497, 2014.) (e) Schematic representation of photocurrent patterns in bioelectrochemical cells with electrolyte under static condition and under forced convection. (Inspired from Friebe, V.M. et al., *Adv. Funct. Mater.*, 26, 285–292, 2016.)

dual electron transfer pathways in opposite directions are a common occurrence in many cells that permit unfavorable electron recombination reactions.[53] A typical example of this in most liquid-electrolyte bioelectrochemical cells is the appearance of sharp transient photocurrent upon switching the illumination on and the photocurrent reversal observed upon switching the illumination off. Most cells exhibit an initial spike of "transient photocurrent," the intensity of which attenuates over short time scales (typically ranges from a few seconds to several minutes), to a lower, steady-state current. In some cases there is also a reverse photocurrent spike before the zero/steady-state dark current is reached, after the illumination is turned off [9,39–49] (Figure 6.2e). This is because the reduced charge carrier produced during the period of illumination can be reoxidized at the photocathode, resulting in a decline in the overall cathodic photocurrent; upon switching the illumination off, this process of reoxidation persists for a short time scale, the duration of which depends on the recombination kinetics and also on the mass transport of the charge carrier, which in turn results in a net anodic current. Reports suggest that the photocurrent attenuations occurring during the initial stages of illumination are due to the limitation imposed by slow mediator diffusion. This has also been corroborated by photocurrent measurements with a rotating disk electrode that provides mixing in the electrolyte solution, which results in a forced convection facilitating the transport of the reduced charge carriers away from the photoelectrode surface.[41,42,54,55] As opposed to the static conditions, the forced convection in the electrolyte solution has been proven to result in a higher photocurrent (devoid of spikes) and virtually a zero photocurrent after the light source is switched off.

Notwithstanding the fact that there have been a number of design improvements and material modifications in the conventional bioelectrochemical cells over the years, there are also concerns on the poor photoelectrochemical power generation in these cells based on several reports that underline the drawback of current output being limited by slow diffusive processes rather than by the light-harvesting ability and charge-separation efficiency of the photosynthetic proteins.[41,42,54,55] In this chapter, we discuss the prospects and perspectives in applying a number of new approaches from electronics, photonics, and device physics to the photo-bioelectrochemical cells.

6.3 ELECTRONIC AND BAND STRUCTURE APPROACHES

A number of major developments in the mainstream photovoltaics such as organic photovoltaics (OPVs) and perovskite solar cells can be owed to materials engineering, particularly thanks to the fine-tuning of the electronic properties of the materials. Interface morphology, interfacial electronic structure, and band-alignment between the various functional layers in the device are some of the main parameters that are given careful consideration in the design of any OPV. The conventional biophotoelectrochemical cells being predominantly liquid-based and their current output being diffusion-controlled, the device physics is often determined only by the choice of the redox potential of the electrolyte and by the mode of immobilization (coating/functionalizing) of the photoactive biological components. However, adopting an electronic/band-structure approach in designing these devices opens up new possibilities in improving the photovoltaic performance. A major advantage this approach brings forth is the ability to control the energy level alignment at various interfaces in the device and hence to have a more precise control over the charge transport pathways in the device.[58–60] Applying the band-structure approach in biohybrid devices would essentially mean that every component of the device is to be treated as an electronically functional material.[60,61] As in most optoelectronic devices, the "function" stems from the various interfaces of materials in the device.[60,62,63] Taking the example of an electroluminescent device, while the electrons are injected from one electrode to the electron transport layer (ETL), the holes are injected from the other electrode into the hole transport layer (HTL), after which the two carriers recombine to emit light.[64–66] Another case where the interfaces play a crucial role is in the organic solar cells where the interface between the organic layer and the metal electrode results in a Schottky barrier, an energy barrier resulting from the band bending at the interface, where the electron-hole pairs generated upon photoabsorption get separated.[60,67–70] The interfacial electronic structure is hence a decisive factor affecting the performance of any optoelectronic device. The band-structure approach, though extensively used in the design and construction of inorganic optoelectronic devices, is still an emerging concept in modern optoelectronics where new organic materials are concocted to constitute the functional layers in the devices replacing their inorganic counterparts, in light of the multifarious benefits ranging from low material cost to ease of property tunability in the organic materials.[63,71,72] In recent years, there has been a great focus on characterizing the energy-level alignment and interfacial electronic structure at organic/organic interfaces and at organic/ metal interfaces in order to understand and improve the charge transport processes in organic optoelectronic devices.[59,73–75] The approach lately has gained immense impetus in the whole gamut of emerging optoelectronic devices such as organic light-emitting diodes, organic photovoltaics, organic field-effect transistors, and perovskite solar cells. Designing biophotovoltaic devices by drawing insights from the band-structure approach is hence a promising route to achieve higher power output from photosynthetic proteins and to possibly move closer to the theoretical efficiency limits.

6.3.1 Interfacial Electronic Structure

Unlike in the other branches of optoelectronics, energy-level alignment and inter-facial electronic structure are the least studied and rather new in biophotovoltaics. A feature common to most biophotovoltaic devices is that there is always at least one interface that is formed between the photoactive biomolecules involved with an electrode. All the physical criteria deciding the nature of band bending and the resulting energy barrier that applies for a metal/organic interface are also applicable in determining the interfacial electronic structure at a metal/biomolecule interface. However, studies investigating the interfacial electronic structure in the biophotovoltaic devices are often sparse.

As the interfacial electronic structure of the bulk heterojunctions in organic solar cells is widely studied, it is worthwhile to compare and contrast some of the structural and functional similarities that the natural photosystems and the organic bulk heterojunctions have in common. Organic Photovoltaics (OPVs) are composed of active light-absorbing layers with domains of conjugated polymers/molecules acting as electron acceptors and donors. As discussed in the earlier chapter (Chapter 3), upon illumination, the photogenerated excitons dissociate at the donor/acceptor interface into individual charge carriers (electrons and holes), which then get further separated by moving into the donor and acceptor domains.[6] Analogous to this, in natural photosynthesis, the photosynthetic pigments present in the light-harvesting antenna complexes absorb sunlight, reach excited state, and funnel the excitation energy into a reaction center where the exciton is separated into positive and negative charges. The role of the reaction center in a natural photosystem is akin to the donor/ acceptor interface in an organic photovoltaic cell.[6,16,69] While the natural photosynthetic architecture in plants and bacteria is highly intricate with the presence of a highly ordered assembly of pigments and proteins in super-complexes (Figure 6.3a), it is difficult to achieve such an order in organic photovoltaics.[6,78,79] In contrast to the

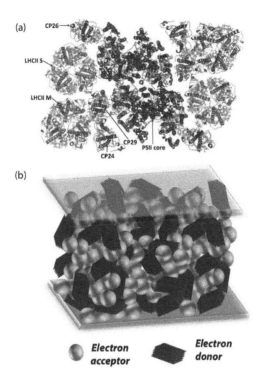

FIGURE 6.3 Photosynthetic supercomplex and organic photovoltaics—Structural differences: (a) Architecture of PS2-LHC2 super complex as seen from the stromal side of the membrane. (Reproduced with permission from *Biochim. Biophys. Acta*, 1858, Xu, P. et al., 815–822, Copyright 2017, Elsevier.) (b) Cartoon of a bulk heterojunction polymer solar cell showing only the active layer; the active layer is composed of randomly mixed domains of electron acceptors (shown as spheres) and donors (shown as rectangular flakes); the two rectangular substrates on either side of the active layer are just a representation of neighboring layers that can be either electrodes or cathodic/anodic interlayers used for charge extraction and transport. (Inspired from Guo, X. et al., *Nat. Photonics*, 7, 825–833, 2013.)

molecular circuitry of the light harvesters and the charge-carrying cofactors in the natural photosystems, the acceptor and donor domains in OPVs exist as a disordered mixture (Figure 6.3b).[6,16,63,69,77]

The charge transport and exciton transport are two separate processes in a photosynthetic complex carried out through dedicated networks; however, in an OPV, the two functions are not separated[6,16,63,69] (Figure 6.4a, b). The high efficiency of light-induced charge generation and charge separation is another feature in natural photosystems that is distinctly different from OPVs. Photogeneration of charge carriers in a natural photosynthetic apparatus is a result of a redox relay or cascade,[69] as shown in Figure 6.4a. Driven by light absorption, there is a formation of a short-lived molecular singlet excited state (lasting typically for a few nanoseconds) in the primary donor, which is typically the pair of excitonically coupled chlorophyll (or bacteriochlorophyll) molecules, followed by charge separation that results from a sequence of energetically downhill electron transfer reactions from the donor excited state to the neighboring acceptor molecules[16,31,83] (Figure 6.5a, b). After the initial charge separation, there are secondary electron transfer reactions that result in a long-lived charge separated state that has a long life in the range of a few seconds[16,31,69] (Figure 6.5b). There have been several reports in literature on the electron transfer dynamics and recombination pathways in the molecular mimics of photosynthetic proteins involving molecular donor/acceptor redox relays; however, most of the studies were limited to dilute solutions.[69] In contrast, the donor and acceptor molecules in OPVs are typically solid films, which gives rise to percolation pathways providing an electrical "wiring" of the photogenerated charges at the donor/acceptor interface to the device electrodes.[69,84,85] As opposed to the architecture of a photosynthetic reaction center complex, where there is a cascade of electron flow reactions through multiple donor/acceptor sites, in an OPV device, only one type of donor and acceptor materials form the interface, which rules out the possibility of such redox relays (Figure 6.4b). In natural photosynthesis, the redox relay effectively prevents any recombination of the photogenerated charge carriers from coulombic attraction whereas in an OPV, this is possible only if the energy offset between the donor and acceptor lowest unoccupied molecular orbital (LUMO) levels exceeds the coulombic binding energy of the photogenerated exciton, which would enable energetically downhill electron transfer.[69,86] Nonetheless, in reality, since the donor and acceptor

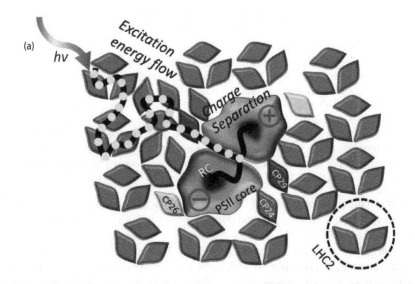

FIGURE 6.4 Working of a photosynthetic supercomplex compared to that of an organic photovoltaic system: (a) Cartoon showing the migration of excitation energy from the antenna complexes to the reaction center in a PS2-LHC2 supercomplex. (The position and arrangement of the antenna complexes and the cofactors are not drawn to precision; the cartoon is created based on the structural information of PS2 supercomplexes reported in literature. (From Dekker, J.P. and Boekema, E.J., *Biochim. Biophys. Acta*, 1706, 12–39, 2005; Fleming, G.R. et al., *Faraday Discuss.*, 155, 27–41, 2012; Jurić, S. et al., Electron transfer routes in oxygenic photosynthesis: Regulatory mechanisms and new perspectives, In *Photosynthesis*, InTech, 2013.))   *(Continued)*

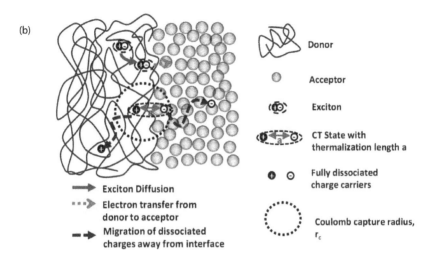

(b)

Donor

Acceptor

Exciton

CT State with
thermalization length a

Fully dissociated
charge carriers

➡ Exciton Diffusion

┅┅▷ Electron transfer from
donor to acceptor

➡ Migration of dissociated
charges away from interface

Coulomb capture radius,
r_c

FIGURE 6.4 (Continued)   Working of a photosynthetic supercomplex compared to that of an organic photovoltaic system: (b) Cartoon showing exciton migration and charge dissociation at the donor/acceptor interface in a plastic solar cell. On light absorption, the exciton generated diffuses to the interface, where the electron transfer to the acceptor occurs, resulting in a charge transfer (CT) state. For clarity, the CT state in the cartoon is shifted down along the vertical axis of the page. The electron and hole are initially separated by a distance called thermalization length "a." Theoretical predictions indicate the dependence of the probability of full charge dissociation on the ratio $a:r_c$ where r_c is the coulomb capture radius, which is represented by a circle (spherical in 3D) for simplicity neglecting the anisotropy. (From Clarke, T.M. and Durrant, J.R. *Chemical Reviews*, 110, 6736–6767, 2010.) (Adapted with permission from Ravi, S.K. et al., *Adv. Funct. Mater.*, 2017. Copyright 2017, John Wiley & Sons.)

molecules are physically close to each other at the charge separation interface, the spatial separation between the two charge carriers in the electron-hole pair is limited and is often in the same order of magnitude as the size of the molecules concerned (0.5–1 nm); this places a serious restriction in completely overcoming the coulombic attraction[69,87] (Figure 6.5c, d).

In order to overcome this limitation in OPVs, a number of studies in recent years point to the need to understate and engineer the interfacial electronic structure and to control the energy-level alignment at the interfaces in the device.[58,89,90] As there is more focus lately on developing solid-state devices in biophotovoltaics (BPVs), discerning the interfacial electronic structures at electrode/biomolecule interfaces and devising ways to tune the band alignment in BPVs have become crucial. The nature of an interface formed by a natural photosystem or any biomolecule can be approached with the same governing principles established by band theory as that for an interface formed by a simple organic molecule, despite the level of complexity. One important aspect of an interface the organic layer forms with the electrode in the device is the interfacial energy barrier, which is widely studied in OPVs.[91–93] It is known that when two materials of different work functions are brought in contact, there results an interfacial band bending because of the non-equilibrium state; this condition also applies to an OPV where an interfacial band bending results at the

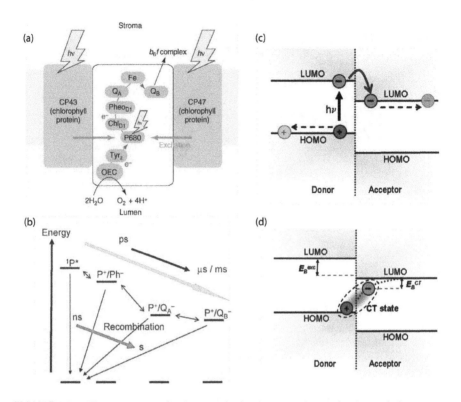

FIGURE 6.5 Charge transport in photosynthetic systems and organic photovoltaic systems: (a) Schematic representation of the structure of PS2 reaction center. (b) Schematic showing the energetics and kinetics of charge separation in the reaction center. (c) Energy level diagram of a donor/acceptor interface showing a simplified representation of photoexcitation of an electron into the donor LUMO followed by electron transfer into the acceptor LUMO and migration of the separated charges away from the interface. (d) Energy level diagram of the donor-acceptor interface in a plastic solar cell showing interfacial electron-hole pairs in charge-transfer (CT) state; the energy of the CT state depends on the coulombic attraction between the two charge carriers and hence on their spatial separation, as shown by the dotted curve. E_B^{exc} and E_B^{CT} are the binding energies associated with the exciton and CT states. (Figure 6.5a is reproduced with permission from *Curr. Opin. Struct. Biol.*, 14, Iwata, S. and Barber, J., 447–453, Copyright 2004, Elsevier and Figure 6.5 b–d are reproduced with permission from Clarke, T.M. and Durrant, J.R. *Chemical Reviews*, 110, 6736–6767, 2010, Copyright 2010, American Chemical Society.)

interface of a thick organic layer with an electrode.[60,94,95] So as to reach an electrical equilibrium, in which case the Fermi levels of the two materials are to be at the same level, charge redistribution occurs around the metal/organic interface.[60,96–98] Until the Fermi energies in the bulk of the materials are aligned, flow of charges into either side of the interface continues, resulting in a diffusion layer with band bending.[60,94,95] This leads to a built-in potential in the device. While the same effect is in principle possible with a protein/electrode interface, it is not straightforward to study the interfacial electronic structure, given the complexity of the interface.

Since photosynthetic complexes are composed of chemically different constituents such as pigments, polypeptides, and other cofactors, each having a distinct Fermi level, it is hard to model the system to a single work function as it greatly depends on the uniformity of the protein orientation on the surface and on the resulting surface charges. When protein complexes are interfaced just by physical adherence or coating on the electrode, it is practically hard to control what cofactors of the protein are in contact with the electrode. Though the interfacial structure of an electrode with a single protein can be modeled, it is challenging to characterize the interface in the case of randomly oriented protein coating. However, though it is relatively easier to characterize the interface in those devices employing ordered monolayers of protein complexes immobilized on electrodes through chemical linkers and genetic tags, such device architectures often suffer low photocurrent output owing to the limitation on the protein loading.[16] It is hence not straightforward to treat a protein/electrode interface as a simple organic/electrode interface especially when thick multilayers of randomly oriented proteins are used in the device. The interfacial electronic properties (particularly the interfacial energy barrier) are often probed by various types of in-device photoelectron spectroscopies under ultra-high vacuum (UHV).[60,93] Such studies have so far not been reported in BPVs because of the challenges in preserving the structural integrity of the protein complexes under the test conditions.

6.3.2   EXCITON TRANSPORT AND CHARGE TRANSPORT MODES

Light harvesting and charge carrier transport are the two fundamental processes in any energy conversion system, though the extent to which they are controlled varies in different systems.[6] For instance, in inorganic photovoltaics such as crystalline silicon solar cells, the research emphasis is not on controlling the light absorption as the photogeneration of charge carriers occurs essentially instantaneously upon illumination; instead, most of the performance optimizations are realized by improving the charge transport properties in the system.[6] In contrast, in photosynthesis, the system involves a sophisticated pigment-protein architecture for optimized and efficient light harvesting with high photoexcitation rate whereas the emphasis on charge transport is lesser and is carried out through a simple sequence of well-defined electron transfer reactions coupled with proton translocation.[6] It has been suggested that the materials in organic photovoltaics fall in between the limits of inorganic crystalline solar cells and the natural photosystems, and the transport properties are limited by both structural and energetic disorder.[6,99] As photosynthetic proteins are integrated in solid-state devices such as OPVs, it becomes important to understand how the excitation energy transport and the charge transport turn out to be in the resulting device. As the transport properties in biohybrid photovoltaic devices are often not sufficiently characterized unlike the other conventional photovoltaics, this section presents a basic overview of the different modes of energy transport and charge transport that are possible in these systems. Principles governing these transport modes are important to be understood as the transport properties strongly vary with the environment—that is, the transport modes in a biomolecular system in vivo (in the native environment) will differ from that in a device environment. This aids in designing new biohybrid systems with better control over the transport modes in the device.

The photochemical energy transduction in photosynthetic systems starts with light-induced electron transport reactions followed by slow dark reactions that result in the production of energy-rich molecules such as sugars.[100] At the very beginning of this process is the photoexcitation of the chromophores such as chlorophyll molecules present in the light-harvesting complexes.[31,100] The excited state lifetime ($\approx$4 ns in vivo[101,102]) of such chromophores is often short compared to that of most other biological processes. Nevertheless, the photoexcitation is immediately followed by even faster electronic energy transfer (EET) reactions in order to effectively transmit the excitation energy to the reaction center before the chromophore returns to ground state. This EET was initially thought to be carried out by a series of incoherent jumps governed by Förster theory.[78,103–108] EET is prevalent in all light-harvesting complexes to convert electronic excitation into charge separation with high efficiency.[31,100] The probability of converting an absorbed photon to a charge separated state is known as quantum efficiency and is known to be close to 100% in photosynthetic systems.[100] Photosynthetic chromophores are found to be capable of mediating rapid EET reactions, which is characterized by large Förster radius (60–100 Å).[100,109,110] For a pair of photosynthetic chromophores, the Förster radius is the characteristic distance between the donor and accepter at which the electronic energy transfer efficiency drops by 50%.[100] This high efficiency is a result of a number of factors such as the size of the antenna complexes, the arrangement of chromophores in the antenna complexes, the excited-state lifetime of those chromophores, and by the light conditions.[100] Deciphering the design principles of photosynthetic light harvesting has been a topic of research for a long time now. However, studying the mechanistic aspects of light harvesting and energy transfer and figuring out the role of coherence in the dynamics of photosynthetic light harvesting have gained immense attention in recent years.[6,111–116] Different models have been put forth to give a mechanistic description of photosynthetic light harvesting. The first one is by Förster theory, the theory of electronic energy transfer applicable within the limit of very weak donor-acceptor electronic coupling in which the energy transfer proceeds by incoherent hopping or jumps.[100,117] From several recent observations, the role of coherent electronic energy transfer is also believed to be effective as opposed to the incoherent hopping model.[118–120] In principle, the electronic energy transfer from an excited-state donor molecule to a ground-state acceptor molecule depends on the coupling strength between the donor de-excitation and acceptor excitation and hence also on their spectral properties.[100] The electronic coupling between the chromophores[121,122] results in delocalized excited states called excitons.[100] These are delocalized excited states comprising a superposition of excited states at different molecular sites.[100,123–127] The idea of "excitons" is typically relevant in organic materials only; in inorganic semiconductors, such a concept is rare because the binding energy of the electron and hole to stay as an exciton is very small (for instance, it is about 15 meV[128] in the case of Si and much smaller in several other inorganic semiconductors).[129] These excitons are specifically known as Wannier excitons in inorganic semiconductors, and they are known to completely dissociate into electrons and holes at room temperature.[129] However, in the organic world (including photosynthesis and OPVs), the idea of excitons is prominently relevant as the binding energy is greater than the thermal energy at room temperature.[129,130] While incoherent hopping was believed to be the only mechanistic explanation for excitation energy transport in photosynthesis, the first indication of coherent transport was witnessed when Fleming and coworkers reported quantum coherence in bacterial photosystems at cryogenic temperatures.[118,131,132] It was explained that as chlorophyll pigment molecules absorb the incident photons, excitons are generated—which evolve in a coherent manner—as a superposition of electron quantum states, and the excitons have a lifetime long enough to coordinate the energy transfer to the reaction center.[132] This process was described to be analogous to a quantum computation, in which all possible paths for energy transfer are simultaneously surveyed before selecting the optimal path.[132] Subsequently, evidences of quantum coherence at room temperature were also reported.[119,120,132,133] The primary origin of electronic interaction between an excited-state molecule and a nearby ground-state molecule is the long-range coulombic interaction between transition densities,[121] modified by the interaction of the optical dielectric properties of the medium (screening).[100] In a majority of antenna complexes, the electronic coupling between chromophores is in the range of ≈ 0.5 cm^{-1} to ≈ 500 cm^{-1}, after taking screening into account.[134–136] An example of strong electronic coupling can be found in LH2 antenna complex of purple bacteria. The densely packed and highly ordered arrangement of the bacteriochlorophyll (BChl a) molecules in the B850 ring (Figure 6.6) allows the chromophores to work cooperatively in light harvesting.[137] Upon absorption of photons, excited states are formed, leading to a red shift in the absorption spectrum and delocalization of the excitation energy, forming a clear distinction between the BChl a molecules in the B850 ring and those in the B800 ring in which excitation tends to be localized.[100] This results in an ultrafast energy-funneling rate from the B800 to the B850 ring, an order of magnitude faster than that is predicted based on localized states.[100,104,138]

It is still intriguing how natural photosynthetic systems have developed such a range of aggregation states and strong electronic couplings, and what is more puzzling is how such systems avoid concentration quenching.[100] Concentration quenching is a common cause for drop in quantum yield in organic systems; the high concentration of fluorophores in a solution of organic dyes results in aggregate formation leading to quenching.[100] For example, the fluorescence emission of dissolved chlorophyll a is significantly quenched at a concentration of 0.1 M.[140,141] However, in the light-harvesting antenna complexes, such quenching is effectively avoided despite the high concentration. For instance, an effective concentration of chlorophyll in LHCII complex is 0.25 M[142] but still with no significant change in the excited-state lifetime compared to that of monomeric chlorophyll a. In the case of green sulfur bacteria, aggregated bacteriochlorophylls in the light-harvesting organelles, called chlorosomes, are present at a concentration as high as ≈ 2 M.[143] These examples point to the fact that there are much more unknown aspects in the design of photosynthetic light harvesting, which are often not considered by EET theories.[100]

If and how coherence plays a role in rendering these light-harvesting systems efficient in the energy transfer has been a question of great research interest in recent times. The effect of coherence on charge transfer is also debatable but less argued. The word coherence can be used in different connotations in literature, and there are different types of coherence with different interpretations in classical physics and quantum mechanics, a comprehensive account of which can be found elsewhere.[100,144]

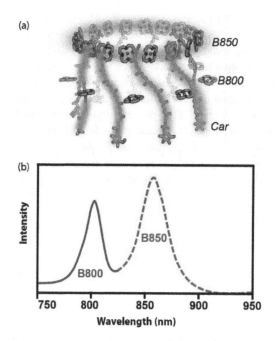

FIGURE 6.6 Optical properties of LH2 antenna complex: (a) Arrangement of the bacterio-chlorophyll (Bchl a) and carotenoid (Car) pigments in the LH2 antenna complex of a purple bacterium (structure from Rps. acidophila, 2FKW); The rings of the B850 and B800 BChls are arranged respectively perpendicular and parallel to the plane of the membrane. (Adapted with permission from Sipka, G. and Maróti, P., *Photosynth. Res.,* 136, 17–30, 2018. Copyright 2017, Springer Nature.) (b) Ensemble absorption spectrum (schematic) of LH2 with the characteristic B800 band (solid line) and B850 band (dashed line) in the near-infrared range. (Inspired from Hildner, R. et al., *Science,* 340, 1448–1451, 2013.)

To say if coherence is relevant in a system, there are two limiting scenarios (i.e., weak electronic coupling and strong electronic coupling) (Figure 6.7a–c).[6] There is an incoherent transport when states (which can be excitations or charges) are localized and hop randomly from site to site.[6] Likewise, when states are delocalized over sites to form extended eigen states, the transport proceeds stochastically in a disordered system through population relaxation.[6] In other words, population relaxes incoherently from state to state because of meager interactions with the environment. But the interesting case is the intermediate of these two, where coherence is found and where delocalization competes with localization.[6] When free evolution (electronic coupling that drives delocalization) interplays with energy fluctuations that tend to localize excitation, the ensuing transport dynamics are often complex.[6] At times, excitons tumble down a ladder of energy states while at other times collective excitations jump through space (Figure 6.7c).[6] During dynamic evolution, there can also be a change in the exciton/charge-carrier size. For instance, an initial semi-localized state "jumps" into a manifold of delocalized states (Figure 6.7c) that eventually localize to result in a final localized state that is remote from the initial state.[6] The intermediate regime

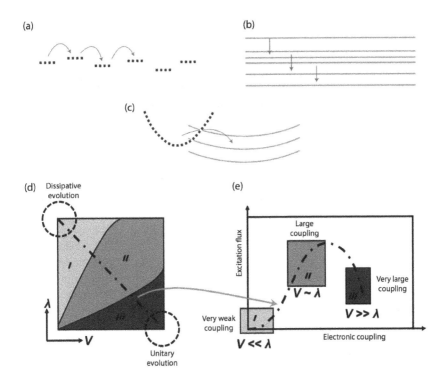

FIGURE 6.7   Coherence in energy transfer: (a–c) Schematics of free energy (vertical axis) versus a schematic representation of position, or site (horizontal axis), comparing limiting model cases for transport. (a) Weak electronic coupling: incoherent hopping transport among localized states. (b) Strong electronic coupling: incoherent relaxation among delocalized states. (c) Intermediate case: competition between timescales of localization and transport; (quasi-)localized states can transfer population to delocalized states. In each case, localized or pseudo-localized levels or free-energy curves are represented by dotted lines, while delocalized levels are shown by solid lines. (d) The regimes of electronic energy transfer (EET), specifically (I) incoherent Förster transfer, (II) the intermediate coupling regime (coherent EET), and (III) the Redfield excitonic regime dominated by relaxation. (e) Illustration of the dependence of the rate of a general excitation energy transfer process on the electronic coupling V for a representative system-bath interaction λ. (Figure 6.7a–c are adapted with permission from Bredas, J.L. et al., *Nat. Mater.*, 16, 35–44, 2017. Copyright 2016, Springer Nature and Figure 6.7d, e are inspired from Chenu, A. and Scholes, G.D., *Annu. Rev. Phys. Chem.*, 66, 69–96, 2015.)

is characterized by competition of timescales, where the coherent dynamics often dominate only for short times and convert to incoherent transport.[6]

Models beyond Förster theory that explain coherence also take into account the interactions of the chromophores with the environment (i.e., system-bath interactions).[100] The effect of the environment around the chromophores in antenna complexes is indicated by Stokes shift, which is the energy difference between the absorption maximum and the fluorescence maximum.[100] Stokes shift is known to be twice the reorganization energy λ, a metric indicating how strongly the electronic transitions of the chromophores are coupled to their environment. In an LHCII antenna complex, the Stokes shift of chlorophyll a is 100 cm^{-1}, whereas in a solution, it is higher in the range of 135–200 cm^{-1}, depending on the solvent polarity.[145,146] The reduction in the Stokes shift in the antenna complex indicates that the reorganization energies in the antenna complexes have evolved to be lower than those in solution environments.[100]

According to Förster theory, the energy transfer rate is directly proportional to $|V|^2$, where V is the electronic coupling.[100] The energy transfer rate increases quadratically with the electronic coupling when it is very small compared to the reorganization energy (λ) of the environment (Figure 6.7d and e). In this regime, the transport occurs by incoherent hopping.[100] On the other hand, when V is very large, the dynamics convert to relaxation between exciton levels; relaxation dominates instead of EET. Intermediate to these limiting cases is the fastest energy transfer— that is, coherent EET. As per the concept of process coherence, a process can be said to be coherent or incoherent depending on the degree to which the evolution of an open quantum system is dominated by the unitary part or the dissipative part.[144] In multichromophoric systems such as those in photosynthetic light-harvesting proteins, the process can be more coherent when the chromophores are more strongly coupled to each other than to the environment.[144] The Förster transfer is said to be incoherent as the donor and acceptor are more strongly coupled to their environment than the strength of coupling between each other, which renders slow transport.[144] On the other extreme, when the coupling between chromophores is very large, relaxation dominates instead of EET. Coherent EET occurs somewhere intermediate to these two limiting cases.

Similarly, the limiting cases for coherent and hopping charge transport have been put forth. Studying the charge-carrier mobilities and understanding the transport mechanisms in π-conjugated materials have gathered immense interest.[6,147–150] Coherence in the case of electron/hole transfer is associated with low-friction transport while the incoherent electron/hole hopping is known to occur in the high-friction limit.[6] In conjugated materials, the transport mechanism is determined by the morphology and structural disorder such as chain twists.[6] The intermolecular interactions are decisive of the nature of transport. For example, in the case of covalent bonding, the transport will predominantly be intra-chain whereas in the case of weak van der Waals links between molecules, inter-chain transport will be dominant.[6] A strong connection between the electronic and geometric structure is an essential characteristic of the π-conjugated systems; in other words, there is a strong electron-vibration coupling.[6] To determine if a system can assume coherent transport in the band regime or incoherent transport in the hopping regime depends largely on the relative strengths of electronic couplings and electron-vibration couplings.[6] Coherent transport with high mobilities has been observed in highly ordered and structurally perfect π-conjugated chains, such as polydiacetylene or ladder polyparaphenylene chains, where the intra-chain electronic couplings are much larger than the geometry relaxation energies.[6,151] On the other hand, in the polymeric materials with a significant degree of disorder or in organic semiconductor thin films, hopping transport is evident as charge carriers jump from one chain (or molecule) to another.[6] Here, the transport depends on the inter-chain couplings which, because of the weak wave function overlap, are at least an order of magnitude lower than the intra-chain couplings.[6]

Structural disorder or presence of any impurities producing trap states further limits the transport.[6,152] In contrast to these scenarios, high-mobility molecular crystals offer a peculiar example that lies intermediate to these limiting cases.[6] Despite the high degree of order in the structure, the transport is found to be intermolecular (akin to inter-chain).[6] Studies suggest the coexistence of localized incoherent states and delocalized coherent states, revealing the potential for coherent transport.[6,149] In the case of conjugated oligomers, the mode of transport depends on the length of molecule; charges are found to tunnel quantum mechanically through chains that are of a length of five repeating units or less and beyond which charge transport occurs by incoherent hopping.[6] It is hence possible in thin films of π-conjugated systems—when there is some degree of local order and there are large electronic couplings—that there can be a combination of different transport regimes becoming operational, adding coherent processes to the incoherent.[6]

In organic photovoltaics, coherence aids in explaining the rapid rate of charge separation. Charge separation in conjugated-molecule/fullerene blends takes place at an ultrafast rate and is suggested that it probably involves delocalized acceptor and/or donor states.[6] It is intriguing how the electron and hole could separate at such a high speed.[6] One explanation is that the electron coherently transits deep into the fullerene domain preceding the photon cloud (Figure 6.8)—that is, the relaxation of the molecular structure lags behind the change of electronic state.[6] This also holds vital implications for the reverse reaction (i.e., geminate recombination).[6] When the photon cloud catches up with the electron (in other words, the molecular relaxation stabilizes the charge), the electron gets localized at some distance from the interface, which reduces the electron-hole attraction owing to the remoteness from the interface.[6] Furthermore, the reverse electron-transfer is suppressed, as the electron now must be transported with the photon cloud, which requires hopping transport. This is classically analogous to having ballistic forward transport and backwards transport subject to high friction.[6] In the view of quantum mechanics, the electron wave function can be strongly delocalized on short timescales, aided by coherence effects, then turn to be localized, trapping the electron remotely from the interface.[6] Studies also suggest that coupling to intermolecular vibrations probably has a vital role in facilitating the conversion of delocalized states to separated electron-hole pairs.[6,153]

With the major goal of deciphering the "design principles" of photosynthetic light harvesting, numerous studies are being carried out to identify the energy transfer and charge transfer routes in the photosynthetic systems. Still, there is no consensus on which mode among the two major transport modes (hopping and coherence) is actually adopted by nature to effect in high quantum efficiencies in photosynthesis. However, it is worthwhile to emulate these transport modes in the biohybrid and biomimetic photovoltaics systems to explore the possibilities of improving the device-level efficiency.

6.3.3 PHOTOSYNTHETIC MIMICS AND PHOTOVOLTAIC MIMICS

As a development over the conventional bioelectrochemical cells, a number of recent reports[38,154–160] focus on constructing solid-state multilayered devices where the charge transfer is determined mainly by the band structure and energy-level alignment. Though the in-device interfacial electronic structure has so far not been characterized

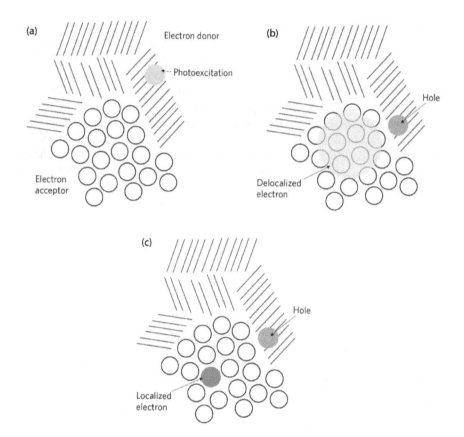

FIGURE 6.8 Coherence at donor–acceptor interfaces: (a) Illustration of an instance of photoexcitation in the donor domain of an OPV bulk heterojunction migrating to donor/acceptor interface. (b) Electron transfer to an initial delocalized electron state in the acceptor domain, leaving a (probably localized) hole in the donor. (c) Rapid localization of the electron away from the interface, which suppresses recombination. (Reproduced with permission from Bredas, J.L. et al., *Nat. Mater.,* 16, 35–44, 2017, Copyright 2016, Springer Nature.)

in detail in biophotovoltaics, design principles based on bandgap theory have been utilized in a few reports, which focus more on the light-harvesting ability and photonics in the device than on the device electronics. Some of these devices still retain the basic liquid electrochemical cell design but superimposed with a few principles of photonics and band theory. These devices are discussed in the Section 6.4.

First, electronic/band-structure approaches are of importance in solid-state hybrid photovoltaic cells that incorporate design principles both from photosynthesis and from conventional photovoltaics. An example of these hybrid devices is the biophotovoltaic cells (BPVs) that integrate biological complexes in an OPV device architecture either as a photoactive layer or any other electronically functional layer. To lay out new routes by which the design principles of BPVs and OPVs can be combined, it is vital to understand the individual research trends in the BPVs and OPVs. A number of recent reviews present comprehensive accounts of the research progress and the emerging trends in these fields.[3,16,18,63,161–164] Although the idea of designing BPVs with a device architecture adopted from OPVs is new, the urge to enhance performance in conventional photovoltaics by borrowing design principles from natural photosynthetic systems has been felt for long. As a matter of fact, the whole field of dye-sensitized solar cells (DSSCs) emerged from a simple design inspiration from natural photosynthesis.

6.3.3.1 Photosynthetic Mimics in Photovoltaics

The working of a DSSC is in many ways comparable to that of the natural photosystems. The functions of light harvesting and charge separation are performed respectively by the antenna complexes and reaction center in a photosynthetic system, whereas the two functions are achieved respectively by a dye and a semiconductor in a DSSC.[16,165] Photosystems in plants and bacteria have a well-structured array of pigments in close proximity to the reaction center so as to aid in an efficient excitation energy transfer, whereas in a DSSC, a nanoporous semiconductor layer is used to increase the number of dye molecules in contact per unit volume, which loosely mimics the design of the photosynthetic protein complexes. In photosynthesis, the array of the pigments (in the antenna complexes) absorbs light and funnels the excitation energy into the reaction center, which is comparable to the process of dye molecules injecting the electrons from their excited state into the conduction band of the semiconductor, in the case of a DSSC.

While the field of organic photovoltaics is still emerging, the idea of bioinspiration has already gained attention in the field, and there are new efforts to emulate the light-harvesting principles of photosynthesis in OPVs with the scope of improvement in the overall device efficiency. In photosynthesis, the light harvesting is driven by the transfer of electronic excitation energy stored (within nanoseconds) in the excited-state chromophores (antenna pigments) to the target chromophores or energy traps (reaction center).[16,31,78,166] To artificially create such an arrangement in a light-harvesting device is practically challenging as the timescale largely constrains the size of the chromophore arrays attached to the trap/target reactive site.[78] In OPVs, there is a limitation on how far the excitation energy can travel in the organic films, which is decided by the exciton diffusion length.[78,167,168] The solar energy harvesting in the natural photosystems is more efficiently carried out than that of any OPV because of the more sophisticated structural arrangement of chromophores as opposed to a disordered mixture of donor and acceptor molecules in any OPV.

To mimic the energy transfer kinetics of the natural photosynthetic system in an organic photovoltaic cell, phycobilisome-photosystem (Figure 6.9a) has recently been studied based on which an artificial system was built emulating a few of its design features.[169] The ability of certain cyanobacterial species to carry out photosynthesis even in those locations with low light flux such as in the deep aquatic zones has been an inspiration in designing artificial photosystems for OPVs. While the light-to-electrical conversion during the initial phases of photosynthesis takes place with an efficiency close to 100%, it is practically hard to achieve a similar efficiency in OPVs, a possible reason for which could be the poor charge carrier generation upon exciton dissociation. Addressing this has been the main focus in a recent work on P3HT-CNT-based bioinspired OPV where poly(3-hexyl)thiophene (P3HT) was

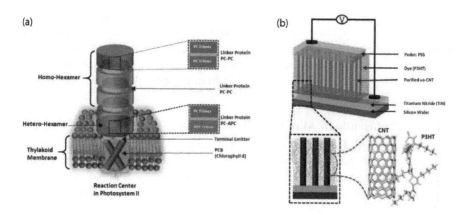

FIGURE 6.9 Organic Photovoltaics mimicking photosynthetic systems: (a) Cartoon showing the structural architecture of the Phycobilisome (PBS) antenna complex found in the cyanobacteria "*Acaryochloris marina*" (b) Schematic structure of a P3HT-va-CNT OPV device (va-CNT: vertically aligned carbon nanotube) (Reproduced with permission from Ravi, S.K. et al., *Adv. Funct. Mater.*, 2017. Copyright 2017, John Wiley & Sons.)

used as the photoactive donor and vertically aligned single-walled carbon nanotubes as the acceptor. The phycobilisome (PBS) antenna complex from the cyanobacteria "*Acaryochloris marina*" was taken as a model for the study. PBS performs the primary light harvesting followed by downhill excitation energy transfer into the reaction center of the photosystem 2 (PS2) protein. The light-harvesting efficiency is about 95%, which is a result of the architecture of the antenna complex encompassing a well-structured and ordered array of pigments. The PBS antenna system has a rod-like architecture that is composed of a stack of hexameric disks of pigment proteins, with non-pigment linker proteins connecting the disks (Figure 6.9a). Three of the hexamers in the stack are composed only of Phycocyanin (PC), while the fourth is a heterohexamer that contains both PC and Allophycocyanin (APC).[169–171] The structure of each hexamer/heterohexamer involves a connection of two trimers through C3 symmetry where the unpigmented protein linkers are located; these unpigmented proteins are also known to affect the absorption and emission characteristics of nearby pigments.[172,173] Although not precisely, the design of the P3HT-CNT system is found analogous to the PBS photosystem, forming organized arrays of photoactive donors (i.e., P3HT). The biological analogues of P3HT are the PC and the APC pigments in the PBS photosystem (Figure 6.9b).[169] Though the device architecture loosely resembled the PBS system, the P3HT-CNT system results in an efficiency only in the range of 10%–15%, which is still not significantly higher compared to that of the conventional organic solar cells.[10,169]

   The formation of excitons and the transfer of excitation energy from the PBS antenna complex to the reaction center within the PS2 of the cyanobacteria are shown in Figure 6.10a. The PC pigments initially absorb the incident light. What follows next is a downhill excitation energy transfer from PC to RC through an intermediate in the order APC→PBS-TE→RC, where PBS-TE is the terminal emitter in the PBS system. It is the lowest energy state in the PBS antenna system that funnels the excitation energy into the reaction center of PS2 and hence is called the terminal emitter. The PBS absorbs light between 550 and 660 nm and forwards it via successively lower energy chromophores after which the excitation energy finally migrates from the terminal emitter of PBS to the chlorophyll in the reaction center (Figure 6.10b). *Acaryochloris marina* has a chlorophyll d (Chl d) instead of a

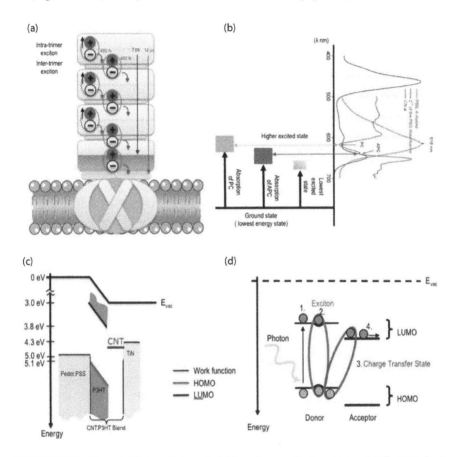

FIGURE 6.10 Organic Photovoltaics mimicking photosynthetic systems: (a) Cartoon showing the exciton generation and migration through the PC and APC trimers toward the reaction center. (b) Illustration of downhill excitation energy migration in PBS; After excitation of PC, the absorbed excitation energy is transferred from PC to APC and further from APC to the low-energy state in the PBS (c) Energy level diagram of the P3HT-va-CNT OPV. (d). Exciton migration and charge separation in the OPV 1. Photoexcitation of an electron into the donor LUMO creates a hole in HOMO. 2. Formation of an exciton as the photogenerated electron and hole are coulombically bound. 3. Hopping of electron onto the LUMO of the acceptor as it has a higher electron affinity while the hole still remains at the donor HOMO. There is a formation of the geminate pair together with the electron existing in the acceptor molecule. (From Ogren, J.I. et al., *Chem. Sci.*, 2018.) Complete dissociation of exciton into charge carriers followed by polaron hopping toward the respective electrodes (electrons → anode and holes → cathode). (Reproduced with permission from Nganou, C. et al., *ACS Appl. Mater. Interfaces*, 9, 19030–19039, 2017. Copyright 2017, American Chemical Society.)

chlorophyll a (Chl a) in its reaction center; the difference in absorption spectrum between the two is shown in Figure 6.8b. The Chl d has an optical absorption in the range of 660–680 nm where it absorbs the excitation energy from the terminal emitter (Figure 6.10b).

While in the bioinspired OPV system, P3HT acts as a dye, absorbs the incident light, and gains energy to push an electron from the highest occupied molecular orbital (HOMO) to the lowest unoccupied molecular orbital (LUMO) leading to an excited state (i.e., an exciton). In the exciton, the electron and the hole are bound by a coulombic attraction; the binding energy holding the carriers together in the exciton should be overcome to enable charge separation. In the OPV, CNT acts as the electron acceptor and P3HT acts as the donor. The exciton dissociates at the P3HT/CNT interface, as CNT has an ionization potential higher than that of the excited electron (Figure 6.10c). The dissociation is induced by the π-electronic valley of CNT; the π-electron induces a coulombic force on the dipole moment of the exciton, which is greater than the coulombic attractive force binding the electron and the hole within the exciton. The splitting of an exciton into individual charge carriers occurs in multiple steps. Since the acceptor molecule (CNT) has a higher electron affinity, at the donor-acceptor interface, it causes the electron to hop from the LUMO of the donor (P3HT) toward the LUMO of the acceptor; an electrostatic potential gradient is formed at the P3HT/CNT interface; this drives the electron into the CNT LUMO while the hole remains in the P3HT HOMO. The electron that hopped from P3HT LUMO to CNT LUMO forms a geminate pair (interacting by coulombic forces) with the hole in the P3HT HOMO (Figure 6.10d). Further separation of the two charge carriers in the geminate pair is driven by thermal activation and electric fields. As they separate from each other with a distance exceeding the coulomb radius, they fully dissociate and relax into polarons because of their large effective mass. Subsequently, these polarons polarize their neighborhood and hop toward the outer electrodes, where the respective charge carriers are finally collected.

Transport of carriers takes place by hopping in this case as organic solids do not favour high charge carrier mobility. This is because the mean free path of the charge carriers is in the same order of magnitude as that of the lattice constant in these organic solids. To mimic the carrier transport in photosynthesis, the hopping distance has to be minimized. This has been attempted by employing vertically aligned CNTs as electron acceptors as they are expected to reduce the mean free path in the OPV because of the ballistic charge transport properties along the CNT sidewall. Several profound conclusions have been drawn on the exciton generation and migration in the P3HT-CNT artificial photosynthetic system and how it differs from that in the natural PBS photosynthetic system, based on time-resolved spectroscopic studies.

It has been found that, though the time taken for exciton formation in both the natural and artificial systems can roughly be equaled, the subsequent downhill energy transfer into the RC in the natural PBS systems takes place at a speed three orders of magnitude faster than that in the P3HT-CNT system. Exciton trapping at the donor/acceptor interface has been found to be the limiting factor affecting the OPV efficiency; and the need for photovoltaic systems with more precise mimicking of photosynthesis is also greatly felt.

6.3.3.2 Photovoltaic Mimics in Biohybrid Devices

Besides the use of fully artificial photosynthetic systems in OPVs, direct integration of certain components from natural photosynthetic complexes in OPVs has also been attempted. Such biohybrid devices may be referred to as photovoltaic mimics as they adopt the basic device architecture of conventional OPVs. Recently, a biohybrid OPV has been reported, in which the active layers are composed of photosynthetic pigments.[38] A linear Carotenoid (Car) pigment lycopene was used as the electron donor and two different derivatives of Chlorophyll (Chl1: methyl $3^2,3^2$-dicyanopyropheophorbide-a and Chl2: methyl 13^1-deoxo-13^1-(dicyanomethylene)pyropheophorbide-a) as electron acceptors (Figure 6.11). Unlike the P3HT-CNT system discussed earlier, this study adopted a simple OPV device structure with no special focus on ordered arrangement of donors and acceptors. The active layer used is simply a blend of the donor and acceptor materials, which is typical to a special class of OPVs called Bulk-heterojunction (BHJ) OPVs, a more detailed account of which is presented in Section 6.3.4. The use of hole-extracting and electron-extracting interlayers such as MoO_3 and Ca is another typical feature of OPV that has been adopted in this biohybrid device (Figure 6.11a).[174] Low work function metals such as Ca, Ba, and Mg are commonly used as cathode interlayers in OPVs as they help in reducing the overall work function of the electrode in contact thereby facilitating efficient electron extraction.[174] Having a layer of these materials on the active layer also prevents any penetration of the cathode material (typically Al or Ag) into the active material during the cathode deposition.[174] In the same way, anode interlayers are used to reduce the energy barrier for hole transport at the interface as direct contact of the organic photoactive layer with the anode typically results in substantial band bending with a Schottky barrier; transparent layers of transition metal oxides such as MoO_3, V_2O_5, and WO_3 are *n*-type semiconductors that are commonly

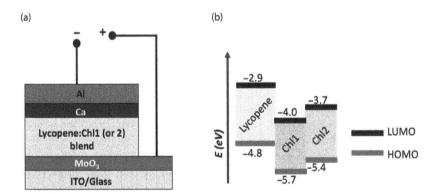

FIGURE 6.11 A biohybrid solar cell mimicking organic photovoltaic device structure: (a) Schematic showing the device structure of the BPV with lycopene as donor and chlorophyll derivatives (Chl1 or Chl2) as acceptor, Ca and MoO_3 as cathodic and anodic interlayers. (b) Energy level diagram of the BPV. (Adapted with permission from Zhuang, T. et al., *RSC Adv.*, 5, 45755–45759, 2015. Copyright 2015, Royal Society of Chemistry.)

used for this purpose.[174,175] Two different biohybrid devices have been constructed mimicking a BHJ device structure, one using Lycopene:Chl1 as the active layer and the other using Lycopene:Chl2.[38] It is important to note that there is one basic design principle from the band-structure approach that has been followed in device design. In both devices, the energy offset between the donor and acceptor LUMO levels was ensured to be greater than the exciton binding energy, which is typically in the range of 0.3–0.5 eV (Figure 6.11b).[169] Based on this, though, both the cases can be expected to have efficient exciton dissociation; the device with Chl2 as electron acceptor was found to have better photovoltaic performance than the one with Chl1, as Chl2 favored a higher electron mobility than Chl1.[38] Carrier mobility is hence another important factor that affects the device performance. Both carrier mobility and exciton binding energy are to be optimized, and their interplay is to be studied in any Bio-OPV device for a deeper understanding and a better performance. Bulk heterojunctions in OPVs aided better control of these two factors; this lately has also been used with photoproteins integrated into the design.

6.3.4 Bilayer and Bulk Heterojunction Biophotovoltaic Cells

Carrier mobility is the speed at which the charge carrier traverses through a medium under an electric field.[176–178] The strength of interaction between the two charge carriers coulombically bound within the exciton is referred to as exciton binding energy.[176,179–181] Both these parameters play crucial roles in deciding the OPV efficiency by influencing carrier recombination. There are three major types of recombination—namely radiative, non-radiative, and Auger—that are common in optoelectronics; these are discussed in detail in a number of reviews.[176,177,182] Most OPVs suffer losses stemming from each of these recombination types, and thus reducing these recombination losses is crucial for high performance. These losses can be avoided if the active layer is defect-free, however, it is challenging to acheive an active layer without any defects. These defects lead to new energy states within the bandgap of the active material, which are known as electronic traps.[176,183] These traps act as potential recombination sites, and it is hence crucial to have the defect density as low as possible.[184,185]

The density of traps (or defect density) cannot be reduced beyond an extent in any OPV device. However, there is an alternative approach called "heterostructuring," where the recombination losses are minimized by separating the two charge carriers into two different phases formed by intermixing/blending of the donor and acceptor materials.[176] Bulk heterojunctions formed in such blends enable rapid exciton dissociation/charge separation at interfaces, thereby reducing radiative recombination losses.[176,186,187] This idea of introducing bulk heterojunctions in OPVs has shown a great advantage in the device performance compared to the conventional bilayer heterojunctions. This concept has also gathered interest in other branches of optoelectronics. In recent years, there have been many efforts to employ the BHJ approach in biophotovoltaic devices.

In terms of the materials and the stages of operation used, bulk heterojunction (BHJ) organic solar cells do not differ from the conventional bilayer OPVs (Figure 6.12a)—that

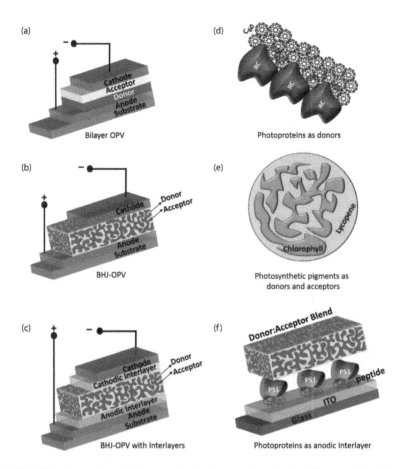

FIGURE 6.12 Integration of photosynthetic pigments/proteins in bilayer and bulk hetero-junction devices: (a) A simple bilayer OPV with donors and acceptors as separate layers. (b) A BHJ OPV with the donors and acceptors intermixed. (c) A BHJ OPV with additional interfacial materials on either of the active BHJ layers. Different approaches in utilizing photosynthetic pigments/proteins in a BHJ OPV. (d) Photoproteins used as a donor in a bilayer OPV with C60 as an acceptor and ETL. (e) Photosynthetic pigments used as both acceptors and donors in a BHJ architecture. (f) Use of photoproteins as an interlayer in a BHJ that has a separate donor/acceptor concoction (The use as "anodic interlayer" is specified considering a conventional OPV structure; the same protein layer would act as a "cathodic interlayer" in an inverted OPV structure." (Adapted with permission from Ravi, S.K. et al., *Adv. Funct. Mater.*, 2017. Copyright 2017, John Wiley & Sons.)

is, both BHJ-OPV and bilayer-OPV use an electron donor and an electron acceptor and follow the same four stages of operation shown in Figure 6.10d. However, the feature unique to the BHJ-OPV is that the donor and acceptor materials are blended together (Figure 6.12b). Besides the use of photosynthetic pigments in BHJ devices, there have also been attempts to directly integrate antenna complexes, reaction center complexes, or photosystem complexes in BHJ-OPVs. Various reports have approached such direct biointegration in different ways and to serve different functions in a photovoltaic device. Such approaches are as follows:

1. One basic approach has been to employ photoproteins/pigments as a photoactive layer or the electron donor in a bilayer-OPV structure (Figure 6.12a) with a conventional electron acceptor or an electron transporting layer interfacing it.[188]
2. Another approach is to use biological components for both donors and acceptors; for example, a blend of two different photosynthetic pigments/proteins are used in a bulk heterojunction structure (Figure 6.12b).[38]
3. Another recent approach is to use the photosynthetic complexes as cathodic or anodic interlayers in the device instead of employing them as the primary photoactive layer.[157,158] The use of such interlayers is common in BHJ OPVs to enhance the charge extraction and transport (Figure 6.12c); they control the interfacial energy-level alignment, adjust the built-in electric field, and also regulate the surface energy and surface recombination.[174]

The use of photoproteins in an OPV device structure has been reported more than a decade back, and the device employed a typical bilayer-OPV architecture (Figure 6.12d).[188] This is an example of the first approach mentioned earlier. The second approach has been evident in those BHJ devices employing photosynthetic pigments such as lycopene and chlorophyll as electron donors and acceptors (Figure 6.12e, also refer to the earlier section—Figure 6.11).[38] With the third approach, natural photosystems with peptide linkers have been used in BHJ-OPVs to function as an anodic interlayer (Figure 6.12f).[158]

The use of the first approach (bilayer-OPV type) could be found in the article (R. Das et al., 2004)[188] where purple bacterial photosynthetic reaction centers (RCs) were used as the photoactive donor layer in the OPV with fullerene (C_{60}) as a separate electron acceptor layer coated on it (Figure 6.12d). The device fabrication (Figure 6.13a) involved: (i) Use of an ITO-coated glass as the substrate; (ii) Deposition of Au anode on the substrate by thermal evaporation with Cr as an intermediate buffer layer to promote adhesion with the substrate; (iii) Chemical functionalization of the anode surface with a self-assembled monolayer of Nickel-Nitrilotriacetic acid (Ni^{2+}-NTA); (iv) Immobilization (Figure 6.13b) of the RC complexes on the anode (the RC proteins were modified with polyhistidine tags that selectively bind with the Ni^{2+}-NTA in such a way that the RCs are oriented with their special pair P facing the anode, so the photooxidized special pair can accept the electrons reentering the circuit); (v) Deposition of the C_{60} acceptor layer on the proteins by thermal evaporation; (vi) Coating of a protective organic interlayer on the protein layer, which is a thin layer of layer of 2,9-dimethyl-4,7-diphenyl-1,10-phenanthroline (bathocuproine, or BCP) by thermal evaporation; and (vii) Cathode deposition: thermal evaporation of silver on the BCP interlayer.

In this device structure, the RC proteins serve as the electron donor and C_{60} Fullerene serve as the electron acceptor. C_{60} had been employed as the acceptor as it has a relatively deep LUMO of 4.7 eV that enhances the electron transfer from the quinone Q_B (which is the final electron acceptor site in the reaction center). The fullerene layer accepts the photogenerated electrons from the RC complexes, and its preferential electron transporting tendency enables it to forward the accepted electrons to the BCP interlayer (Figure 6.13c). The BCP is a thin layer that suffers significant damage to

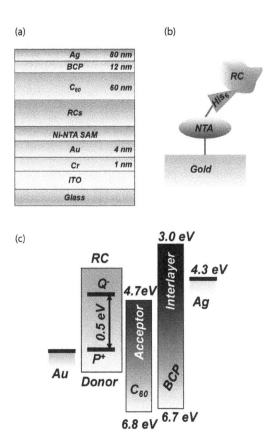

FIGURE 6.13 A Bilayer Biohybrid-photovoltaic device: (a) Device architecture of the bilayer bio-OPV device. (b) Immobilization route for orienting the reaction center protein on the Au electrode. (c) Energy level diagram of the device. (Inspired from Das, R. et al., *Nano Lett.*, 4, 1079–1083, 2004.)

itself while protecting the underlying active layers during cathode deposition. Damage to the BCP layer facilitates electron extraction and its deep HOMO aids in preventing the injection of holes into the device, which significantly improves the device performance.

With similar bilayer-OPV type device structures, the use of photosystem 1 (PS1) has also been reported in two different reports, where the protein served as the sole photoactive layer. PS1 proteins were immobilized on Au-coated ITO, and a device fabrication route similar to that in Figure 6.13b had been used with a few modifications.[188] The PS1 layer served as the electron donor. To serve as the electron acceptor, an organic semiconductor tris(8-hydroxyquinoline) aluminum (Alq$_3$) was used, which was also a protective electron transporting layer interfacing the PS1 layer with the silver cathode.[188] In this report, though significant advancement in photocurrent compared to the wet electrochemical cells was put forward, the effect of PS1 on the open-circuit voltage was unclear.

Recently, in a similar PS1-based OPV device, a high open-circuit voltage of 0.76 V was achieved.[157] The device employed a dense layer of PS1 proteins without the use of any immobilization technique to orient the proteins on the electrode (Figure 6.14a). A transparent semiconducting polymer, poly triarylamine (PTAA), was used as a hole-conducting medium. Unlike the conventional OPV structure where the photogenerated electrons are driven toward the Al/Ag electrode, the biohybrid OPV device adopted an inverted OPV structure, the working mechanism of which involved the following steps: (a) Absorption of light by the PS1 protein; (b) Photoexcitation of pigments and subsequent charge separation in the PS1 reaction center resulting in electron and holes; (c) Electron transport to the ITO electrode through the titanium oxide layer and simultaneous hole transport to the Al electrode through the passage PS1→PTAA→MoO$_3$→Al. While PTAA served as the hole-transporting layer, the additional MoO$_3$ layer aided in better hole extraction by reducing the energy barrier for hole transport.[157] The electron transfer in the route PS1→TiO$_x$→ITO was facilitated by the descending order of LUMO levels as the electron traverses from PS1 to ITO (Figure 6.14b).[157]

This sums up how the first approach has been adopted in different reports. Section 6.3.3.1 may be referred to for an account of the second approach (BHJ-type OPV) put to use.

The third approach of using proteins as interlayers has been put to use in a BHJ device where PS1 proteins were used to modify the electrode work function and in turn to tune the open-circuit voltage of the device. This was achieved by establishing a particular ordered orientation of the proteins on the electrode. In an earlier report, PS1 proteins were found to naturally orient themselves with a reasonable uniformity even without any special immobilization methods. In a BHJ device structure of ITO/PS1/MEH-PPV:PCBM/(LiF or MoO$_3$)/Al, most proteins, though not 100% of them, oriented naturally with the P700 site facing up and F$_B$ site contacting the ITO. In this device, the BHJ was formed by the blend of the conjugated polymer MEH-PPV (poly[2-methoxy-5-(2′-ethylhexyloxy)-p-phenylene vinylene]) and the fullerene derivative PCBM ([6,6]-phenyl-C$_{61}$-butyric acid methyl ester)[157,158] (Figure 6.14c and d). Two different BHJ devices were constructed: one with conventional and the other with inverted OPV architecture differing only in the type of interlayer used (electron-extracting LiF or hole-extracting MoO$_3$) and hence in the direction of charge transport. The role played by the PS1 proteins, however, caused significant differences in the device performance. This can be explained by treating the proteins on the ITO electrode as a layer of electric dipoles. Upon illumination, the light absorption renders a charge-separated state in the protein with electrons staying at the F$_B$ site and the holes at the P700 site with a definite spatial separation between the opposite charges, analogous to electric dipoles.[157] The presence of electric dipoles on a conductive surface modifies its surface potential and hence its work function. Since the work function difference between the two electrodes in the OPV is a main factor affecting its open circuit voltage, the presence of PS1 dipoles had different effects in the two device structures (case A, ITO/PS1/MEH-PPV:PCBM/LiF/Al and case B, ITO/PS1/MEH-PPV:PCBM/MoO$_3$/Al) because of the difference in the resultant work function difference between the electrodes.[157] The PS1 dipole orientation (with F$_B$ site contacting electrode) causing electrons to accumulate at the ITO side had a

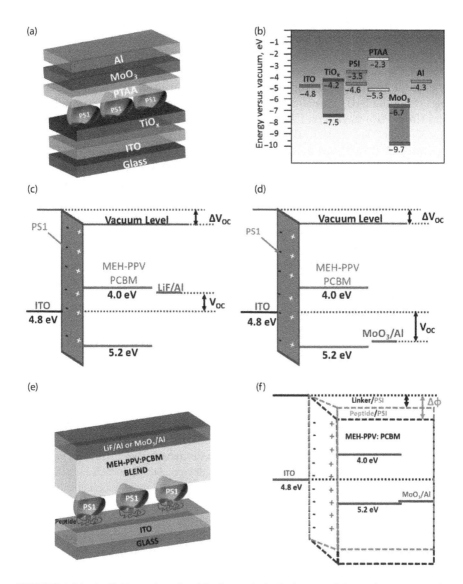

FIGURE 6.14 Bulk Heterojunction Biophotovoltaic devices: (a) Schematic representation of a PS1-integrated BHJ-OPV where PS1 is the only photoactive layer. (b) Energy level diagram of the PS1-BHJ-OPV. (c to f) - Effect of employing PS1 layer in the BHJ-OPV not as the primary photoactive layer but as an anodic interfacial layer: Variation in open-circuit voltage in MEH-PPV PCBM BHJ devices with PS1 (without immobilization) used as an interfacial layer between the BHJ and ITO, with LiF (c) and MoO$_3$ (d) as cathodic interfacial layers. (e) Use of oriented PS1 in a MEH-PPV PCBM BHJ device to serve as an anodic interfacial layer. (f) Effect of the PS1 interlayer on the cathode work function. (Reproduced with permission from Ravi, S.K. et al., *Adv. Funct. Mater.*, 2017. Copyright 2017, John Wiley & Sons.)

favorable effect on the "case B" (the inverted OPV structure). In this case, the photogenerated electrons from the BHJ were preferably driven toward the ITO electrode due to the presence of the high work function MoO_3 interlayer at the other electrode. The PS1 dipole layer of same orientation had a negative effect on the device performance in "case A" resulting from an unfavorable reaction of the photogenerated holes (from the BHJ) traversing to ITO, annihilating with the photogenerated electrons (from PS1) staying on ITO.[157] The dipole effect from the PS1 layer has varied effects on the "electrode work function difference ($\Delta\varphi$)" in the two devices. The presence of PS1 in the particular orientation reduces the work function of ITO electrode in both the cases; however, such a reduction in ITO work function increases the $\Delta\varphi$ between the ITO and MoO_3/Al electrodes in case A and decreases that between ITO and LiF/Al in case B, thus negatively affecting the latter.[157]

The same effect was confirmed in another recent report by using a fully oriented PS1 layer in the same BHJ structure. Peptide anchors were employed to orient the PS1 proteins with FB site facing ITO and P700 site facing the BHJ (Figure 6.14e). Almost 100% uniform orientation was achieved using phage display technique which is popularly used in biochemistry and bioinformatics.[158] The presence of peptides resulted in a greater work function shift (Figure 6.14f) and enhanced the open-circuit voltage of the device when an inverted structure was employed (i.e., with MoO_3/Al as the second electrode).[158]

To summarize, this section presented the basic concepts from electronics and band-structure approaches that are relevant for understanding the device physics of the emerging protein-based biohybrid photovoltaics and for developing new device architectures. With a background of discussion on interfacial electronic structure and exciton/charge transport modes, the recent efforts to understand the "design principles" in photosynthetic light harvesting were highlighted, and some of the recent attempts to mimic photosynthetic systems in organic photovoltaics and counter-mimic organic photovoltaics in biophotovoltaics were discussed. Band structure approach is a crucial field of study in any optoelectronic device. The approach aids in understanding and improving the device architectures in emerging optoelectronics such as OPVs, where controlling interfacial electronic structures, energy-level alignment, electrode work functions, and tuning exciton/charge transport modes are gaining immense research interest. It is hence worthwhile to adopt similar approaches in biophotovoltaics to better the design, performance, and understanding of the devices.

6.4   PHOTONIC APPROACHES

The previous sections focused primarily on energy-level alignment and transport properties in the devices. With the background of band-structure approach and interfacial electronic structure, different architectures of solid-state biohybrid devices were discussed with a focus on charge transport route and general device physics in each device. The devices discussed in these sections adopted the approach of improving the charge transport properties in the device in order to improve the device performance. In the coming sections, the approach of improving device performance in biohybrid photovoltaics through enhanced light harvesting will be of primary focus. While the previous sections focused on solid-state OPV-type biohybrid devices controlling energy-level alignment and charge transport, the following sections will cover approaches of enhancing the light harvesting and employing auxiliary light harvesting in both biohybrid wet-electrochemical cell and solid-state devices.

6.4.1 SEMICONDUCTOR-PROTEIN HYBRIDS

Enhancing the overall light harvesting in the device has been achieved by a number of techniques in biohybrid photovoltaic cells and bioelectrochemical cells. One of the common approaches is the use of a secondary light-harvesting material in the device that serves as an auxiliary photoactive component, supplementing the photogeneration of charge carriers by the primary active material (i.e., the photosynthetic proteins) in the device. Semiconductors have been used as secondary light harvesters in a number of different approaches. Cascading the photoreactions of the primary and secondary light harvesters is one such approach. This approach aids in enhancing the open-circuit voltage of a photoelectrochemical cell integrated with photosynthetic pigment-protein by cascading the light-harvesting reaction of the protein with that of a semiconductor. Recently, this has been achieved by the use of highly oxidizing redox electrolytes as a junctioning medium connecting the two photoreactions, enabling the cascade effect. This approach has been demonstrated with a purple bacterial RC-LH1 protein and an n-type Si (n-Si) semiconductor.[189] Upon incidence of light, the pigments in the LH1 antenna complex and reaction center reach excited states and following this photoexcitation, the special pair of bacteriochorophylls in the RC protein (denoted as P) initiates a metastable charge separation, which is a four-step electron transfer reaction spanning across the RC and ending at a cofactor called ubiquinone (Q_B), resulting in a radical pair $P^+Q_B^-$ (Figure 6.15a and b). In any bio-photoelectrochemical cell, the open-circuit voltage is typically limited by the potential difference between the molecular species receiving charge carriers from one electrode and the species receiving the opposite charge carrier from the electrode or in other words, donating the same charge carriers to the electrode. In this respect, the open-circuit voltage of any RC-based bioelectrochemical cell was estimated to be dependent on the potential gap between the P/P^+ couple that interfaces with the cathode and the electron transport mediator or the redox electrolyte that interfaces with the anode. This estimation proved effective in controlling the open-circuit voltage simply by means of manipulating the electrolyte redox potential.[46] Nevertheless, the design still suffered losses stemming from recombination reactions. These are futile electron transfer reactions from the electrolyte to the P^+ state (marked by the dashed arrow in Figure 6.15b). In the earlier cell designs, the choice of electrolytes in regime I (Figure 6.15b), where the redox potential of the electrolyte lies in between the Q_B^- and P^+ states (Regime II, Figure 6.15b), has been an obvious factor favoring the recombination losses. However, the choice was also restricted by the work function of the counter electrode chosen. As a way to overcome these losses and simultaneously enhance the light harvesting, the cascade approach seemed promising.

This was realized by choosing electrolytes whose redox potenital lie below the P^+ state, which not only renders the recombination reactions improbable but also serves to bridge the photoinduced charge separation in the protein complexes with

(a)

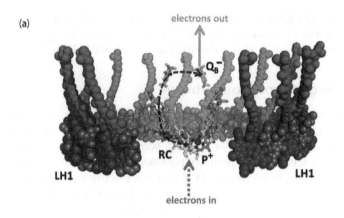

(b)

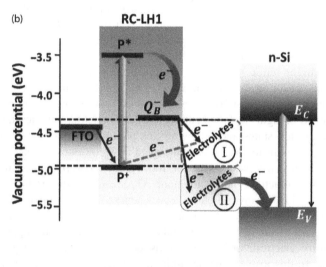

FIGURE 6.15 RC-LH1/n-Si Hybrid: (a) Illustration of charge separation in purple bacterial reaction center complex (with its surrounding light-harvesting antenna complex). On photoinduced charge separation through a series of electron transfer reactions (dashed arrow) to result in $P^+Q_B^-$, electrons enter the complex by means of reduction of P^+ (dotted arrow) and exit the complex by oxidation of Q_B^- (solid arrow). (b) The working of a cascade-mechanism in the hybrid bio-photoelectrochemical cell: Regime I electrolytes: In conventional bio-photoelectrochemical cells, the redox potentials of the electrolytes typically lying in between those of P/P^+ and Q_B/Q_B^-, the possibility of recombination of electrons from the electrolyte to the P^+ cannot be ruled out. Regime II electrolytes: Futile recombination reactions are averted. Steps in the cascade reactions: Incident photon initiates a primary photochemical reaction in the RC-LH1 complex, which involves photoexcitation of the special pair ($P \rightarrow P^*$) and charge-separation to form P^+ and Q_B^-. Remnant light unabsorbed by the protein triggers an auxiliary photoexcitation in n-Si, resulting in excitation of an electron into the conduction band (E_C) while leaving a hole in the valence band (E_V). The two photoreactions are cascaded by the highly oxidizing electrolytes which replenish the photogenerated holes in the n-Si valence band with those electrons collected from the RC-LH1 complex. (Reproduced with permission from Singh, V.K. et al., *Adv. Funct. Mater.*, 1703689, 2017. Copyright 2017, John Wiley & Sons.)

the concurrent phototransition in an n-Si anode/counter electrode.[189] Upon illumination, the remnant light reaching the back electrode (after photoabsorption at the protein layer) excites the n-Si, as a result of which there are photogenerated holes in its valence band and photogenerated electrons in the conduction band. The holes in the silicon's valence band are at a more oxidizing potential than the P/P+ couple in the RC. In the device, the protein-coated FTO photoelectrode (cathode) and the n-Si anode were connected by one of three electrolytes, which are: (A) TEMPO (2,2,6,6-tetramethyl-1-piperidinyloxy), (B) Ferrocene/ferrocenium, and (C) Iodide/triiodide (I−/I3−) couple.[189] The redox potentials of all the three electrolytes are such that they are more oxidizing than P/P+. This prevents undesirable electron transfer reactions between the oxidizing and reducing cofactors of the RC protein or between the RC and the FTO. The cascade mechanism in the cell is illustrated in Figure 6.15b. The cascade effect involves the following steps: (1) Photoexcitation and charge-separation at the protein; photogeneration of electrons at the protein, leaving photooxidixed P+ state; (2) Concurrent photoexcitation of n-Si with photogenerated electrons in the conduction band and their corresponding holes in the valence band; (3) Migration of the photogenerated electrons from the protein to fill the photogenerated holes in the Si valence band, facilitated by the electrolyte; (4) Flow of the electrons at the n-Si conductor band through the electrode-contact to the external circuit, reaching the FTO photoelectrode where the P+ state in the RC protein gets rereduced, thereby completing the circuit.

To better the overall light harvesting in the device, surface modifications to back electrode materials have been attempted. Texturizing the silicon surface (Figure 6.16a and b) proved effective both in improving the overall photoabsorption and in improving the charge transfer at the electrolyte/electrode interface by increasing the contact area. Since the surface of a polished planar Si-wafer is highly reflective, a significant fraction of light gets reflected and lost through scattering in the electrolyte (Figure 6.16c). To minimize the losses due to reflection, the surface of the silicon was textured with micropyramids (Figure 6.16b) that increased the Si light absorption by means of local scattering and re-incidence[189] (Figure 6.16d). The increased surface area ensuing from texturing also resulted in reduced charge transfer resistance at the electrode/electrolyte interface. In this device architecture, the open-circuit voltage was predicted to be the energy-level difference between the P/P+ couple in the RC and the conduction band of the n-Si, which amounts to 0.7 eV. A photovoltage of 0.6 V was generated in the device with planar Si anode, which was in good agreement with the theoretical prediction; further to this, an increment of 0.1 V was achieved by replacing the planar Si anode in the device with a textured Si.[189]

A similar approach of cascaded photoreactions has also been used in bioelectrochemical cells for water splitting, using PS2 proteins.[160] PS2 proteins were loaded onto a high-surface area semiconductor nanostructure. Hierarchical nanotubular titania was synthesized by a sol-gel technique using natural cellulose fibers as scaffolds (Figure 6.17a). A device architecture similar to a three-electrode photoelectrochemical cell illustrated in Figure 6.1d was adopted. An ITO photoelectrode modified with the semiconductor nanostructures integrated with the PS2 proteins served as the working electrode while a platinum wire and a saturated calomel electrode (SCE) served respectively as the counter and reference electrodes.[160] The three

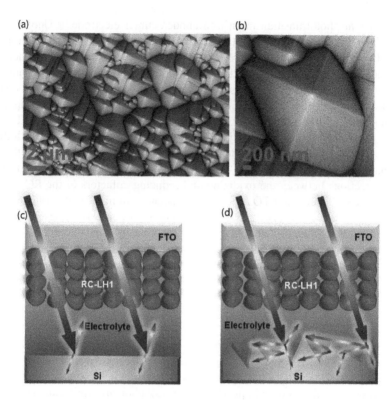

FIGURE 6.16 Enhanced light harvesting by minimizing reflection losses: Effect of back electrode surface modification: (a) Scanning electron microscopy image of the textured n-Si electrode. (b) Micron-scale pyramidal structures in the textured Si. (c) Cells with planar polished Si have reflection losses (a considerable fraction of the incident light gets reflected back into the electrolyte and lost due to scattering). (d) Reduced reflection loss and higher light absorption by replacing a plain Si with a textured Si (the pyramidal structures scatter the incoming light back to the surface facilitating multiple instances of light absorption). (Reproduced with permission from Singh, V.K. et al., *Adv. Funct. Mater.*, 1703689, 2017. Copyright 2017, John Wiley & Sons.)

electrodes were immersed in an electrolyte buffer solution containing 2,5-dichloro-1,4-benzoquinone (DCBQ), which served as an electrode transfer mediator.[160] A cellulose filter paper was used as a template for the nanotubular titania synthesis, as it has a well-defined hierarchical nanofibrous structure; with one cycle of sol-gel deposition, the surface of cellulose nanofibers gets coated with a titania gel film of 0.5 nm thickness; the thickness increased as the cycles were repeated n times ($n = 5$, 10, 20), resulting in titania films of varied thickness around the cellulose fibers in the filter paper; after calcination, all organic constituents in the composite sheet were removed, transforming the titania thin films into anatase-phase titania with hierarchical nanotubular structures ((TiO_2)$_n$-NTs) (Figure 6.17a).[160] The PS2 proteins were able to be integrated in the nanotubular titania-modifed ITO photoelectrode with high protein loading and sound electrical contact between the protein and the semiconductor.[160] The cascade of photoelectric reactions was possible because of the low

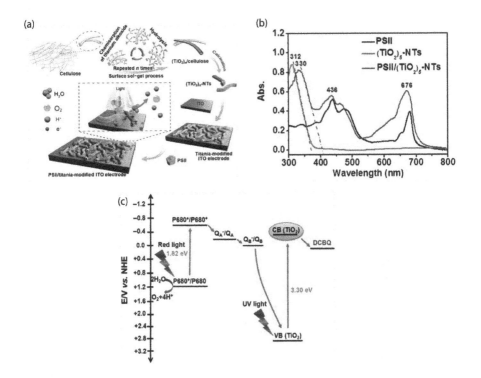

FIGURE 6.17 PS2/TiO$_2$ Hybrid: (a) Cartoon showing synthesis of nanotubular titania and fabrication of PS2/TiO$_2$ hybrid photoelectrode. (b) UV-vis spectra of PS2-coated ITO, Titania nanotubes coated ITO and PS2/Nanotubular Titania hybrid ITO photoelectrode. (c) Cascaded photoinduced electron transfer reactions. (Reproduced with permission from Li, J. et al., *J. Mater. Chem.* A, 4, 12197–12204, 2016. Copyright 2016, Royal Society of Chemistry.)

visible-light absorption (and high UV-light absorption) of the titania semiconductor, which was complemented by the high visible-light absorption (and low UV-light absorption) of the PS2 protein (Figure 6.17b).

The photocurrent achieved with the ITO photoelectrode with PS2-integrated (TiO$_2$)$_n$-NTs was 2.5 times higher than the sum of photocurrents obtained with PS2-coated ITO and (TiO$_2$)$_n$-NTs coated ITO, without the use of any electron transport mediator in the electrolyte buffer solution.[160] The contribution of the TiO$_2$ photoabsorption to the photocurrent of the PS2/TiO$_2$ hybrid was estimated to be less than 40% and even after subtracting the TiO$_2$ contribution from the photocurrent of the hybrid, the remnant value was still higher than the photocurrent of PS2-coated ITO (devoid of TiO$_2$), which indicated that there is a synergic effect between TiO$_2$ and PS2 in the hybrid system.[160] Photoabsorption and charge-carrier generation occurred both in the PS2 and in the TiO$_2$ under illumination. In TiO$_2$, the electrons get excited to the conduction band, leaving behind holes in the valence band and in PS2; electrons excite from P680$^+$/P680 to P680*/P680$^+$ and after charge separation get injected into the TiO$_2$ valence band from Q$_A$ or Q$_B$ donor sites, facilitating further carrier-generation in TiO$_2$ (Figure 6.17c).[160] The presence of a soluble electron transport mediator in the electrolyte further enhances the photocurrent by facilitating better electron transport from the PS2/TiO$_2$ hybrid to the counter electrode. While illumination with red light weakened TiO$_2$ contribution, thus making PS2 contribution higher, white illumination resulted in an overall higher photocurrent resulting from the synergistic effect of the photocascade reactions, due to the availability of the UV component for TiO$_2$ absorption.

6.4.2 Bio-Sensitized Solar Cells

Another classic approach is in enhancing the light harvesting to use a device structure of a dye-sensitized solar cell. Dyes have been replaced with photosynthetic proteins or light-harvesting complexes in a number of reports to construct biohybrid DSSCs or bio-sensitized solar cells (BSSCs). A comprehensive account of the working of dye-sensitized solar cells have been outlined in the earlier chapter (Chapter 2), which forms the basis for biohybrid DSSCs. Many attempts have been made to replace the conventional synthetic organic dyes in the DSSCs with natural dyes and bio-complexes with little changes to the overall device structure.[190–199] However, while the conventional DSSCs hit power conversion efficiencies as high as 12%, the efficiency in bio-DSSCs often does not exceed 2%.[196,200] This is because of the poor charge transfer between the semiconductor and any natural/bio dye used. The steric hindrance stemming from the chemical groups in the structure of the natural/bio dye prevents a sound bonding of the dyes with the oxide surface (e.g., TiO$_2$), thereby rendering the electron transfer from the dye to the semiconductor conduction band ineffective. However, efforts are still made to develop more efficient bio-DSSCs in view of the economic and environmental benefits attached. Photosynthetic pigments and proteins have been used for sensitizing different semiconductors such as TiO$_2$[192,201] ZnO,[202,203] Fe$_2$O$_3$,[204] etc., in Bio-DSSCs.

The hybrid devices with cascade effect discussed in the earlier Section 6.4.1 are not to be confused with BSSCs, which might employ the same combination of semiconductors, proteins, and redox electrolytes. The BSSCs are basically in biohybrid analogues of dye-sensitized solar cells, and the working does not involve any cascade effect discussed previously. One primary difference between a BSSC and a protein-semiconductor hybrid is the nature of electron transfer from the protein to the semiconductor. In a protein-semiconductor hybrid, the photogenerated electrons from the proteins are injected into the valence band of the semiconductor (Figure 6.17c) whereas in a BSSC, the electrons from the photoexcited protein or pigment are directly injected into the conduction band of the semiconductor (Figure 6.18a, b). Similar to that in any typical DSSC, an electron gets injected into the semiconductor conduction band, as the sensitizer (protein/dye/pigment) gets photoexcited and the photogenerated hole in the sensitizer gets filled by electron transfer from the redox electrolyte.

For any DSSC, in order to have a good anchorage of the dye molecules on the semiconductor structure, the dye should have anchoring groups such as -COOH, -H$_2$PO$_3$, -SO$_3$H, etc.[192] To firmly bind the dye onto the semiconductor surface, the standard anchoring group that is required in the sensitizers is carboxylic acid (-COOH), which reacts with the surface hydroxyl groups to form chemical bonds.[192,205] Besides the use

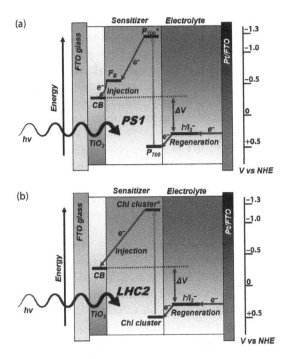

FIGURE 6.18 General working mechanism of a BSSC: (a) Energy level diagram of a PS1 protein-BSSC. (b) Energy level diagram of an LHC2 antenna complex-BSSC. (Inspired from Yu, D. et al., *Sci. Rep.*, 5, 9375, 2015.)

of natural pigments as sensitizers, it has been possible to use photosystems and antenna complexes as sensitizers in BSSCs, as it is likely that the assembly of PS1 or LHC2 complexes may be facilitated by the many carboxyl residues such as aspartic or glutamic acid in the protein sequences of PS1 or LHC2, which can facilitate easy anchorage to the surface of the TiO_2.[192] The carboxylic acid group can bind to TiO_2 either by coordinate covalent bond or carboxylate bond or by hydrogen bonds.[192,195] In both PS1 trimer and LHC2 trimer, the stromal side surface tends to preferentially adhere to the TiO_2 surface due to the presence of relatively more carboxyl groups.[192]

Comparing the performance of PS1-BSSC with that of LHC2-BSSC (Figure 6.18), both the photocurrent density and the overall efficiency were higher in the case of PS1-BSSC.[192] This is because of the high efficiency of the excitation energy transfer and the charge separation steps in the PS1 protein. The PS1 protein has an antenna system encompassing 90 Chlorophyll-a molecules and 22 carotenes, the function of which is to capture light and transfer the excitation energy to an electron transfer chain (ETC) at the center of the PS1 protein.[192] Each pigment molecule in the antenna system absorbs a photon and transfers the excitation energy through multiple pigments to elevate the energy level of a single electron in the special pair of chlorophyll (P700) found in the reaction center of the PS1 protein.[192,206] At room temperature, following the excitation of any of the antenna chlorophylls, the chance that the energy is successfully transferred to the P700 site and subsequent charge separation taking place is 99.98%.[207] Charge separation and the subsequent electron-transfer reactions are carried out by the ETC, where light-energy/excitation-energy excites an electron at the P700 site, which then proceeds through the ETC and reaches the terminal iron-sulfur complex F_B.[192,208] This process has a remarkably high quantum yield of close to 1.[209] In LHC2, chlorophylls in each monomeric subunit form several clusters of strongly excitonically coupled pigments, and intra-monomer excitation energy transfer rates are extremely fast.[192,210,211] In the LHC2 trimer and its aggregate, the energy transfer from Chl b to Chl a takes place at a high efficiency; however, the efficiency of energy transfer from carotenoid to Chl a is only ~70%.[192,212]

In PS1-BSSC, there is a high efficiency in the various stages such as energy transfer in the antenna system, charge separation and transfer in the ETC, and electron injection from F_B to the conducting band of TiO_2 film.[192] Similarly, the concurrent charge regeneration at the photooxidized P700 by electron transfer from the redox couple occurs with greater ease and efficiency.[192] Whereas, in the LHC2-BSSC, the processes of energy transfer, charge injection into semiconductor, and charge regeneration take place at much lower efficiencies compared to that of PS1-BSSC. However, the open-circuit voltages of both the devices were close to each other.[192] This similarity is because the open-circuit voltage in the BSSC devices is approximately indicated by the potential gap between the TiO_2 Fermi level, and the chemical potential of the redox electrolyte used and the other sensitizer-specific factors are relatively less dominant.

Recently, a BSSC was reported with anthocyanin (AC) pigment as the sensitizer and PS1 proteins as a complementary absorption layer and an electrochemical modifier (Figure 6.19a).[200] Anthocyanins are plant pigments that exhibit vibrant colorations in leaves, stems, fruits, etc. These pigments also exhibit high chemical affinity for the metal oxides, which is crucial for DSSC photoelectrodes.[200] Importantly, the purple, blue, and red absorbance of PS1 complements the green absorbance of ACs, thereby expanding the absorption cross section of the device and facilitating better utilization of the solar spectrum (Figure 6.19b).[200] Moreover, the presence of PS1 layer in the device also aids in reducing the recombination losses.[200] Electrolytic recombination, a process by which excited states in the adsorbed dye are oxidized by solubilized redox mediators, is a major factor that lowers the photovoltage and thereby the device efficiency, as it reduces the number of electrons available for injection into the semiconductor conduction band.[200] The electrolytic recombination reactions can be curbed either by decreasing the concentration of oxidized states (O) of the redox molecule at the dye-sensitized photoanode or by augmenting the dye reduction reactions by increasing the concentration of reduced states (R) of the redox molecule within the photoanode.[200] The photoinduced kinetics of a PS1 layer were coupled to the BSSC photoanode to increase the photovoltage.[200] The photoinduced kinetic activity of a PS1 multilayer film increases the concentration of R and decreases the concentration of O, thereby facilitating an increased rate of dye reduction and a decreased rate of electrolytic recombination in the AC-sensitized photoanode (Figure 6.19c).[200] This resulted in an enhanced rate of electron injection into TiO_2 and hence an improved photovoltage.[200] Thus, the PS1 protein layer

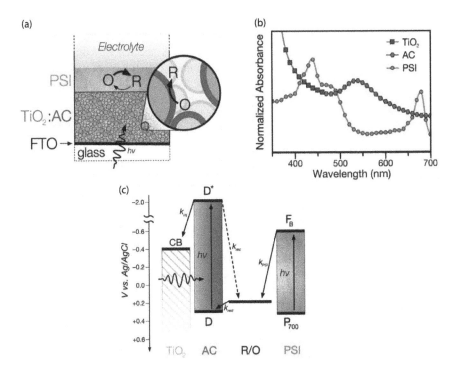

FIGURE 6.19   Working mechanism of a BSSC with natural dyes and PS1 proteins: (a) PS1 multilayer film assembled on top of a mesoporous film of TiO_2 nanoparticles sensitized by natural anthocyanin (AC) pigment molecules in a hierarchical BSSC photoanode. (b) Enhanced light harvesting in BSSC with complementary absorption from PS1 and AC. (c) Energy diagram of the BSSC. F_B and P_{700} are respectively the excited and low-energy electronic states in the PS1 protein. R and O are respectively the reduced and oxidized states of the water-soluble mediator. D* and D are the excited and low-energy electronic states of each AC molecule, respectively. CB denotes the conduction band of TiO_2. k_{rec}, k_{inj}, k_{red}, and k_{PSI} denote the rate constants for electrolytic recombination, electron injection, reduction of AC, and reduction of O by F_B, respectively. (Adapted with permission from Robinson, M.T., *ACS Appl. Energy Mater.*, 2018., Copyright 2018, American Chemical Society.)

facilitated nearly a twofold increase in the photovoltage of the BSSC, relative to the unmodified equivalent.[200]

6.4.3   PROTEIN-QUANTUM DOT HYBRIDS

Device architectures with better photoelectric performance would be possible by controlling the mode and rate of electronic energy transfer (EET) possible in the molecular circuitry of the device. In semiconductor-protein hybrids, where the two photoactive materials with complementary absorbing characteristics are employed, the overall light harvesting is improved by cascading the two charge transport pathways. Performance enhancement from expanded light harvesting can also be achieved by excitonically coupling two photoactive species of complementary absorption characteristics, which is the subject matter of this section. Unlike the protein-semiconductor hybrids where the two active materials individually photo-generate charge carriers—which are brought together by cascading the two charge transport pathways—in this section, the systems discussed involve linking of the excitation energy transfer pathways of the two photoactive materials, ultimately resulting in a single charge-carrier generation process.

In a photosynthetic apparatus, the excitation energy absorbed by a pigment molecule is transferred to another molecule separated by distances up to several tens of angstroms by a process of resonance energy transfer. Depending on the electronic coupling between the pigment molecules and the coupling of the photosynthetic protein with its environment, the energy transfer mode could be an incoherent EET (Förster energy transfer), a coherent EET, or a relaxation dominant mode.[100] This principle can be used in designing a biohybrid solar cell by engineering the molecular circuitry by linking different natural and synthetic molecules for improved power conversion efficiency. The Förster resonance energy transfer (FRET) has been utilized in different hybrid systems of photosynthetic biomolecules linked with fluorophores of complementary absorption characteristics. Biohybrid systems with FRET coupled molecules are in general designed to follow two main criteria: (1) An optimum proximity between the light-harvesting biomolecule (the excited state donor) and the ground-state acceptor molecule, close enough to enable the short-range interaction and far enough to prevent the overlapping of molecular orbitals, thus avoiding the quenching of excitation states; (2) A sizeable spectral overlap between the donor emission profile and the acceptor absorption profile.

Based on this principle, a number of artificial antenna systems have been developed using supramolecular chemistry with dendrimers incorporating porphyrins or other organic fluorophores or organometallic complexes.[214,215] Though the excitation energy transfer in these systems was efficient, the use of organic fluorophores in light-harvesting systems has limitations of narrow spectral windows for light absorption and lack of photostability.[214,216] Inorganic nanocrystals such as quantum dots, however, were found to harvest light over a wide spectral window and were suggested to have efficient excitation energy transfer.[217–220] Hence, developing hybrid materials in which light energy harvested by the inorganic nanocrystals may be transferred to a photosynthetic protein is promising for enhancing the efficiency of the photosynthetic system in the device. It has been demonstrated that the photoluminescent quantum dots (QDs) of selected photoluminescence (PL) wavelengths can be tagged with a photosynthetic reaction center (RC) in such a way that FRET from the QD to the RC is realized.[213]

This approach aims at enhancing the light harvesting and making the energy transfer from QD to RC more, which could pave the way for the application of the RC-QD hybrid in biophotovoltaics.[213] In its native environment, each purple bacterial reaction center has two membrane-spanning branches, which are respectively the active branch (A) and the inactive branch (B).[213] Each branch includes one quinone

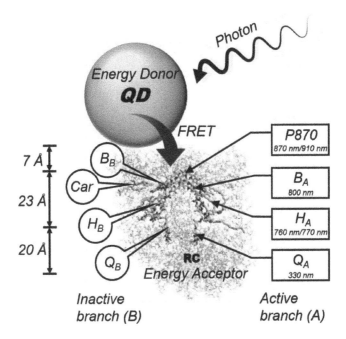

FIGURE 6.20 Protein-quantum dot hybrids: Organization and functionality of a hybrid system composed of a purple bacterial reaction center (from *Rhodobacter sphaeroides*) and a QD; the diagram is presented to scale. Active (A) and inactive (B) electron-transfer branches in the protein are shown. The positions of the absorption/photoluminescence maxima for the BChl special pair (P870), BChl monomer (B), bacteriopheophytin (H), and quinone (Q) are indicated for the active branch (A). Photons are absorbed both by the RC and the QD. An exciton from the QD is transferred to the RC by FRET. Car denotes carotenoid pigment (Adapted with permission from Nabiev, I. et al., *Angew. Chem. Int. Ed.*, 49, 7217–7221, 2010. Copyright 2010, John Wiley & Sons.)

($Q_{A/B}$), one bacteriopheophytin ($H_{A/B}$), and one bacteriochlorophyll ($B_{A/B}$).[213] The two branches are connected by two bacteriochlorophyll molecules that are excitonically coupled, which together are known as the special pair (P or P870) (Figure 6.20).[213] Each of the cofactors of the reaction center can be identified from the absorption spectra of a solution containing the RCs. Achieving a strong coupling between the QDs and the absorbing species is crucial for developing an efficient FRET-based nano-biohybrid system.[213] This has been realized by carefully choosing the diameters of the QDs (which determine the PL colors) to ensure optical coupling to the pigment chromophores in the reaction centers.[213] As RCs are naturally surrounded by light-harvesting antenna complexes in their native environment, the purity of the RCs (to be devoid of the any attached antenna complexes) is important to ensure an unhindered contact between the QDs and the RC and hence to realize efficient energy transfer.[213]

The energy diagram showing the energy relaxation (Figure 6.21a) for the QD-RC hybrid illustrates the working mechanism of the energy transfer in the system.[213]

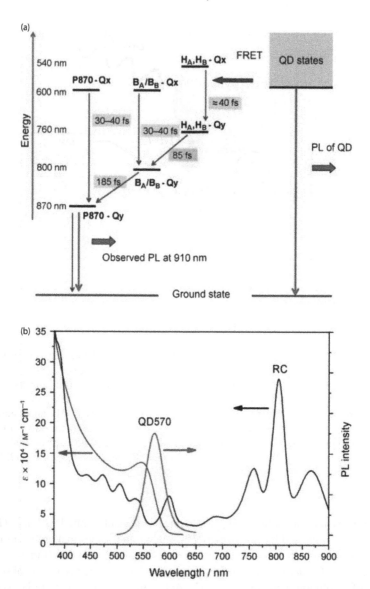

FIGURE 6.21 Protein-quantum dot hybrids—light harvesting and energy transfer: (a) Energy flow QD-RC hybrids. QDs transfer the absorbed photonic energy to any of the RC cofactors by FRET. The excitation quickly relaxes to the P870-Qy level, where the exciton is split into constituent carriers (in natural environment) or it decays with a characteristic emission at ~910 nm (under experiment conditions). (b) Comparison of optical properties of reaction centers (RCs) and CdTe QDs. The extinction coefficient of QDs dominates over the intrinsic absorption of RCs in the wavelength range of 400–570 nm. The high extinction coefficient of RCs ensures sufficient coupling between QD570 PL band and RC absorption for efficient energy transfer to occur. Both of these facts suggest that optical enhancement of RC excitation is possible in RC-QD hybrids. (Reproduced with permission from Nabiev, I. et al., *Angew. Chem. Int. Ed.*, 49, 7217–7221, 2010. Copyright 2010, John Wiley & Sons.)

Upon irradiation with light, the QDs absorb the photonic energy and donate the energy to one of the RC cofactors by means of FRET.[213] The excitation within the reaction center decays within a very short span to the lowest excited level (P8700), which corresponds to an exciton reaching the special pair.[213] At this stage, in the native environment, it would be expected that the exciton will be split into an electron and a hole (charge separation).[213,221] Such charge separation, however, did not take place in the QD-RC hybrid in the experimental condition (involving the use of sodium ascorbate molecules as a source of electrons to result in a closed-state RC).[213] The sodium ascorbate supplied electrons to the photooxidized P870$^+$ species, promoting the reduction reaction P870$^+$ → P870.[213,221] The presence of sodium ascorbate rendered a so-called "closed state" of the RC, 9P870/$Q_A^-Q_B^-$, where the quinones are fully reduced.[213] As the closed-state RC absorbs a photon, there is no charge separation; instead, there is a recombination in the P870 unit, which results in a photoluminescent band at 910 nm (Figure 6.21a).[213,221] The exciton decayed with a characteristic emission at 910 nm, the intensity of which was used to gauge the potential photosynthetic efficiency of the QD-RC hybrid. This energy structure reflects the absorption spectrum of the reaction center (Figure 6.21b).[213] The feasibility of optical enhancement of the RC absorption can be determined by comparing the extinction spectra of QDs and RCs (Figure 6.21b).[213] As it can be seen that at comparable molar concentrations, the QD570 (CdTe QDs emitting at 570 nm) absorption in the wavelength range of 400 to 570 nm is stronger than that of the RC, which indicates the strong possibility of optical enhancement of the RC absorption.[213,221] The RC-QD hybrid exhibited nearly a threefold increase in the rate of generation of excitons compared to an unmodified RC.[213,221] Furthermore, theoretical predictions point to the possibilities of enhancement of light harvesting by as much as five times in properly optimized hybrids.[213,221]

6.4.4 PLASMON-ENHANCED BIOHYBRID CELLS

Another popular approach of enhancing the light-harvesting capability in biophotovoltaic devices is to facilitate broadband optical absorption by integrating plasmonic nanostructures in the devices. This approach, though closely related to the band theory and photonics, is a separate field per se. Plasmonics, a branch of nanophotonics, deals with confinement of an electromagnetic field over a dimension of the order of the wavelength of light and its interaction with the free electrons in a metal or metallic nanostructures.[222] Using plasmonic nanostructures to complement the photoactivity of light-harvesting complexes has become a popular and a promising strategy in biophotovoltaics in recent years. Strong enhancement of electromagnetic fields generated through surface plasmon resonances (SPRs) in metal films and nanoparticles (NP) has recently gathered a great deal of research attention due to their versatility in affecting absorption, fluorescence, and excitation energy transfer (EET) of molecular systems in proximity.[223] A number of hybrid light-harvesting devices have been developed by integrating pigment-protein complexes with metal nanoparticles.[223] In these hybrid systems, the net change in the fluorescence is the result of a subtle balance among different competitive effects.[223] In general, metal nanoparticles enhance the radiative decay rates of acceptors as well as the electronic absorption of the donors.[223] They also tend to act as competitive energy acceptors and they can directly affect the electronic coupling, which in turn determines the EET.[223] All these processes, besides getting affected to different extents by the characteristics of the metal nanoparticle like its nature, shape and dimension, might also depend significantly on its position and orientation with respect to the pigments in the protein as well as on the environment (e.g., type of solvent).[223] Multiscale models have been developed that explain these factors and their specific contribution in the whole process of light harvesting and energy transfer.[223]

A number of reports in the past few years have attempted to enhance the output of the biohybrid solar cells through the use of surface plasmons.[42,156,159] A nano-biohybrid cell has been recently reported with silver (Ag) nanoparticles (NP) integrated in the device, aiding in photocurrent enhancement assisted by surface plasmon effect.[10,156] The device architecture involved a typical structure similar to that in Figure 6.12f where the photosynthetic complexes served as interlayers and not as the primary photoactive layers. The plasmon enhancement was demonstrated using LHC2 antenna complexes in an inverted BHJ structure ITO/ZnO/Interlayer/ PIDTT-DFBT:PC$_{71}$BM/MoO$_3$/Ag where LHC2-Ag NP nano-biohybrids served as the interlayer. PIDTT-DFBT:PC$_{71}$BM blend formed the BHJ where PIDTT-DFBT (poly(indacenodithieno[3,2-b]thio-phene-difluorobenzothiadiazole) served as the donor polymer and PC$_{71}$BM ([6,6]-phenyl-C$_{71}$-butyric acid methyl ester) as the electron acceptor (Figure 6.22a). As the nanoparticles were incorporated into the light-harvesting complexes, the photoactivity of the LHC2 antenna complex was remarkably enhanced due to the localized surface plasmon resonance of the Ag NPs. These nanoparticles enhanced the device performance by means of two main factors: (1) broadband optical absorption enhancement caused by the complementary absorption of the Ag NPs, and (2) increased light harvesting by the LHC2 complexes due to the LSPR effect[10,156] (Figure 6.22b).

Moreover, the nanoparticles also acted as nano-optical antennas, which will act as a center for electromagnetic coupling for the proteins and nanoparticles, resulting in enhanced light absorption over the entire spectrum. Based on this same approach, a self-assembly of purple bacterial proteins (RC-LH1) on silver nanostructured substrate yielded a 2.5-fold improvement in current density in a recent report.[10,42] The device structure involved Ag nanostructures loaded with RC-LH1 complexes, with cytochrome c as an electron transfer mediator.[10] The charge transfer mechanism involved the transfer of electrons from the silver substrate to the cytochrome c and further to the reaction center and then getting captured in the quinol oozing out of the protein. Plasmon effect increased the overall number of photogenerated electrons hence resulting in high photocurrents in the device.[10,42]

6.4.5 Biohybrid Tandem Cells

While most of the reported bio-photoelectrochemical cells devices focus on photocurrent enhancement by improving the electron transfer in three-electrode or two-electrode cells interfacing the proteins with an electrolyte or electron transporter,[16, 154,188] the idea of enhancing photocurrent by photonic approaches such as increasing the light-harvesting ability and the spectral range of the protein-integrated devices

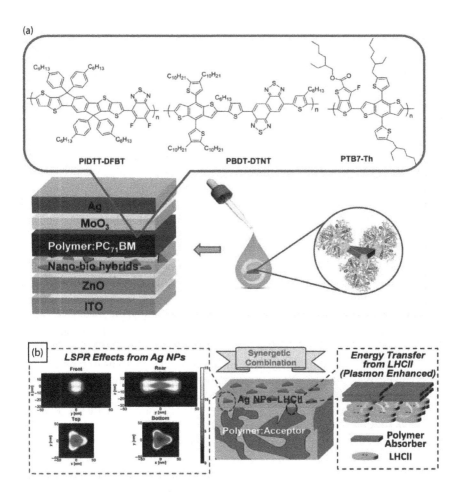

FIGURE 6.22   Plasmon-enhanced Biohybrid OPV: (a) An Inverted BHJ device with Ag-NP-LHC2 nano-biohybrids as an interlayer. (b) The synergetic effect of the two factors contributing to the enhanced photocurrents. (Reproduced with permission from Yao, K. et al., *J. Mater. Chem. A*, 4, 13400–13406, 2016. Copyright 2016, Royal Society of Chemistry.)

has gathered momentum in recent research. Use of surface plasmon effect in biophotovoltaics discussed in the earlier Section 6.4.4 is one such approach that aims to broaden the light absorption range. Other approaches include expansion of the optical absorption cross section of the photosynthetic reaction centers by means of tagging tailored molecular fluorophores and photoluminescent quantum dots to the protein complexes, though not scaled up at a device level for photocurrent generation.[213,224,225] While the enhancement in light absorption has been realized by Förster resonance energy transfer (FRET) from the attached fluorophore to the core reaction center complex,[213] it is still challenging to realize the same with an RC-LH1 complex, which if made possible, could lead to a remarkable enhancement in photocurrent generation as a result of the spectral response broadened by the fluorophore complementing the role of the LH1 protein.[10,154]

An alternative approach to achieve this is to have a stacked device structure where pigments of complementary absorption characteristics can be incorporated into the proteins at different layers of the device, rather than all into a single protein.[154] This architecture would need a transparent rear/counter electrode so as to let the incident light reach the complementary absorption layer positioned underneath. Recently, a proof-of-principle bio-tandem cell was reported employing two variants of RC-LH1 complexes with one having the native red carotenoids in the LH1 protein (RC-LH1$_{red}$) while the other being engineered to have green carotenoids in the LH1 (RC-LH1$_{green}$) to demonstrate the enhancement in light absorption and hence in the photocurrent (Figure 6.23).[154] The two pigment-proteins having optically complementary absorption characteristics in the visible spectrum (Figure 6.23e) were contained in two subcells connected in parallel so as to realize addition of photocurrents in the tandem-structured cell (Figure 6.24) where the front and rear electrodes for each subcell were respectively FTO and PEDOT:PSS.[154]

There are two possible tandem architectures—series and parallel (Figure 6.25). Though theoretically both are capable of resulting in high light absorption cross section for a given footprint, the series combination of subcells is limited by stringent current-matching criteria.[154,226] To avoid current losses in a parallel-connected tandem cell, the constituent subcells should ideally have equal photovoltage so as to avoid any stray current resulting from the potential difference, which could counteract the photocurrent of the tandem cell. Similarly, in the case of a series tandem cell, the constituent subcells are to have equal photocurrents so as to minimize the voltage losses. While the open-circuit voltage of the biohybrid photoelectrochemical cells is often energy-level dependent, achieving approximately equal V_{oc} in the two subcells is easier than achieving equal J_{sc}, since V_{oc} is not as sensitive as J_{sc} to the photo-absorption characteristics (e.g., light intensity dependence) of the proteins.[154] Hence, the parallel-connected tandem architecture was suggested to be a better alternative in enhancing the photocurrent generation without altering the footprint of the cell device.[10,154] Though ideally the photocurrent of the parallel-connected tandem cell can be 100% of the sum of the two subcell photocurrents, there was ≈10% loss in the overall photocurrent of the tandem cell. This loss was attributed to the reduced incident light intensity reaching the bottom subcell and also to any minor difference in the open-circuit voltage between the two subcells that would result in an undesirable circulating current, reducing the overall photocurrent output.[154] The device employed two electron transport mediators TMPD (N,N,N′,N′-tetramethyl-p-phenylenediamine) and Q0 (ubiquinone-0) and the working mechanism involved the following steps: (I) photoinduced charge separation in the reaction center; (II) migration of electrons from the Q_B site to the PEDOT:PSS counter electrode through the Q0 electrolyte; (III) charge regeneration in the protein—electron entering the device from the external circuit is used by the TMPD mediator to reduce the photooxidized special pair P+ (Figure 6.26).[154]

The use of PEDOT:PSS film as the counter electrode served as a better alternative to the conventional metal electrodes besides facilitating the tandem device construction by being a transparent conductive polymer device.[10,154] The electron transfer from the Q0 electrolyte to PEDOT:PSS takes place with greater ease than that from Q0 to Pt, which is due to the closeness of PEDOT:PSS work function to

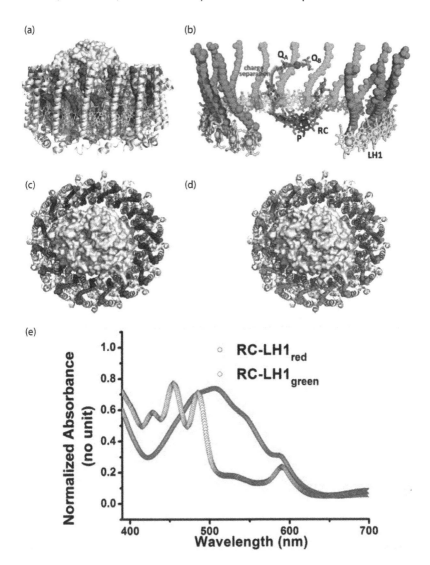

FIGURE 6.23 Proteins with complementary absorption characteristics for bio-tandem cells: (a) RC-LH1$_{red}$ complex viewed parallel to the photosynthetic membrane, with the 16 LH1 carotenoids carotenoid shown as red spheres, LH1 BChls in yellow, and all other components in white. The RC is shown as a solid object and LH1 proteins as ribbons. (b) The LH1 carotenoids (green) and BChls (yellow) power charge separation in the central RC by passing excited state energy to the P BChls (orange carbons). The nearest four BChls and two carotenoids have been removed. Views of (c) RC-LH1$_{red}$ and (d) RC-LH1$_{green}$ complexes perpendicular to the photosynthetic membrane; only the carotenoid pigments differ between complexes. (e) Visible region absorbance spectra of RC-LH1$_{red}$ and RC-LH1$_{green}$ complexes in solution, normalized to BChl absorbance at 875 nm. (Reproduced with permission from Ravi, S.K. et al., *Adv. Energy Mater.*, 7, 2017. Copyright 2016, John Wiley & Sons – protein color coding can be found in the original version of the figure in Ravi, S.K. et al., *Adv. Energy Mater.*, 7, 2017.)

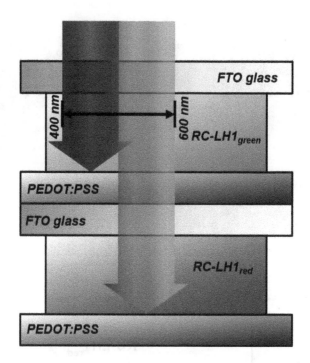

FIGURE 6.24 Schematic illustration of a biohybrid tandem cell: Two proteins (RC-LH1$_{green}$ and RC-LH1$_{red}$) of complementary absorption characteristics in different layers of the device. (Inspired from Ravi, S.K. et al., *Adv. Energy Mater.*, 7, 2017.)

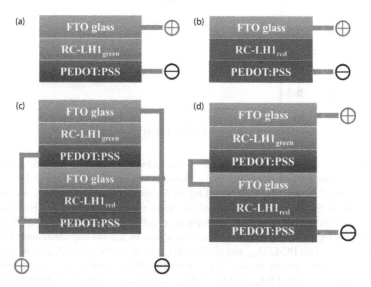

FIGURE 6.25 Tandem cell configurations: Schematic showing the two terminals in (a) a RC-LH1$_{green}$ subcell, (b) a RC-LH1$_{red}$ subcell, (c) a parallel tandem cell, (d) a series tandem cell. (Reproduced with permission from Ravi, S.K. et al., *Adv. Energy Mater.*, 7, 2017. Copyright 2016, John Wiley & Sons.)

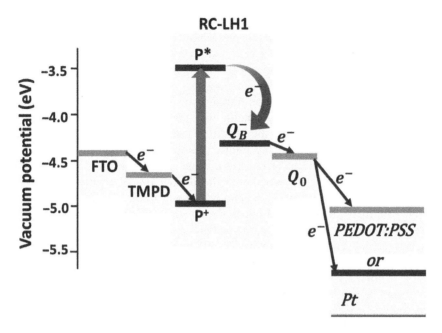

FIGURE 6.26 Energy level diagram and mechanism of photocurrent generation. (Adapted with permission from Ravi, S.K. et al., *Adv. Energy Mater.*, 7, 2017. Copyright 2016, John Wiley & Sons.)

the vacuum potential of Q0 as compared to Pt device.[10,154] The use of PEDOT:PSS resulted in a 12-fold improvement in photocurrents over the conventional Pt electrode, and a maximum of 88% photocurrent addition has been demonstrated in the tandem cell with a parallel configuration.[154] The study highlighted the photocurrent enhancement possible by integrating different pigment-proteins at different layers of a photovoltaic device in a fashion determined by the band theory—that is, the photoactive layer with the biggest bandgap (shortest wavelength) is to be positioned on top and lower bandgap materials take positions at the bottom in a multilayer device.[10,154]

6.5 DEVICE ARCHITECTURES FOR IMPROVED STABILITY

Despite the enormous efforts to improve the photoelectric performance of the protein-based biophotovoltaic devices through a variety of approaches, the useful lifetime of the devices is still much inferior compared to the inorganic photovoltaics.[16] Reports on high photocurrents from photoprotein-integrated hybrid devices are growing in numbers in recent years; however, it is still sparse to see how stable the reported devices are. These biohybrid devices are short-lived, and it is common to find a huge dip in the performance within days—and there would hardly be any photocurrent a week after device fabrication; this is indicative of degradation of proteins in the non-native environment over time.[227] As the major photovoltaic components in these devices are biomolecular complexes, it is important to understand their vulnerabilities in a foreign environment. The biomolecular complexes often lack a protective environment in the device environment, which deteriorates their functionalities, resulting in a short life span.[16] The stability of the protein complexes needs to be improved to devise a more useful and realistic biohybrid solar cell. As the protein complexes are isolated from their native environment, they are prone to conformational changes since the stabilizing effect offered by the membrane lipids is lost.[16] Lipids play a crucial role in affecting the biophysical and electron-transfer properties of the protein; they promote structural stability and flexibility, binding the light-harvesting cofactors and filling the intra-protein cavities.[34] The stability of these complexes is affected mainly by two main stress factors—light and temperature.[228] Both these stress factors contribute to protein denaturation, which involves a loss of structural integrity due to the separation of secondary structural subunits and unfolding of domains outside the membrane.[229]

The stability of the protein-based photoelectrochemical cells has been found to last only for a few hours on continuous illumination at room temperature.[16] When stored in dark conditions at low temperatures, the devices have exhibited extended lifetimes, as the denaturation is prevented by minimizing both the stress factors.[16] One major approach to improve the stability of the proteins in the devices is to achieve a protein-compatible environment, which can be best achieved only by mimicking the native membrane of RCs.[16] As opposed to the isolated core reaction centers, the photosynthetic membranes used as the photoactive components in the devices exhibited better resistance to the stress factors, and the functionality of the embedded proteins was maintained for three days when continuously illuminated.[230] The presence of a light-harvesting antenna complex surrounding the reaction center core has also been found to increase its robustness and improve its resistance to intense lights, relative to an isolated reaction center.[230] While one way to improve the protein stability is to make the material environment more conducive to the biomolecules, another approach is to make the proteins more robust and resistant to harsh environments and stress factors.[16] An example of the latter approach is to increase the carotenoid content in the protein complex, as the carotenoids are known to play photoprotective roles and improve the robustness of the proteins. The first approach is the topic of interest in this section.

Concerns of poor stability in the conventional bio-photoelectrochemical cells have always intrigued possibilities of developing new device architectures. Progression from liquid- to solid-state device architectures has been promising for enhancement of photocurrent output and elimination of photocurrent decline due to diffusional limitations. Solid-state architectures are also the key to create a near-native environment for proteins integrated in devices. The first report on a solid-state biohybrid device employed peptide surfactants to stabilize the proteins in the device. However, there were stability concerns because of the thermal evaporation step involved in the device fabrication to interface the electron acceptor material to the proteins.[50,188] Interfacing proteins to a fully solid-state material often required a coating step involving high-velocity impinging atoms or conditions involving denaturing temperatures.[16,50] It is hence important to develop a soft interface with the proteins akin to the native environment where the proteins are held in well-defined orientations by the lipid-bilayer membrane. Recently, a biohybrid device with a solid-state electrolyte forming a soft interface with the proteins was reported.[50] This was achieved by means of a mechano-responsive gel interfaced with the protein multilayer at room temperature, creating a soft near-native environment without any potential denaturing step in the fabrication.

Proteins in the multilayers were connected to the electrodes using a solid/gel interface based on succinonitrile ($N\equiv C\text{-}CH_2\text{-}CH_2\text{-}C\equiv N$).[50] Succinonitrile (SCN) is a highly polar organic plastic crystalline material, which due to lattice defects and rotational vacancies, can provide a non-conducting matrix for a conducting salt.[50] The SCN matrix was suffused by an equimolar mixture of the N-tetramethylammonium ($^+$NMe4) salt of 5-mercapto-1-methyltetrazole (T^-) and di-5-(1-methyltetrazole) disulfide (T_2), producing a plastic gel-phase material with a high ionic and molecular diffusivity.[50] While gels are typically liquefied by heating, crucially for work with thermally labile pigment-proteins, it was discovered that this material undergoes a reversible gel-to-liquid transition under mechanical vibration (Figure 6.27).[50] As sonication did not produce significant heating of the succinonitrile/electrolyte mix, this provided a means of permeating layers of photoactive protein with the electrolyte matrix at room temperature.[50]

Using natural and engineered variants of photosynthetic reaction centers and light-harvesting complexes, different multilayer devices were constructed.[50] It was found

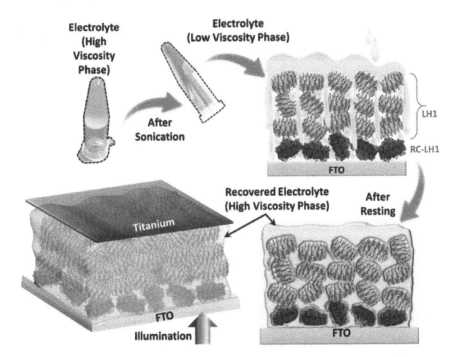

FIGURE 6.27 Solid-state biophotovoltaic device with protein-gel interface: To achieve device fabrication, the gel-phase succinonitrile/T-/T2 electrolyte was liquefied by sonication and applied to a protein multilayer that had been spin-coated on the working electrode. During the subsequent resting period, the electrolyte soaked into the protein layer after which the counter electrode was placed on the gel surface and the cell sealed with epoxy resin. (Reproduced with permission from Ravi, S. K. et al., *Adv. Mater.*, 30, 2018. Copyright 2017, John Wiley & Sons.)

that different layers in the device played well-defined light-harvesting (antenna) and charge-separation (transducer) roles, with clear evidence of directional energy transfer.[50] The report discusses a "satellite dish effect" in the bioelectrochemical devices whereby an array of natural light-harvesting "antenna" complexes absorbs light from a wide expanse and concentrates the excitonic energy to the base protein that acts like an "energy trap" (Figure 6.28a).[50] The photocurrent generation in the device involved photoexcitation of the pigment-protein, which produced electron donation to the FTO working electrode from a sufficiently reducing excited or anion state (Figure 6.28b, arrows marked by square and pentagon), with re-reduction by the Ti counter electrode of the resulting oxidized pigment(s), most probably P+.[50] As the vacuum potential of the T_2/T^- redox couple was much deeper than that of FTO or Ti, it was concluded that the T_2/T^- electrolyte facilitated electron transfer from the counter electrode to the photooxidized species in the protein coating (Figure 6.28b,

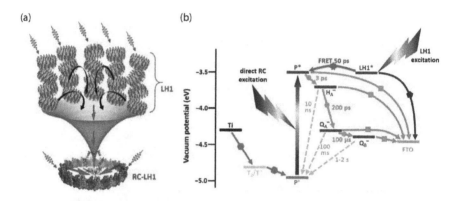

FIGURE 6.28 Working mechanism of the device: (a) Energy transfer through multilayers: In natural photosystems, light energy harvested by an extended antenna pigment-protein system is concentrated by directional energy transfer onto a smaller number of photovoltaic reaction center pigment-proteins, where energy is trapped through charge separation. In this model, this is mimicked in three dimensions by coating a base layer of RC-LH1 proteins with multilayers of LH1 antenna proteins (not drawn to scale). This demonstrates the possibility of expansive collection of photons by extended layers of light-harvesting antennae that concentrate the excitonic energy to a smaller number of energy traps, which is analogous to the mechanism of a satellite dish that collects weak signals from a wide space and concentrates them on a sensor at a focal point. (b) Charge transfer routes: Mechanism of photocurrent generation in cells with an FTO-glass working electrode. Direct excitation of the RC, or excitation of LH1 pigments followed by FRET to the RC (arrows marked with hexagons), triggers charge separation by promoting a pair of bacteriochlorophyll cofactors in the RC (P) into their first singlet excited state (P* - rainbow arrow). Charge separation (arrows marked with circles) proceeds through the radical pairs P^+H_A, P^+Q_A and P^+Q_B. At each stage rapid forward electron transfer (arrows marked with circles) outcompetes slow radical pair recombination (dashed arrows). Arrows marked by squares and arrows marked by pentagons indicate possible processes for reduction of the working electrode by RCs or LH1 complexes respectively, some or all of which can operate depending on which protein complex makes up the base coating of the device. (Adapted with permission from Ravi, S. K. et al., *Adv. Mater.*, 30, 2018., Copyright 2017, John Wiley & Sons.)

arrows marked by hexagons).[50] The devices exhibited an enhanced current stability and a maximal photoresponse of ≈860 µA cm[-2], which is at least fivefold larger than the photocurrents in most of the earlier reports on biohybrid devices with purple bacterial proteins.[50]

In addition to enabling very stable photocurrent densities during short periods of continuous illumination, stability studies on sealed and dummy cells indicated long-term stability of the RC-LH1 complex in the biohybrid device.[50] The stability of the proteins was found to be enhanced by embedding them in the succinonitrile/T_2/T^- gel.[50]

Over 28 days of storage at room temperature with a continuous ambient illumination of ~2 W m[-2], a transparent dummy cell (with proteins embedded in the gel electrolyte sandwiched between two FTO glasses) exhibited only a minimal absorbance (at 875 nm) shift and a modest 39% drop in absorbance (at 875 nm) (Figure 6.29a, c).[50] This is a strong indication that the degradation of the LH1 protein is slowed down

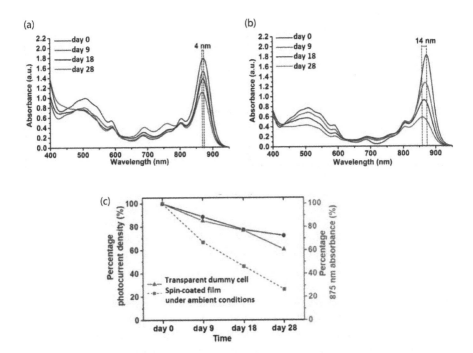

FIGURE 6.29 Device stability—Stability of RC-LH1 complexes under continuous ambient illumination. Decay of the native absorbance spectrum of RC-LH1 complexes: (a) in a transparent dummy RC-LH1/T_2/T^- cell constructed using two FTO-glass electrodes; (b) in a spin-coated RC-LH1 film on FTO-glass not incorporated into a cell. Pigment-protein degradation gives rise to absorbance decreases at 420–570 nm for carotenoid and at 590 and 875 nm for BChl. The appearance of BChl breakdown products produces broad absorbance increases in the region between 650 and 800 nm. The drop in LH1 absorbance at 875 nm is accompanied by a blue shift of the absorbance band due to increasing overlap with underlying RC absorbance at 800 nm (visible) and 865 nm (not visible). (c) Protein stability (i.e., absorbance) and photocurrent stability over 28 days at ambient light intensity and temperature. (Reproduced with permission from Ravi, S. K. et al., *Adv. Mater.*, 30, 2018. Copyright 2017, John Wiley & Sons.)

significantly in the gel environment.[50] In good agreement with this, the photocurrent obtained from an equivalent cell with a Ti counter electrode showed a 27% decrease in current density after 28 days (Figure 6.29c).[50] For a spin-coated RC-LH1 film on FTO-glass (not embedded in the gel electrolyte) the 875 nm absorbance dropped by 73% over the same period (Figure 6.29b, c), suggesting a protective effect of the gel electrolyte.[50]

6.6 SUMMARY

Capturing solar energy with intricate processes of energy transfer and charge transfer through incredibly efficient photosynthetic systems has become routine by nature since time immemorial. Deciphering the light-harvesting design principles of natural photosynthesis has constantly been a huge research interest with the enticement of reaching new heights in photovoltaic efficiency. This has led to two main roads of applied research, namely artificial photosynthetic systems and biophotovoltaic systems. Biophotovoltaic systems constructed with photosynthetic proteins were predominantly liquid electrochemical cells that suffered a number of limitations both in performance and stability.

Although there is a reasonably good understanding of the structure and function of photosynthetic proteins in vivo and the biochemical aspects of them, the same could not be extended to the proteins integrated in photovoltaic devices. With a brief historical note on the approaches adopted in the field a decade back, this chapter aimed to highlight two broad approaches in designing biophotovoltaic devices, namely the electronic and photonic approaches. The electronic approach aims at designing device architectures that focus on performance enhancement by tweaking the charge transport processes in the device. This was substantiated with principles and ideas from band theory and solid-state physics. The new promising trend of developing solid-state biophotovoltaics with device physics adopted from organic photovoltaics was highlighted. A comprehensive discussion on the energy and charge transfer processes in natural photosynthetic and organic photovoltaic systems was presented to provide a more holistic view on the working of a solid-state biohybrid device. While the field of protein-biophotovoltaics aims at designing efficient solid-state devices, in recent times, OPVs have also been eying bio-inspiration and adapting photosynthetic proteins for better performance. The efforts to develop solid-state biohybrid solar cells are now being extended from both the fields. Though the use of bandgap approach/band-structure approach in device design and construction is common in the field of OPVs, the approach is almost alien to BPVs. The chapter hence outlined the ideas of interfacial electronic structure and energy-level alignment between the device layers (which are based on the band theory of solids) that would be crucial for designing any solid-state biophotovoltaic device.

While the primary focus of the devices discussed in the first half of the chapter (i.e., the electronic approaches) is on controlling the charge transport processes, the latter half presented works using photonic approaches, where the prime focus is to improve the light harvesting in the device. This section discussed the scope of different hybrid device architectures in expanding the spectral window of the device and in enhancing light harvesting by combining photoproteins with secondary/auxiliary light harvesters in different fashions. Finally, the challenges in improving protein stability in a device environment were highlighted, and the recent attempts to enhance the device stability were reviewed.

REFERENCES

1. Ball, P. *Nature* **2011**, 474, (7351), 272.
2. Fassioli, F.; Dinshaw, R.; Arpin, P. C.; Scholes, G. D. *Journal of The Royal Society Interface* **2014**, 11, (92).
3. Operamolla, A.; Ragni, R.; Milano, F.; Roberto Tangorra, R.; Antonucci, A.; Agostiano, A.; Trotta, M.; Farinola, G. *Journal of Materials Chemistry C* **2015**, 3, (25), 6471–6478.
4. Ogren, J. I.; Tong, A. L.; Gordon, S. C.; Chenu, A.; Lu, Y.; Blankenship, R.; Cao, J.; Schlau-Cohen, G. *Chemical Science* **2018**, 9, 3095–3104.
5. Scholes, G. D.; Mirkovic, T.; Turner, D. B.; Fassioli, F.; Buchleitner, A. *Energy & Environmental Science* **2012**, 5, (11), 9374–9393.
6. Bredas, J. L.; Sargent, E. H.; Scholes, G. D. *Nature Materials* **2017**, 16, (1), 35–44.
7. Shukla, M.; Kumar, S. *Renewable and Sustainable Energy Reviews* **2018**, 82, 402–414.
8. Zhang, Z.; Liao, M.; Lou, H.; Hu, Y.; Sun, X.; Peng, H. *Advanced Materials* **2018**, 30, 1704261.
9. Tan, S. C.; Yan, F.; Crouch, L. I.; Robertson, J.; Jones, M. R.; Welland, M. E. *Advanced Functional Materials* **2013**, 23, (44), 5556–5563.
10. Ravi, S. K.; Udayagiri, V. S.; Suresh, L.; Tan, S. C. *Advanced Functional Materials* **2017**, 28, 1705305.
11. Giardi, M. T.; Scognamiglio, V.; Rea, G.; Rodio, G.; Antonacci, A.; Lambreva, M.; Pezzotti, G.; Johanningmeier, U. *Biosensors & Bioelectronics* **2009**, 25, (2), 294–300.
12. Krassen, H.; Schwarze, A.; Friedrich, B.; Ataka, K.; Lenz, O.; Heberle, J. *ACS Nano* **2009**, 3, (12), 4055–4061.
13. Sekar, N.; Jain, R.; Yan, Y.; Ramasamy, R. P. *Biotechnology and Bioengineering* **2016**, 113, (3), 675–679.
14. Sekar, N.; Umasankar, Y.; Ramasamy, R. P. *Physical Chemistry Chemical Physics* **2014**, 16, (17), 7862–7871.
15. Wenzel, T.; Härtter, D.; Bombelli, P.; Howe, C. J.; Steiner, U. *Nature Communications* **2018**, 9, (1), 1299.
16. Ravi, S. K.; Tan, S. C. *Energy & Environmental Science* **2015**, 8, (9), 2551–2573.
17. Leonova, M. M.; Fufina, T. Y.; Vasilieva, L. G.; Shuvalov, V. A. *Biochemistry-Moscow* **2011**, 76, (13), 1465–1483.
18. Friebe, V. M.; Frese, R. N. *Current Opinion in Electrochemistry* **2017**, 5, 126–134.
19. Hillier, W.; Babcock, G. T. *Plant Physiology* **2001**, 125, (1), 33–37.
20. Golbeck, J.; Est, A., *The Biophysics of Photosynthesis*. Springer Science & Business Media: New York, **2014**; Vol. 11.
21. Nelson, N.; Junge, W. *Annual Review of Biochemistry* **2015**, 84, 659–683.
22. Ort, D. R.; Yocum, C. F., *Oxygenic Photosynthesis: The Light Reactions*. Springer Science & Business Media: New York, **1996**; Vol. 4.
23. Tel-Vered, R.; Willner, I. *Chemelectrochem* **2014**, 1, (11), 1778–1797.
24. Wang, F.; Liu, X.; Willner, I. *Advanced Materials* **2013**, 25, (3), 349–377.
25. Sekar, N.; Ramasamy, R. P. *Journal of Photochemistry and Photobiology C: Photochemistry Reviews* **2015**, 22, 19–33.
26. Xie, X.; Crespo, G. A.; Mistlberger, G.; Bakker, E. *Nature Chemistry* **2014**, 6, (3), 202–207.
27. O'Connor, C. M.; Adams, J. U. *Essentials of Cell Biology*. NPG Education: Cambridge, MA, **2010**.
28. Guo, Z.; Liang, D.; Rao, S.; Xiang, Y. *Nano Energy* **2015**, 11, 654–661.
29. Schrantz, K.; Wyss, P. P.; Ihssen, J.; Toth, R.; Bora, D. K.; Vitol, E. A.; Rozhkova, E. A.; Pieles, U.; Thöny-Meyer, L.; Braun, A. *Catalysis Today* **2017**, 284, 44–51.
30. Bora, D. K.; Rozhkova, E. A.; Schrantz, K.; Wyss, P. P.; Braun, A.; Graule, T.; Constable, E. C. *Advanced Functional Materials* **2012**, 22, (3), 490–502.

31. Blankenship, R. E., *Molecular Mechanisms of Photosynthesis*. John Wiley & Sons: New York, **2013**.
32. Blankenship, R. E. *Molecular Mechanisms of Photosynthesis*. Wiley-Blackwell: UK, **2002**; 11–25.
33. Hsin, J.; Gumbart, J.; Trabuco, L. G.; Villa, E.; Qian, P.; Hunter, C. N.; Schulten, K. *Biophysical Journal* **2009**, 97, (1), 321–329.
34. Jones, M. R. *Progress in Lipid Research* **2007**, 46, (1), 56–87.
35. Pandit, A.; Morosinotto, T.; Reus, M.; Holzwarth, A. R.; Bassi, R.; de Groot, H. J. M. *Biochimica et Biophysica Acta (BBA) - Bioenergetics* **2011**, 1807, (4), 437–443.
36. Contreras-Martel, C.; Matamala, A.; Bruna, C.; Poo-Caamaño, G.; Almonacid, D.; Figueroa, M.; Martínez-Oyanedel, J.; Bunster, M. *Biophysical Chemistry* **2007**, 125, (2), 388–396.
37. Jones, M. R., Bacterial photosynthesis. *Photobiological Sciences Online* (KC Smith, Ed.) American Society for Photobiology, http://www.photobiology.info/ 2009.
38. Zhuang, T.; Sasaki, S.-i.; Ikeuchi, T.; Kido, J.; Wang, X.-F. *RSC Advances* **2015**, 5, (57), 45755–45759.
39. Ham, M.-H.; Choi, J. H.; Boghossian, A. A.; Jeng, E. S.; Graff, R. A.; Heller, D. A.; Chang, A. C.; Mattis, A.; Bayburt, T. H.; Grinkova, Y. V. *Nature Chemistry* **2010**, 2, (11), 929–936.
40. den Hollander, M.-J.; Magis, J. G.; Fuchsenberger, P.; Aartsma, T. J.; Jones, M. R.; Frese, R. N. *Langmuir* **2011**, 27, (16), 10282–10294.
41. Caterino, R.; Csiki, R.; Lyuleeva, A.; Pfisterer, J.; Wiesinger, M.; Janssens, S. D.; Haenen, K.; Cattani-Scholz, A.; Stutzmann, M.; Garrido, J. A. *ACS Applied Materials & Interfaces* **2015**, 7, (15), 8099–8107.
42. Friebe, V. M.; Delgado, J. D.; Swainsbury, D. J.; Gruber, J. M.; Chanaewa, A.; van Grondelle, R.; von Hauff, E.; Millo, D.; Jones, M. R.; Frese, R. N. *Advanced Functional Materials* **2016**, 26, (2), 285–292.
43. Yaghoubi, H.; Lafalce, E.; Jun, D.; Jiang, X.; Beatty, J. T.; Takshi, A. *Biomacromolecules* **2015**, 16, (4), 1112–1118.
44. Kondo, M.; Iida, K.; Dewa, T.; Tanaka, H.; Ogawa, T.; Nagashima, S.; Nagashima, K. V. P. et al. *Biomacromolecules* **2012**, 13, (2), 432–438.
45. Tan, S. C.; Crouch, L. I.; Jones, M. R.; Welland, M. *Angewandte Chemie-International Edition* **2012**, 51, (27), 6667–6671.
46. Tan, S. C.; Crouch, L. I.; Mahajan, S.; Jones, M. R.; Welland, M. E. *Acs Nano* **2012**, 6, (10), 9103–9109.
47. Mirvakili, S. M.; Slota, J. E.; Usgaocar, A. R.; Mahmoudzadeh, A.; Jun, D.; Mirvakili, M. N.; Beatty, J. T.; Madden, J. D. W. *Advanced Functional Materials* **2014**, 24, (30), 4789–4794.
48. LeBlanc, G.; Chen, G.; Gizzie, E. A.; Jennings, G. K.; Cliffel, D. E. *Advanced Materials* **2012**, 24, (44), 5959–5962.
49. Ciesielski, P. N.; Faulkner, C. J.; Irwin, M. T.; Gregory, J. M.; Tolk, N. H.; Cliffel, D. E.; Jennings, G. K. *Advanced Functional Materials* **2010**, 20, (23), 4048–4054.
50. Ravi, S. K.; Swainsbury, D. J.; Singh, V. K.; Ngeow, Y. K.; Jones, M. R.; Tan, S. C. *Advanced Materials* **2018**, 30, (5).
51. Seibert, M.; Janzen, A. F.; Kendalltobias, M. *Photochemistry and Photobiology* **1982**, 35, (2), 193–200.
52. Janzen, A. F.; Seibert, M. *Nature* **1980**, 286, (5773), 584–585.
53. Plumeré, N.; Nowaczyk, M. M., Biophotoelectrochemistry of Photosynthetic Proteins. In *Biophotoelectrochemistry: From Bioelectrochemistry to Biophotovoltaics*, Springer: Cham, Switzerland, 2016; pp. 111–136.
54. Katz, E. *Journal of Electroanalytical Chemistry* **1994**, 365, (1–2), 157–164.
55. Takshi, A.; Madden, J. D.; Beatty, J. T. *Electrochimica Acta* **2009**, 54, (14), 3806–3811.

56. Pinhassi, R. I.; Kallmann, D.; Saper, G.; Dotan, H.; Linkov, A.; Kay, A.; Liveanu, V.; Schuster, G.; Adir, N.; Rothschild, A. *Nature Communications* **2016**, 7, 12552.

57. Kato, M.; Zhang, J. Z.; Paul, N.; Reisner, E. *Chemical Society Reviews* **2014**, 43, (18), 6485–6497.

58. Atxabal, A.; Braun, S.; Arnold, T.; Sun, X.; Parui, S.; Liu, X.; Gozalvez, C.; Llopis, R.; Mateo-Alonso, A.; Casanova, F.; Ortmann, F.; Fahlman, M.; Hueso, L. E. *Advanced Materials* **2017**, 29, (19).

59. Hu, Z.; Zhong, Z.; Chen, Y.; Sun, C.; Huang, F.; Peng, J.; Wang, J.; Cao, Y. *Advanced Functional Materials* **2016**, 26, (1), 129–136.

60. Ishii, H.; Sugiyama, K.; Ito, E.; Seki, K. *Advanced Materials* **1999**, 11, (8), 605–625.

61. Tang, J.; Lee, C.; Lee, S.; Xu, Y. *Chemical Physics Letters* **2004**, 396, (1), 92–96.

62. Muccini, M. *Nature Materials* **2006**, 5, (8), 605.

63. Mazzio, K. A.; Luscombe, C. K. *Chemical Society Reviews* **2015**, 44, (1), 78–90.

64. Zhang, Q.; Tsang, D.; Kuwabara, H.; Hatae, Y.; Li, B.; Takahashi, T.; Lee, S. Y.; Yasuda, T.; Adachi, C. *Advanced Materials* **2015**, 27, (12), 2096–2100.

65. Farinola, G. M.; Ragni, R. *Chemical Society Reviews* **2011**, 40, (7), 3467–3482.

66. Wang, Q.; Ma, D. *Chemical Society Reviews* **2010**, 39, (7), 2387–2398.

67. Liu, Z.; Kobayashi, M.; Paul, B. C.; Bao, Z.; Nishi, Y. *Physical Review B* **2010**, 82, (3), 035311.

68. Wagenpfahl, A.; Rauh, D.; Binder, M.; Deibel, C.; Dyakonov, V. *Physical Review B* **2010**, 82, (11), 115306.

69. Clarke, T. M.; Durrant, J. R. *Chemical Reviews* **2010**, 110, (11), 6736–6767.

70. Davis, R. J.; Lloyd, M. T.; Ferreira, S. R.; Bruzek, M. J.; Watkins, S. E.; Lindell, L.; Sehati, P.; Fahlman, M.; Anthony, J. E.; Hsu, J. W. *Journal of Materials Chemistry* **2011**, 21, (6), 1721–1729.

71. Fu, H. Organic photonic devices. In: Hu, W. (Ed.) *Organic Optoelectronics.* Wiley-VCH Verlag GmbH & Co. KGaA: Germany, **2013**; 351–374.

72. Clark, J.; Lanzani, G. *Nature Photonics* **2010**, 4, (7), 438–446.

73. Ostroverkhova, O. *Chemical Reviews* **2016**, 116, (22), 13279–13412.

74. Akaike, K.; Oehzelt, M.; Heimel, G.; Koch, N. In A comprehensive and unified picture of energy level alignment at interfaces with organic semiconductors, SPIE Organic Photonics+ Electronics, 2016; International Society for Optics and Photonics: pp. 99410N-99410N-7.

75. Zhao, J.; Feng, M.; Dougherty, D. B.; Sun, H.; Petek, H. *ACS Nano* **2014**, 8, (10), 10988–10997.

76. Xu, P.; Roy, L. M.; Croce, R. *Biochimica et Biophysica Acta (BBA)-Bioenergetics* **2017**, 1858, (10), 815–822.

77. Guo, X.; Zhou, N.; Lou, S. J.; Smith, J.; Tice, D. B.; Hennek, J. W.; Ortiz, R. P.; Navarrete, J. T. L.; Li, S.; Strzalka, J. *Nature Photonics* **2013**, 7, (10), 825–833.

78. Scholes, G. D.; Fleming, G. R.; Olaya-Castro, A.; van Grondelle, R. *Nature Chemistry* **2011**, 3, (10), 763–774.

79. Croce, R.; van Amerongen, H. *Nature Chemical Biology* **2014**, 10, (7), 492–501.

80. Dekker, J. P.; Boekema, E. J. *Biochimica et Biophysica Acta (BBA) - Bioenergetics* **2005**, 1706, (1), 12–39.

81. Fleming, G. R.; Schlau-Cohen, G. S.; Amarnath, K.; Zaks, J. *Faraday Discussions* **2012**, 155, 27–41.

82. Jurić, S.; Vojta, L.; Fulgosi, H. Electron transfer routes in oxygenic photosynthesis: regulatory mechanisms and new perspectives. In: Dubinsky, Z. (Ed.) *Photosynthesis*, InTech: **2013**.

83. Knör, G. *Coordination Chemistry Reviews* **2015**, 304, 102–108.

84. Su, M.-S.; Kuo, C.-Y.; Yuan, M.-C.; Jeng, U. S.; Su, C.-J.; Wei, K.-H. *Advanced Materials* **2011**, 23, (29), 3315–3319.

85. Kim, J. S.; Lee, Y.; Lee, J. H.; Park, J. H.; Kim, J. K.; Cho, K. *Advanced Materials* **2010**, 22, (12), 1355–1360.

86. Bittner, E. R.; Ramon, J. G. S.; Karabunarliev, S. *The Journal of Chemical Physics* **2005**, 122, (21), 214719.

87. Muntwiler, M.; Yang, Q.; Tisdale, W. A.; Zhu, X. Y. *Physical Review Letters* **2008**, 101, (19), 196403.

88. Iwata, S.; Barber, J. *Current Opinion in Structural Biology* **2004**, 14, (4), 447–453.

89. Zheng, Z.; Awartani, O. M.; Gautam, B.; Liu, D.; Qin, Y.; Li, W.; Bataller, A.; Gundogdu, K.; Ade, H.; Hou, J. *Advanced Materials* **2017**, 29, (5).

90. Oehzelt, M.; Koch, N.; Heimel, G. *Nature Communications* **2014**, 5, 4174.

91. Steim, R.; Kogler, F. R.; Brabec, C. J. *Journal of Materials Chemistry* **2010**, 20, (13), 2499–2512.

92. Ratcliff, E. L.; Garcia, A.; Paniagua, S. A.; Cowan, S. R.; Giordano, A. J.; Ginley, D. S.; Marder, S. R.; Berry, J. J.; Olson, D. C. *Advanced Energy Materials* **2013**, 3, (5), 647–656.

93. Correa Baena, J. P.; Steier, L.; Tress, W.; Saliba, M.; Neutzner, S.; Matsui, T.; Giordano, F. et al. *Energy & Environmental Science* **2015**, 8, (10), 2928–2934.

94. Ishii, H.; Hayashi, N.; Ito, E.; Washizu, Y.; Sugi, K.; Kimura, Y.; Niwano, M.; Ouchi, Y.; Seki, K. *Physica Status Solidi (a)* **2004**, 201, (6), 1075–1094.

95. Wang, H.; Amsalem, P.; Heimel, G.; Salzmann, I.; Koch, N.; Oehzelt, M. *Advanced Materials* **2014**, 26, (6), 925–930.

96. Hwang, J.; Wan, A.; Kahn, A. *Materials Science and Engineering: R: Reports* **2009**, 64, (1), 1–31.

97. Müller, K.; Seitsonen, A. P.; Brugger, T.; Westover, J.; Greber, T.; Jung, T.; Kara, A. *The Journal of Physical Chemistry C* **2012**, 116, (44), 23465–23471.

98. Yang, H.-H.; Chu, Y.-H.; Lu, C.-I.; Yang, T.-H.; Yang, K.-J.; Kaun, C.-C.; Hoffmann, G.; Lin, M.-T. *ACS Nano* **2013**, 7, (3), 2814–2819.

99. Venkateshvaran, D.; Nikolka, M.; Sadhanala, A.; Lemaur, V.; Zelazny, M.; Kepa, M.; Hurhangee, M.; Kronemeijer, A. J.; Pecunia, V.; Nasrallah, I. *Nature* **2014**, 515, (7527), 384.

100. Chenu, A.; Scholes, G. D. *Annual Review of Physical Chemistry* **2015**, 66, 69–96.

101. Connolly, J. S.; Janzen, A. F.; Samuel, E. B. *Photochemistry and Photobiology* **1982**, 36, (5), 559–563.

102. Mullineaux, C. W.; Pascal, A. A.; Horton, P.; Holzwarth, A. R. *Biochimica et Biophysica Acta (BBA)-Bioenergetics* **1993**, 1141, (1), 23–28.

103. Green, B.; Parson, W. W., *Light-Harvesting Antennas in Photosynthesis*. Springer Science & Business Media: Dordrecht, the Netherlands, **2003**; Vol. 13.

104. Sundström, V.; Pullerits, T.; van Grondelle, R., Photosynthetic light-harvesting: reconciling dynamics and structure of purple bacterial LH2 reveals function of photosynthetic unit. *The Journal of Physical Chemistry B*, ACS Publications: **1999**, 103, (13), 2327–2346.

105. Novoderezhkin, V. I.; van Grondelle, R. *Physical Chemistry Chemical Physics* **2010**, 12, (27), 7352–7365.

106. van Grondelle, R.; van Gorkom, H. *Photosynthesis Research* **2014**, 120, (1–2), 3–7.

107. Renger, T. *Photosynthesis Research* **2009**, 102, (2–3), 471–485.

108. Cheng, Y.-C.; Fleming, G. R. *Annual Review of Physical Chemistry* **2009**, 60.

109. Colbow, K. *Biochimica et Biophysica Acta (BBA)-Bioenergetics* **1973**, 314, (3), 320–327.

110. Van Grondelle, R. *Biochimica et Biophysica Acta (BBA)-Reviews on Bioenergetics* **1985**, 811, (2), 147–195.

111. Anna, J. M.; Scholes, G. D.; van Grondelle, R. *BioScience* **2013**, 64, (1), 14–25.

112. Ishizaki, A.; Calhoun, T. R.; Schlau-Cohen, G. S.; Fleming, G. R. *Physical Chemistry Chemical Physics* **2010**, 12, (27), 7319–7337.

113. Ishizaki, A.; Fleming, G. R. *Annual Review of Condensed Matter Physics* **2012**, 3, (1), 333–361.
114. Romero, E.; Augulis, R.; Novoderezhkin, V. I.; Ferretti, M.; Thieme, J.; Zigmantas, D.; Van Grondelle, R. *Nature Physics* **2014**, 10, (9), 676–682.
115. Paleček, D.; Edlund, P.; Westenhoff, S.; Zigmantas, D. *Science Advances* **2017**, 3, (9), e1603141.
116. Romero, E.; Novoderezhkin, V. I.; van Grondelle, R. *Nature* **2017**, 543, (7645), 355.
117. Leegwater, J. A. *The Journal of Physical Chemistry* **1996**, 100, (34), 14403–14409.
118. Engel, G. S.; Calhoun, T. R.; Read, E. L.; Ahn, T.-K.; Mančal, T.; Cheng, Y.-C.; Blankenship, R. E.; Fleming, G. R. *Nature* **2007**, 446, (7137), 782.
119. Panitchayangkoon, G.; Hayes, D.; Fransted, K. A.; Caram, J. R.; Harel, E.; Wen, J.; Blankenship, R. E.; Engel, G. S. *Proceedings of the National Academy of Sciences* **2010**, 107, (29), 12766–12770.
120. Collini, E.; Wong, C. Y.; Wilk, K. E.; Curmi, P. M.; Brumer, P.; Scholes, G. D. *Nature* **2010**, 463, (7281), 644.
121. Krueger, B. P.; Scholes, G. D.; Fleming, G. R. *The Journal of Physical Chemistry B* **1998**, 102, (27), 5378–5386.
122. Hsu, C.-P. *Accounts of Chemical Research* **2009**, 42, (4), 509–518.
123. Kasha, M. *Radiation Research* **1963**, 20, (1), 55–70.
124. Scholes, G. D.; Rumbles, G. *Nature Materials* **2006**, 5, (9), 683.
125. Bardeen, C. J. *Annual Review of Physical Chemistry* **2014**, 65, 127–148.
126. Spano, F. C. *Accounts of Chemical Research* **2009**, 43, (3), 429–439.
127. Scholes, G. D.; Smyth, C. *The Journal of Chemical Physics* **2014**, 140, (11), 03B201_1.
128. Green, M. A. *AIP Advances* **2013**, 3, (11), 112104.
129. Kirk, A. P.; Ferry, D. K. *Journal of Computational Electronics* **2018**, 17, (1), 313–318.
130. Würfel, P. *CHIMIA International Journal for Chemistry* **2007**, 61, (12), 770–774.
131. Lee, H.; Cheng, Y.-C.; Fleming, G. R. *Science* **2007**, 316, (5830), 1462–1465.
132. Ball, P. *Nature Materials* **2018**, 17, (3), 220.
133. Hildner, R.; Brinks, D.; Nieder, J. B.; Cogdell, R. J.; van Hulst, N. F. *Science* **2013**, 340, (6139), 1448–1451.
134. Scholes, G. D.; Curutchet, C.; Mennucci, B.; Cammi, R.; Tomasi, J. *The Journal of Physical Chemistry B* **2007**, 111, (25), 6978–6982.
135. Renger, T.; Müh, F. *Photosynthesis Research* **2012**, 111, (1–2), 47–52.
136. Müh, F.; Madjet, M. E.-A.; Renger, T. *The Journal of Physical Chemistry B* **2010**, 114, (42), 13517–13535.
137. Cogdell, R. J.; Gall, A.; Köhler, J. *Quarterly Reviews of Biophysics* **2006**, 39, (3), 227–324.
138. Scholes, G. D.; Fleming, G. R. *The Journal of Physical Chemistry B* **2000**, 104, (8), 1854–1868.
139. Sipka, G.; Maróti, P. *Photosynthesis Research* **2018**, 136, (1), 17–30.
140. Beddard, G.; Porter, G. *Nature* **1976**, 260, (5549), 366.
141. Watson, W.; Livingston, R. *The Journal of Chemical Physics* **1950**, 18, (6), 802–809.
142. Barros, T.; Kühlbrandt, W. *Biochimica et Biophysica Acta (BBA)-Bioenergetics* **2009**, 1787, (6), 753–772.
143. Orf, G. S.; Blankenship, R. E. *Photosynthesis Research* **2013**, 116, (2–3), 315–331.
144. Kassal, I.; Yuen-Zhou, J.; Rahimi-Keshari, S. *The Journal of Physical Chemistry Letters* **2013**, 4, (3), 362–367.
145. Hemelrijk, P. W.; Kwa, S. L.; van Grondelle, R.; Dekker, J. P. *Biochimica et Biophysica Acta (BBA)-Bioenergetics* **1992**, 1098, (2), 159–166.
146. Szalay, L.; Tombácz, E.; Singhal, G. *Acta Physica Academiae Scientiarum Hungaricae* **1974**, 35, (1–4), 29–36.

147. Saeki, A.; Koizumi, Y.; Aida, T.; Seki, S. *Accounts of Chemical Research* **2012**, 45, (8), 1193–1202.
148. Pasveer, W.; Cottaar, J.; Tanase, C.; Coehoorn, R.; Bobbert, P.; Blom, P.; De Leeuw, D.; Michels, M. *Physical Review Letters* **2005**, 94, (20), 206601.
149. Fratini, S.; Ciuchi, S. *Physical Review Letters* **2009**, 103, (26), 266601.
150. Blom, P. W.; Mihailetchi, V. D.; Koster, L. J. A.; Markov, D. E. *Advanced Materials* **2007**, 19, (12), 1551–1566.
151. Prins, P.; Grozema, F.; Schins, J.; Patil, S.; Scherf, U.; Siebbeles, L. *Physical Review Letters* **2006**, 96, (14), 146601.
152. Nicolai, H. T.; Kuik, M.; Wetzelaer, G.; De Boer, B.; Campbell, C.; Risko, C.; Brédas, J.; Blom, P. *Nature Materials* **2012**, 11, (10), 882.
153. Bittner, E. R.; Kelley, A. *Physical Chemistry Chemical Physics* **2015**, 17, (43), 28853–28859.
154. Ravi, S. K.; Yu, Z.; Swainsbury, D. J.; Ouyang, J.; Jones, M. R.; Tan, S. C. *Advanced Energy Materials* **2017**, 7, (7).
155. Renugopalakrishnan, V.; Barbiellini, B.; King, C.; Molinari, M.; Mochalov, K.; Sukhanova, A.; Nabiev, I. et al. *The Journal of Physical Chemistry C Nanomaterials and Interfaces* **2014**, 118, (30), 16710–16717.
156. Yao, K.; Jiao, H.; Xu, Y.-X.; He, Q.; Li, F.; Wang, X. *Journal of Materials Chemistry A* **2016**, 4, (35), 13400–13406.
157. Gordiichuk, P. I.; Wetzelaer, G. J.; Rimmerman, D.; Gruszka, A.; de Vries, J. W.; Saller, M.; Gautier, D. A. et al. *Advanced Materials* **2014**, 26, (28), 4863–4869.
158. Gordiichuk, P.; Pesce, D.; Ocampo, O. E. C.; Marcozzi, A.; Wetzelaer, G. A. H.; Paul, A.; Loznik, M. et al. *Advanced Science (Weinheim)* **2017**, 4, (5), 1600393.
159. Yang, Y.; Gobeze, H. B.; D'Souza, F.; Jankowiak, R.; Li, J. *Advanced Materials Interfaces* **2016**, 3, (15), 1600371.
160. Li, J.; Feng, X.; Fei, J.; Cai, P.; Huang, J.; Li, J. *Journal of Materials Chemistry A* **2016**, 4, (31), 12197–12204.
161. Su, Y.-W.; Lan, S.-C.; Wei, K.-H. *Materials Today* **2012**, 15, (12), 554–562.
162. Elumalai, N. K.; Uddin, A. *Energy & Environmental Science* **2016**, 9, (2), 391–410.
163. Hedley, G. J.; Ruseckas, A.; Samuel, I. D. *Chemical Reviews* **2016**, 117, (2), 796–837.
164. Vogelbaum, H. S.; Sauvé, G. *Synthetic Metals* **2017**, 223, 107–121.
165. McConnell, I.; Li, G.; Brudvig, G. W. *Chemistry & Biology* **2010**, 17, (5), 434–447.
166. Olaya-Castro, A.; Scholes, G. D. *International Reviews in Physical Chemistry* **2011**, 30, (1), 49–77.
167. Forrest, S. R. *MRS Bulletin* **2005**, 30, (1), 28–32.
168. Terao, Y.; Sasabe, H.; Adachi, C. *Applied Physics Letters* **2007**, 90, (10), 103515.
169. Nganou, C.; Lackner, G.; Teschome, B.; Deen, M. J.; Adir, N.; Pouhe, D.; Lupascu, D. C.; Mkandawire, M. *ACS Applied Materials & Interfaces* **2017**, 9, (22), 19030–19039.
170. Hu, Q.; Marquardt, J.; Iwasaki, I.; Miyashita, H.; Kurano, N.; Mörschel, E.; Miyachi, S. *Biochimica et Biophysica Acta (BBA)-Bioenergetics* **1999**, 1412, (3), 250–261.
171. Chen, M.; Floetenmeyer, M.; Bibby, T. S. *FEBS Letters* **2009**, 583, (15), 2535–2539.
172. Adir, N. *Photosynthesis Research* **2005**, 85, (1), 15–32.
173. Dai, H. *Accounts of Chemical Research* **2002**, 35, (12), 1035–1044.
174. Lai, T.-H.; Tsang, S.-W.; Manders, J. R.; Chen, S.; So, F. *Materials Today* **2013**, 16, (11), 424–432.
175. Marchal, W.; De Dobbelaere, C.; Kesters, J.; Bonneux, G.; Vandenbergh, J.; Damm, H.; Junkers, T.; Maes, W.; D'Haen, J.; Van Bael, M. K. *RSC Advances* **2015**, 5, (111), 91349–91362.
176. Voznyy, O.; Sutherland, B. R.; Ip, A. H.; Zhitomirsky, D.; Sargent, E. H. *Nature Reviews Materials* **2017**, 2, (6), 17026.
177. Mastria, R.; Rizzo, A. *Journal of Materials Chemistry C* **2016**, 4, (27), 6430–6446.

178. Hubbard, S. Carrier transport. In *Photovoltaic Solar Energy*, John Wiley & Sons: Chichester, UK, **2016**; pp. 47–53.

179. Dvorak, M.; Wei, S.-H.; Wu, Z. *Physical Review Letters* **2013**, 110, (1), 016402.

180. Knupfer, M. *Applied Physics A: Materials Science & Processing* **2003**, 77, (5), 623–626.

181. Rand, B. P.; Burk, D. P.; Forrest, S. R. *Physical Review B* **2007**, 75, (11), 115327.

182. Hubbard, S. Recombination. In *Photovoltaic Solar Energy*, John Wiley & Sons: Chichester, UK, **2016**; pp. 39–46.

183. Verlinden, P. Doping, diffusion, and defects in solar cells. In *Photovoltaic Solar Energy*, John Wiley & Sons: Chichester, UK, **2016**; pp. 21–31.

184. Sandén, S.; Wilson, N. M.; Wang, E.; Österbacka, R. *The Journal of Physical Chemistry C* **2017**, 121, (14), 8211–8219.

185. Wen, X.; Feng, Y.; Huang, S.; Huang, F.; Cheng, Y.-B.; Green, M.; Ho-Baillie, A. *Journal of Materials Chemistry C* **2016**, 4, (4), 793–800.

186. Castet, F.; D'Avino, G.; Muccioli, L.; Cornil, J.; Beljonne, D. *Physical Chemistry Chemical Physics* **2014**, 16, (38), 20279–20290.

187. Archer, M. D. *Nanostructured and Photoelectrochemical Systems for Solar Photon Conversion.* Imperial College Press: London, UK, **2008**; Vol. 3.

188. Das, R.; Kiley, P. J.; Segal, M.; Norville, J.; Yu, A. A.; Wang, L. Y.; Trammell, S. A. et al. *Nano Letters* **2004**, 4, (6), 1079–1083.

189. Singh, V. K.; Ravi, S. K.; Ho, J. W.; Wong, J. K. C.; Jones, M. R.; Tan, S. C. *Advanced Functional Materials* **2017**, 1703689.

190. Amao, Y.; Komori, T. *Biosensors and Bioelectronics* **2004**, 19, (8), 843–847.

191. Janfaza, S.; Molaeirad, A.; Mohamadpour, R.; Khayati, M.; Mehrvand, J. *BioNanoScience* **2014**, 4, (1), 71–77.

192. Yu, D.; Wang, M.; Zhu, G.; Ge, B.; Liu, S.; Huang, F. *Scientific Reports* **2015**, 5, 9375.

193. Thavasi, V.; Lazarova, T.; Filipek, S.; Kolinski, M.; Querol, E.; Kumar, A.; Ramakrishna, S.; Padrós, E.; Renugopalakrishnan, V. *Journal of Nanoscience and Nanotechnology* **2009**, 9, (3), 1679–1687.

194. Syafinar, R.; Gomesh, N.; Irwanto, M.; Fareq, M.; Irwan, Y. *Energy Procedia* **2015**, 79, 896–902.

195. Hug, H.; Bader, M.; Mair, P.; Glatzel, T. *Applied Energy* **2014**, 115, 216–225.

196. Narayan, M. R. *Renewable and Sustainable Energy Reviews* **2012**, 16, (1), 208–215.

197. Calogero, G.; Yum, J.-H.; Sinopoli, A.; Di Marco, G.; Grätzel, M.; Nazeeruddin, M. K. *Solar Energy* **2012**, 86, (5), 1563–1575.

198. Abraham, N.; Rufus, A.; Unni, C.; Philip, D. *Journal of Materials Science: Materials in Electronics* **2017**, 28, (21), 16527–16539.

199. Wongcharee, K.; Meeyoo, V.; Chavadej, S. *Solar Energy Materials and Solar Cells* **2007**, 91, (7), 566–571.

200. Robinson, M. T.; Armbruster, M. E.; Gargye, A.; Cliffel, D. E.; Jennings, G. K. *ACS Applied Energy Materials* **2018**, 1, 301–305.

201. Yu, D.; Zhu, G.; Liu, S.; Ge, B.; Huang, F. *International Journal of Hydrogen Energy* **2013**, 38, (36), 16740–16748.

202. Mershin, A.; Matsumoto, K.; Kaiser, L.; Yu, D.; Vaughn, M.; Nazeeruddin, M. K.; Bruce, B. D.; Graetzel, M.; Zhang, S. *Scientific Reports* **2012**, 2.

203. Petrella, A.; Cozzoli, P. D.; Curri, M. L.; Striccoli, M.; Cosma, P.; Agostiano, A. *Bioelectrochemistry* **2004**, 63, (1), 99–102.

204. Ocakoglu, K.; Krupnik, T.; van den Bosch, B.; Harputlu, E.; Gullo, M. P.; Olmos, J. D. J.; Yildirimcan, S. et al. *Advanced Functional Materials* **2014**, 24, (47), 7467–7477.

205. Hagfeldt, A.; Boschloo, G.; Sun, L.; Kloo, L.; Pettersson, H. *Chemical Reviews* **2010**, 110, (11), 6595–6663.

206. Şener, M. K.; Park, S.; Lu, D.; Damjanović, A.; Ritz, T.; Fromme, P.; Schulten, K. *The Journal of Chemical Physics* **2004**, 120, (23), 11183–11195.

207. Fromme, P.; Grotjohann, I., Structural analysis of cyanobacterial photosystem I. In *Photosystem I*, Springer: Amsterdam, the Netherlands, **2006**; pp. 47–69.
208. Brettel, K.; Leibl, W. *Biochimica et Biophysica Acta (BBA)-Bioenergetics* **2001**, 1507, (1–3), 100–114.
209. Nelson, N.; Ben-Shem, A. *Nature Reviews Molecular Cell Biology* **2004**, 5, (12), 971.
210. Connelly, J.; Müller, M.; Hucke, M.; Gatzen, G.; Mullineaux, C.; Ruban, A.; Horton, P.; Holzwarth, A. *The Journal of Physical Chemistry B* **1997**, 101, (10), 1902–1909.
211. Gradinaru, C. C.; Özdemir, S.; Gülen, D.; van Stokkum, I. H.; van Grondelle, R.; van Amerongen, H. *Biophysical Journal* **1998**, 75, (6), 3064–3077.
212. Magdaong, N. M.; Enriquez, M. M.; LaFountain, A. M.; Rafka, L.; Frank, H. A. *Photosynthesis Research* **2013**, 118, (3), 259–276.
213. Nabiev, I.; Rakovich, A.; Sukhanova, A.; Lukashev, E.; Zagidullin, V.; Pachenko, V.; Rakovich, Y. P.; Donegan, J. F.; Rubin, A. B.; Govorov, A. O. *Angewandte Chemie International Edition* **2010**, 49, (40), 7217–7221.
214. Gust, D.; Moore, T. A.; Moore, A. L. *Accounts of Chemical Research* **2001**, 34, (1), 40–48.
215. Balzani, V.; Credi, A.; Venturi, M. *ChemSusChem* **2008**, 1, (1–2), 26–58.
216. Alstrum-Acevedo, J. H.; Brennaman, M. K.; Meyer, T. J. *Inorganic Chemistry* **2005**, 44, (20), 6802–6827.
217. Govorov, A. O.; Carmeli, I. *Nano Letters* **2007**, 7, (3), 620–625.
218. Govorov, A. O. *Advanced Materials* **2008**, 20, (22), 4330–4335.
219. Wargnier, R.; Baranov, A. V.; Maslov, V. G.; Stsiapura, V.; Artemyev, M.; Pluot, M.; Sukhanova, A.; Nabiev, I. *Nano Letters* **2004**, 4, (3), 451–457.
220. Franzl, T.; Shavel, A.; Rogach, A. L.; Gaponik, N.; Klar, T. A.; Eychmüller, A.; Feldmann, J. *Small* **2005**, 1, (4), 392–395.
221. Rakovich, A.; Donegan, J. F.; Oleinikov, V.; Molinari, M.; Sukhanova, A.; Nabiev, I.; Rakovich, Y. P. *Journal of Photochemistry and Photobiology C: Photochemistry Reviews* **2014**, 20, 17–32.
222. Lindquist, N. C.; Nagpal, P.; McPeak, K. M.; Norris, D. J.; Oh, S.-H. *Reports on Progress in Physics* **2012**, 75, (3), 036501.
223. Andreussi, O.; Biancardi, A.; Corni, S.; Mennucci, B. *Nano Letters* **2013**, 13, (9), 4475–4484.
224. Dutta, P. K.; Lin, S.; Loskutov, A.; Levenberg, S.; Jun, D.; Saer, R.; Beatty, J. T.; Liu, Y.; Yan, H.; Woodbury, N. W. *Journal of the American Chemical Society* **2014**, 136, (12), 4599–4604.
225. Milano, F.; Tangorra, R. R.; Hassan Omar, O.; Ragni, R.; Operamolla, A.; Agostiano, A.; Farinola, G. M.; Trotta, M. *Angewandte Chemie International Edition* **2012**, 51, (44), 11019–11023.
226. Guo, F.; Kubis, P.; Li, N.; Przybilla, T.; Matt, G.; Stubhan, T.; Ameri, T.; Butz, B.; Spiecker, E.; Forberich, K. *ACS Nano* **2014**, 8, (12), 12632–12640.
227. Takshi, A.; Madden, J. D. W.; Mahmoudzadeh, A.; Saer, R.; Beatty, J. T. *Energies* **2010**, 3, (11), 1721–1727.
228. Tokaji, Z.; Tandori, J.; Maroti, P. *Photochemistry and Photobiology* **2002**, 75, (6), 605–612.
229. Hughes, A. V.; Rees, P.; Heathcote, P.; Jones, M. R. *Biophysical Journal* **2006**, 90, (11), 4155–4166.
230. Magis, G. J.; den Hollander, M.-J.; Onderwaater, W. G.; Olsen, J. D.; Hunter, C. N.; Aartsma, T. J.; Frese, R. N. *Biochimica Et Biophysica Acta-Biomembranes* **2010**, 1798, (3), 637–645.

7 Challenges and Opportunities of Photosynthetic Protein-Based Solar Cell

Di Sheng Lee, Yoke Keng Ngeow, and Swee Ching Tan

CONTENTS

7.1 COMPARISON BETWEEN NATURAL AND BIOMIMETIC PHOTOSYNTHETIC DEVICE

Undeniably, the photosynthetic apparatus found in photosynthetic organisms are superior bio-machineries that convert sunlight into useful energy.[1] The architecture of these nanodevices is designed to optimize forward, energy-storing reactions while minimizing backward, energy-dissipating reactions. Amazingly, these photosynthetic machineries have many aspects in common, both structurally and functionally.[2,3] These universal design aspects could inspire and be integrated into artificial photosynthetic devices. In fact, the resemblance between artificial photosynthetic systems and natural photosynthetic systems is obvious.[4] Both systems operate to generate energy by harvesting light, separating charge and catalysis. Most of the time, the structure and function of components in artificial photosynthetic devices are designed to emulate those in natural photosynthetic systems. For example, some aspects of natural photosynthetic design are already similar to current photovoltaic devices, particularly the dye-sensitized solar cells (DSSCs).[5] In natural photosynthesis, light absorption by light-harvesting (LH) systems is followed by charge separation in the reaction center (RC). Remarkably, DSSCs employ a similar mechanism

225

to collect sunlight and convert it into electricity. However, scientists are aware of some major differences between both systems that exist. One example would be the medium of transport for electrons and protons. In natural photosynthetic systems, a membrane serves as the medium of electron transport, but it also causes resistance for the flow of proton. On the other hand, protons are able to flow freely in the artificial photosynthetic cells while the electrons travel through the electrodes. The similarities and differences in both systems will be addressed later in terms of light harvesting, charge separation, catalysis, and photoprotection.

In a natural photosynthetic system, a wide range of pigments are present to optimize the light-harvesting process. The variation in absorption wavelength of these pigments appears to obey certain rules.[8] The pigment absorption spectrum is aligned with the peak photon flux spectrum at the longest available wavelengths such that the low photon energies are capable of supporting reactions such as water oxidation and transport of transmembrane protons. Another absorption peak of the pigment absorption spectrum is aligned at the shortest available wavelengths. The gap between these two peaks explains the green appearance of those photosynthetic organisms.[9] Quantum mechanics is governing the process of light absorption, the first step that is crucial for a photosynthetic system to utilize solar energy.[10] The absorption of solar radiation incident on the photosynthetic organisms is confined to the visible spectrum, which ranges from 400 nm to 700 nm. Thus, photosynthetic organisms can only access ~50% of the sun's energy.[11] On the other hand, a silicon cell has wider light absorption that ranges from 400 nm to 1200 nm, which means a silicon cell has more access to the solar energy as compared to a natural photosynthetic system.[10] The absorption spectra of natural and artificial pigments are compared in Figure 7.1.

The redox reaction occurs in a single-electron manner for both systems, and the cyclic electron transport is present in both purple bacteria and DSSCs (Figure 7.2). In DSSCs, usually only one type of pigment that absorbs light under a wide spectrum is utilized to cover the solar spectrum. Comparing DSSCs to a natural photosynthetic system, natural photosynthesis utilizes a number of pigments for a wider coverage in the solar spectrum to gather sunlight. Both systems utilized the unique characteristics of pigments to maximize the coverage of the solar spectrum in order to maximize the energy yield of the system. As the light quality decreases as light travels from the surface to the bottom of a photosynthetic device, multilayer photosynthetic cells are developed with the incorporation of different pigments in each layer to enable efficient light harvesting. In a natural photosynthetic system, only a fraction of light harvested by the LH antenna is used for charge separation. During the course of evolution, photosynthetic organisms have adapted to various environmental factors, which tend to fluctuate in order to maintain quantum efficiency of the system. The assembly of larger harvesting antenna complexes in green algae is beneficial for light harvesting, but this approach fails to utilize 80% of the photons after absorption.[14] Most solar energy from the antenna is dissipated as heat or in the form of fluorescence, reducing the energy available for production of chemical fuels. Surprisingly, one way to enhance the efficiency of solar energy conversion is to minimize the size of the antenna, which is a possible approach.[15] This approach can be adapted in the making of an artificial photosynthetic system. Furthermore, while

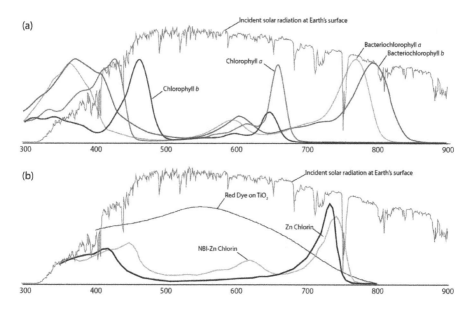

FIGURE 7.1 Absorption spectra of natural and artificial pigments: (a) Absorption spectra of chlorophylls a and b as well as bacteriochlorophylls a and b. (From Blankenship, R.E., *Molecular Mechanisms of Photosynthesis*, John Wiley & Sons, Chichester, UK, 2013.) (b) Absorption spectra of a TiO₂ thin film sensitized with a Ru-based red dye, NBI–Zn–Chlorin, and Zn–Chlorin. The solar spectrum that reaches Earth's surface (air mass 1.5, NREL) is indicated in gray in both panels. (Reprinted from *Chemistry & Biology*, 17, McConnell, I. et al., 434–447, Copyright 2010, with permission from Elsevier; Reprinted with permission from Röger, C. et al., *Journal of the American Chemical Society*, 128, 6542–6543, 2006. Copyright 2006 American Chemical Society.)

nature increases the surface area for light absorption by stacking thylakoids membranes to form grana structures in the chloroplast,[16] DSSCs employ TiO_2 nanoparticles containing film to increase their surface area; a high surface area is crucial because it allows a monolayer of adsorbed sensitizer dye to strongly absorb sunlight for efficient device performance.[16]

In natural PSII protein complex, the process of charge separation in pheophytin and Chl occurs picoseconds after the excitation of RC by sunlight. A redox reaction that involves two redox components, Yz and quinone, that drives electron-transfer further stabilizes charge separation. Overall, the efficiency of the PSII protein complex is increased by the presence of components that facilitate the fast electron-transfer that reduces the chances of back reaction. Similar to natural photosynthesis where the forward electron transfer is significantly faster than the back reaction, the electron injection from the excited sensitizer into the semiconductor membrane in DSSCs is also a rapid process, such that the chances of immediate recombination is reduced.[13,16] The stability of TiO_2 has advantages over the lipid membrane in a natural photosynthetic system because of its ability to support fast electron transfer. Moreover, the majority of the absorbed energy in the natural photosynthetic system was lost during the electron transfer processes in the transmembrane.

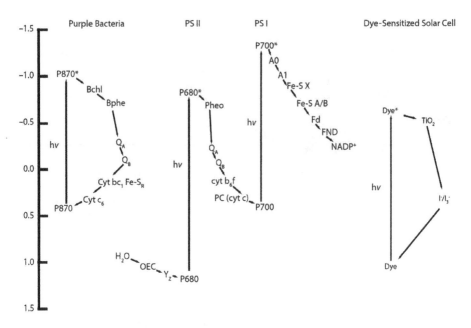

FIGURE 7.2 Reduction potentials in V (versus SHE) in redox intermediates in RCs and DSSCs. Energy-level diagram of purple bacterial, higher plant (photosystems I and II) RCs (From Blankenship, R.E., *Molecular Mechanisms of Photosynthesis*, John Wiley & Sons, Chichester, UK, 2013; Rappaport, F. and Diner, B.A., *Coordin. Chem. Rev.*, 252, 259–272, 2008.), and DSSCs using N3 red dye. (From Grätzel, M., *Inorg. Chem.*, 44, 6841–6851, 2005.) (Reprinted from *Chem. Biol.*, 17, McConnell, I. et al., 434–447, Copyright 2010, with permission from Elsevier.)

Nature has chosen Mn as a water-oxidation catalyst in PSII. There are certainly more options of catalysts to be chosen for artificial photosynthetic systems, but they are usually less cost-effective than Mn.[17,18] The problem with the catalyst found in a natural photosynthetic system was that it was damaged from the oxidation process and required replacement. The desired catalyst needs to be robust in order to overcome this problem. The desired candidate of catalyst also needs to be able to bind and to stabilize components in the systems for a duration to support ligand exchanging. Advancement in encapsulation approaches and innovation of a self-repair system are possible ways to address the issues faced in natural photosynthetic systems. In order to cope with photodamage, a natural antenna system has developed several photoprotection mechanisms. These mechanisms play a role in dissipating excess light excitation energy and facilitating the repair of the system damaged by oxygenic photosynthesis. On the other hand, the components in DSSCs and the structural design of the DSSCs can be designed to optimize the performance under the natural light environment. The natural photosynthetic system can serve as a model to develop DSSCs and even to incorporate these repair mechanisms in DSSCs since DSSCs do not have the renewal ability of chlorophyll in plants.[16]

7.2   FUTURE DIRECTIONS

7.2.1   Biohydrogen Production and Biomass

There are two major approaches for the solar energy storage and conversion: (1) direct conversion of solar energy to electricity; (2) conversion of solar energy to high energy fuels such as molecular hydrogen from water (Figure 7.3). While most of the existing solar cells convert solar energy directly into electricity, natural photosynthesis converts solar power to chemical products. For example, green plants, algae, and cyanobacteria use sunlight to oxidize water, and the resulting electrons are employed to generate fuel such as carbohydrate, which can be directly burnt or converted into ethanol; lipid, which can be converted into biodiesel; or even hydrogen gas, which can be used directly for many applications. In fact, existing technology is able to achieve this by combining photovoltaic solar cells and electrolysis of water. However, the catalysts needed for electrolysis are scarce and expensive; hence, electrolysis of water to produce hydrogen is not favored over conventional ways as our primary energy source. While the search for useful solar-driven catalysts made up of earth-abundant elements for water oxidation and fuel production is important, the answer might already be found in Mother Nature, as many organisms possess metals such as iron and nickel in

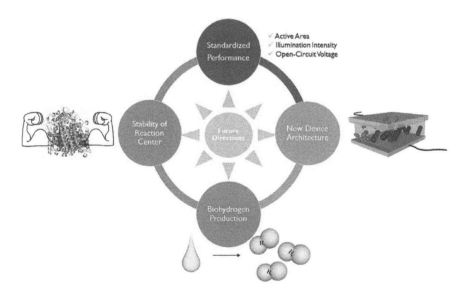

FIGURE 7.3   Future directions of photosynthetic protein-based solar cell. (Top) The disparities in reporting the performance of biohybrid solar cells including the light intensity used for illumination, the active area of the solar cells, and the open-circuit voltage output should be addressed and standardized. (Bottom) The conversion of solar energy to high-energy fuels such as molecular hydrogen from water using photosynthetic proteins is a promising direction. (Left) The stability of reaction center must be improved for further applications. (Right) New device architecture, such as devices consisting of entire photosynthetic organisms, should be conceived in order to improve existing biohybrid devices.

their enzymes to produce hydrogen gas.[19] For example, *Clostridium acetobutylicum* has a hydrogenase enzyme known as CaHydA, which contains a [6Fe-6S] H-cluster active site to produce H_2 from hydrogen ions.[20] This engineering approach has been employed to adsorb CaHydA onto a carbon-felt cathode in a TiO_2-based photoelectrochemical biofuel cell; when the cell is exposed to light, H_2 is produced.[21] Not only does the cell function with negligible overpotential, but the current densities obtained are similar to those of a platinum foil cathode. Therefore, biohydrogen production by biological catalysts made from earth-abundant elements could challenge existing technologies, and to fulfill the mammoth humanity's energy demand in the future, nature's way of biohydrogen production might be the most viable approach.[22] The hydrogen produced could be used directly or to reduce carbon dioxide to other types of fuels such as methane, just like photosynthesis.

In addition, Mother Nature invented photosynthetic water-splitting reaction to supply living organisms with an unlimited amount of "hydrogen" to make organic molecules from carbon dioxide. Water and carbon dioxide, which are available in almost unlimited amounts, are convenient materials for this process, and the products formed are "hydrogen" and oxygen. The "hydrogen" is not readily released as hydrogen gas but is converted into chemical fuels instead. In plants, by coupling a few subsystems together, the photosynthetic apparatus of the chloroplast is able to convert sunlight into biologically useful chemical fuels such as: (1) sugars and amino acids; (2) ammonium; (3) starch; and (4) complex organic compounds.[23] When biomass is burned, the "hydrogen" stored in these chemical fuels combines with atmospheric oxygen, and energy is released. Therefore, these organic chemical fuels represent an approach to store hydrogen in the form of chemical bonds. In nature, the "hydrogen" stored are subsequently used to produce adenosine triphosphate (ATP) and nicotinamide adenine dinucleotide phosphate (NADPH) through a transmembrane proton gradient. The natural catalysts have evolved to such efficiency that after light absorption, all the following steps are exergonic and the accumulation of harmful intermediates is prevented. As such, the catalysts are conserved and are similar in most organisms.

Photosynthesis stores a considerable amount of energy in wood and fibers of trees and plants.[24] Not surprisingly, terrestrial biomass was the major energy source for our ancestors. Since the production and use of terrestrial biomass is considered carbon dioxide neutral, there has been a renewed interest in using biomass and biofuels such as biohydrogen, bioethanol, and biodiesel to replace the use of fossil fuels. Since fuel is used to power ~66% of global energy and most solar technologies can only convert sunlight to heat or electricity, biofuels would become an important player in the energy market in the near future.[25] Therefore, it is imperative to look into nature's molecular mechanisms to convert solar energy to high-energy molecular hydrogen, especially the water-splitting reaction of PSII, which is heralded as the "engine of life" since it solved biology's energy problem.[24,26] Its inception has significantly changed the chemical and biological composition of our planet. PSII is unique compared to other photosystems since it has much sophisticated redox chemistries. As such, there are already many artificial catalytic systems attempting to mimic PSII.[24,27–29] The artificial catalytic systems could also integrate other bio-inspired features to improve hydrogen production yield, such as a LH antenna with smaller size to suppress fluorescence and heat dissipation, which otherwise could lead to loss of ~80% of the collected solar energy.[30]

7.2.2 STABILITY OF PROTEINS

Absorption spectrum is often used to check the structural integrity of the RCs.[43,44] Generally, the absorbance peaks of the RC cofactors change as RCs denature and unfold.[45] RCs are stable up to 70°C in their native lipid environment; however, when isolated, they become less resistant to thermal denaturation.[45] In fact, solar cells based on photosynthetic protein are only able to last for several hours under continuous irradiation; the photocurrent is reduced by 15% after an hour[36] and 60% after 10 hours.[46] Therefore, it is imperative to improve the stability of RCs so that they are robust enough for applications (Figure 7.3). One way to increase the stability of RCs is to make the environment around RCs more compatible to the RCs. For instance, by removing oxygen to create an anaerobic environment, RCs are found to be more stable.[47] Mimicking the native environment of RCs by incorporating photosynthetic membranes is another approach to improve the stability of RCs.[48] With the photosynthetic membranes, the solar cell was found to be more resistant to stress factors, and that the RCs were stable for three days in spite of continuous illumination. Also, by coupling LH1 complex with RCs, RCs exhibited increased stability toward aerobic conditions and intense illumination.[48] What's more, surfactants as well as copolymer-lipid environment were also found to be able to maintain RCs' functionality *in vitro*.[49,50] Another way to improve the stability of RCs is by increasing the robustness of RCs toward stress factors and harsh environment. It has been found that by increasing the carotenoid content, the RCs are better protected against photodamage and hence are more stable.[48] Furthermore, in order to retain the natural function of RCs *in vitro* in photochemical devices, it is important to immobilize the RCs effectively on electrodes (Figure 7.4).[43,51]

7.2.3 NOVEL DEVICE ARCHITECTURE

New device architectures[43,52,53] are conceived to improve existing biohybrid solar cells (Figure 7.3). For example, surfactants have been found to improve the lifetime of a photosynthetic protein-based device for a few weeks; therefore, a solid-state, lipid surfactant-based device is a possible direction for the next generation of photosynthetic biohybrid devices. The electrode materials and redox mediators used should also be considered and designed carefully to ensure energy level match[53,54] for cyclic electron flow and the stability of RCs.[43,44,55] For example, graphene has been found to be a good candidate as a front electrode for the immobilization of RCs since it is transparent to sunlight and has high carrier mobility.[56] Recent biohybrid solar cells made use of Förster resonance energy transfer (FRET) to improve power conversion efficiency; these solar cells have two main properties, which are optimum distance between light-harvesting molecule and the ground-state acceptor molecule[57,58] as well as a large spectral overlap between the donor emission profile and the acceptor absorption profile.[57] Some of the biohybrid systems of this category include QD-LH[59] and QD-polypeptide[57] systems. In fact, DSSCs also made use of

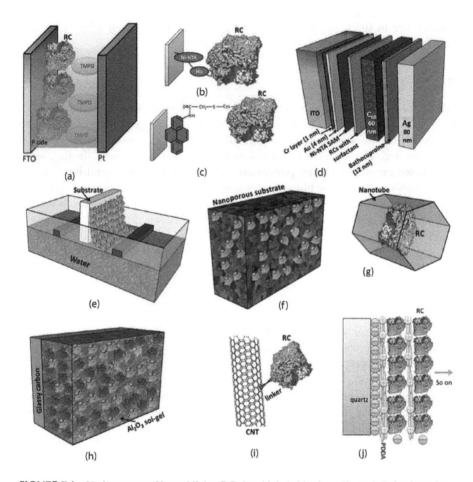

FIGURE 7.4 Various ways of immoblizing RCs in a biohybrid solar cells. (a) RCs in electrolyte. (From Tan, S.C. et al., *Angew. Chem. Int. Ed.*, 51, 6667–6671, 2012; Tan, S.C., *ACS Nano*, 6, 9103–9109, 2012.) (b) Attachment of RCs to the Ni-NTA modified electrode via genetically engineered His-tag. (From Nakamura, C. et al., Self-assembling photosynthetic reaction centers on electrodes for current generation, In *Twenty-First Symposium on Biotechnology for Fuels and Chemicals: Proceedings of the Twenty-First Symposium on Biotechnology for Fuels and Chemicals* Held May 2–6, 1999, in Fort Collins, Colorado, Humana Press, Totowa, NJ, pp. 401–408, 2000.) (c) Attachment of RCs to the electrode via chemical linkers. (From Katz, E., *J. of Electroanal. Chem.*, 365, 157–164, 1994.) (d) RCs stabilized in a solid-state device. (From Das, R. et al., *Nano Lett.*, 4, 1079–1083, 2004.) (e) Monolayers/multilayers of RCs coated on the electrode by the Langmuir–Blodgett (LB) method. (f) Immobilization of RCs on the nanostructured electrode. (From Lu, Y. et al., *Langmuir*, 21, 4071–4076, 2005.) (g) Entrapping RCs inside nanopores and nanotubes. (From Oda, I. et al., *Langmuir*, 26, 13399–13406, 2010; Oda, I. et al., *J. Phys. Chem. B*, 110, 1114–1120, 2006.) (h) Entrapping RCs in sol–gel medium. (From Zhao, J. et al., *J. Photochem. Photobiol.*, 152, 53–60, 2002.) (i) Attachment of RCs to carbon nanotubes (CNT). (From Yang, W. et al., *Nanotechnology*, 18, 412001, 2007.) (j) Immobilization of electrostatically-bound multilayers of RCs on the electrode. (From Zhao, J. et al., *Electrochimica Acta*, 47, 2013–2017, 2002; Giustini, M. et al., *Sens. Actuators B*, 163, 69–75, 2012; Ravi, S.K. and Tan, S.C., *Energy Environ. Sci.*, 8, 2551–2573, 2015. Reproduced by permission of The Royal Society of Chemistry.)

FRET to improve light absorption across wider wavelengths[60]; this is achieved by coupling energy relay dyes, which have stronger absorption at lower wavelengths, to the sensitizing dyes via FRET. In addition, plasmonic nanostructures could be combined with photosynthetic proteins to improve light absorption by plasmon-induced increase in fluorescence of LH complexes.[53,61,62] Although photosynthetic solar cells are still in their infancy, they still hold great promise as better device architectures come into the picture.[63] The next step will be more than photosynthetic proteins but toward devices consisting of entire photosynthetic organisms such as algal cells. Recent studies have found methods to extract electrons directly from intact algal cells,[64] and this will pave the way toward the use of biohybrid devices consisting of algal cells,[65] bacteria, or even living plants.[66] Although plants and algae absorb only in the visible spectrum, it has been proposed to engineer one of the photosystems to use bacteriochlorophylls found in anoxygenic photosynthetic organisms, which possess absorption maxima up to ~1100 nm.[10]

7.2.4 DISPARITIES IN REPORTING THE PERFORMANCE OF BIOHYBRID SOLAR CELLS

Some of the disparities in reporting the performance of biohybrid solar cells include the light intensity used for illumination, the active area of the solar cells, and the open-circuit voltage output (Figure 7.3).[43] Shockingly, previous studies used light intensities inconsistently so much that some are as low as 0.1 mW cm^{-2} while some are 10^5 as great in intensities. This inconsistency should be corrected instantly so that an intensity similar to that of natural sunlight is used instead; this could be done by using a xenon lamp with appropriate light filters.[67] The active area of the solar cells is also seldom reported in the literature, making accurate comparison of photocurrents difficult. Since a larger active area would lead to higher current output, it is important to find the photocurrent per area instead to avoid ambiguity. In addition, without open-circuit voltage, the overall conversion efficiency of any photovoltaic device is unable to be calculated since it depends on both photocurrent density and open-circuit voltage. Scientists tend to concentrate on enhancing the photocurrent density, ignoring the associated open-circuit voltage, which is equally important. In short, standardization of measurement should be practiced by scientists working in this field in order to have better and more meaningful research.

7.3 CONCLUSION

In the long term, we do not have many choices to meet the increasing energy demand of our growing population, which is approaching 10 billion sooner or later. Renewable energies such as wind, geothermal, and hydropower will not be sufficient to replace fossil fuels as our main energy source.[68] While nuclear fusion is enough to meet our huge energy demand, it is far from realization. We already have a nuclear reaction that has been powering our planet for billions of years, which is the sun. The sun will be our ultimate source of energy; although there are existing solar technologies to generate electricity from sunlight, they are still not on par with fossil fuels as our main source of energy. This is in part due to the diurnal nature of sunlight, different sunlight intensity during different weathers and seasons, as well as the diffuse nature of sunlight. This pushes for the development of better photovoltaic devices and alternative device architectures by exploiting emerging nanotechnologies to convert sunlight more efficiently to electricity or even fuels. Moreover, it is also important to develop novel solar cells based on new concepts that are unlike any other conventional ones. One of the directions would be to couple photosynthetic organisms to photovoltaics and to use genetic engineering and synthetic biology to overcome the inefficiencies of natural systems. Although nature's molecular machineries are relatively fragile since they consist of soft matter, subtle changes that occur in them are able to produce profound effects that boost efficiencies of biological reactions. As Charles Darwin noted: "Man can act only on external and visible characters; nature cares nothing for appearances, except in so far as they may be useful to any being. She can act on every internal organ, on every shade of constitutional difference, on the whole machinery of life."[69] Therefore, we should never underestimate the creations of Mother Nature but should instead learn from her.

REFERENCES

1. Barber, J.; Andersson, B. *Nature* **1994**, 370, (6484), 31–34.
2. Schubert, W. D.; Klukas, O.; Saenger, W.; Witt, H. T.; Fromme, P.; Krauß, N. *Journal of Molecular Biology* **1998**, 280, (2), 297–314.
3. Rhee, K.-H.; Morris, E. P.; Barber, J.; Kuhlbrandt, W. *Nature* **1998**, 396, (6708), 283–286.
4. McConnell, I.; Li, G.; Brudvig, G. W. *Chemistry & Biology* **2010**, 17, (5), 434–447.
5. Hagberg, D. P.; Yum, J. H.; Lee, H.; De Angelis, F.; Marinado, T.; Karlsson, K. M.; Humphry-Baker, R. et al. *Journal of the American Chemical Society* **2008**, 130, (19), 6259–6266.
6. Blankenship, R. E. *Molecular Mechanisms of Photosynthesis*. John Wiley & Sons: Chichester, UK, 2013.
7. Röger, C.; Müller, M. G.; Lysetska, M.; Miloslavina, Y.; Holzwarth, A. R.; Würthner, F. *Journal of the American Chemical Society* **2006**, 128, (20), 6542–6543.
8. Kiang, N. Y.; Siefert, J.; Blankenship, R. E. *Astrobiology* **2007**, 7, (1), 222–251.
9. Zinth, W.; Wachtveitl, J. *ChemPhysChem* **2005**, 6, (5), 871–880.
10. Blankenship, R. E.; Tiede, D. M.; Barber, J.; Brudvig, G. W.; Fleming, G.; Ghirardi, M.; Gunner, M. R. et al. *Science* **2011**, 332, (6031), 805–809.
11. Zhu, X.-G.; Long, S. P.; Ort, D. R. *Annual Review of Plant Biology* **2010**, 61, (1), 235–261.
12. Rappaport, F.; Diner, B. A. *Coordination Chemistry Reviews* **2008**, 252, (3–4), 259–272.
13. Grätzel, M. *Inorganic Chemistry* **2005**, 44, (20), 6841–6851.
14. Polle, J. E. W.; Kanakagiri, S.; Jin, E.; Masuda, T.; Melis, A. *International Journal of Hydrogen Energy* **2002**, 27, (11–12), 1257–1264.
15. Melis, A. *Plant Science* **2009**, 177, (4), 272–280.
16. Hagfeldt, A.; Graetzel, M. *Chemical Reviews* **1995**, 95, (1), 49–68.
17. Gersten, S. W.; Samuels, G. J.; Meyer, T. J. *Journal of the American Chemical Society* **1982**, 104, (14), 4029–4030.
18. Hull, J. F.; Balcells, D.; Blakemore, J. D.; Incarvito, C. D.; Eisenstein, O.; Brudvig, G. W.; Crabtree, R. H. *Journal of the American Chemical Society* **2009**, 131, (25), 8730–8731.
19. Gust, D.; Moore, T. A.; Moore, A. L. *Accounts of Chemical Research* **2009**, 42, (12), 1890–1898.
20. King, P. W.; Posewitz, M. C.; Ghirardi, M. L.; Seibert, M. *Journal of Bacteriology* **2006**, 188, (6), 2163–2172.

21. Hambourger, M.; Gervaldo, M.; Svedruzic, D.; King, P. W.; Gust, D.; Ghirardi, M.; Moore, A. L.; Moore, T. A. *Journal of the American Chemical Society* **2008**, 130, (6), 2015–2022.
22. Tachibana, Y.; Vayssieres, L.; Durrant, J. R. *Nature Photonics* **2012**, 6, (8), 511–518.
23. Bogorad, L. *Trends in Biotechnology* **2000**, 18, (6), 257–263.
24. Barber, J. *Chemical Society Reviews* **2009**, 38, (1), 185–196.
25. Kruse, O.; Rupprecht, J.; Mussgnug, J. H.; Dismukes, G. C.; Hankamer, B. *Photochemical & Photobiological Sciences* **2005**, 4, (12), 957–970.
26. Barber, J. *Quarterly Reviews of Biophysics* **2003**, 36, (1), 71–89.
27. Herrero, C.; Lassalle-Kaiser, B.; Leibl, W.; Rutherford, A. W.; Aukauloo, A. *Coordination Chemistry Reviews* **2008**, 252, (3–4), 456–468.
28. Magnuson, A.; Anderlund, M.; Johansson, O.; Lindblad, P.; Lomoth, R.; Polivka, T.; Ott, S. et al. *Accounts of Chemical Research* **2009**, 42, (12), 1899–1909.
29. Eisenberg, R.; Gray, H. B. *Inorganic Chemistry* **2008**, 47, (6), 1697–1699.
30. Melis, A.; Happe, T. *Photosynthesis Research* **2004**, 80, (1), 401–409.
31. Tan, S. C.; Crouch, L. I.; Jones, M. R.; Welland, M. *Angewandte Chemie International Edition* **2012**, 51, (27), 6667–6671.
32. Tan, S. C.; Crouch, L. I.; Mahajan, S.; Jones, M. R.; Welland, M. E. *ACS Nano* **2012**, 6, (10), 9103–9109.
33. Nakamura, C.; Hasegawa, M.; Yasuda, Y.; Miyake, J. Self-Assembling Photosynthetic Reaction Centers on Electrodes for Current Generation. In *Twenty-First Symposium on Biotechnology for Fuels and Chemicals: Proceedings of the Twenty-First Symposium on Biotechnology for Fuels and Chemicals Held May 2–6, 1999, in Fort Collins, Colorado,* Humana Press: Totowa, NJ, 2000; pp. 401–408.
34. Katz, E. *Journal of Electroanalytical Chemistry* **1994**, 365, (1), 157–164.
35. Das, R.; Kiley, P. J.; Segal, M.; Norville, J.; Yu, A. A.; Wang, L.; Trammell, S. A. et al. *Nano Letters* **2004**, 4, (6), 1079–1083.
36. Lu, Y.; Yuan, M.; Liu, Y.; Tu, B.; Xu, C.; Liu, B.; Zhao, D.; Kong, J. *Langmuir* **2005**, 21, (9), 4071–4076.
37. Oda, I.; Iwaki, M.; Fujita, D.; Tsutsui, Y.; Ishizaka, S.; Dewa, M.; Nango, M.; Kajino, T.; Fukushima, Y.; Itoh, S. *Langmuir* **2010**, 26, (16), 13399–13406.
38. Oda, I.; Hirata, K.; Watanabe, S.; Shibata, Y.; Kajino, T.; Fukushima, Y.; Iwai, S.; Itoh, S. *The Journal of Physical Chemistry B* **2006**, 110, (3), 1114–1120.
39. Zhao, J.; Ma, N.; Liu, B.; Zhou, Y.; Xu, C.; Kong, J. *Journal of Photochemistry and Photobiology A: Chemistry* **2002**, 152, (1–3), 53–60.
40. Yang, W.; Thordarson, P.; Gooding, J. J.; Ringer, S. P.; Braet, F. *Nanotechnology* **2007**, 18, (41), 412001.
41. Zhao, J.; Liu, B.; Zou, Y.; Xu, C.; Kong, J. *Electrochimica Acta* **2002**, 47, (12), 2013–2017.
42. Giustini, M.; Autullo, M.; Mennuni, M.; Palazzo, G.; Mallardi, A. *Sensors and Actuators B: Chemical* **2012**, 163, (1), 69–75.
43. Ravi, S. K.; Tan, S. C. *Energy & Environmental Science* **2015**, 8, (9), 2551–2573.
44. Ravi, S. K.; Swainsbury, D. J.; Singh, V. K.; Ngeow, Y. K.; Jones, M. R.; Tan, S. C. *Advanced Materials* **2018**, 30, (5), 1704073.
45. Hughes, A. V.; Rees, P.; Heathcote, P.; Jones, M. R. *Biophysical Journal* **2006**, 90, (11), 4155–4166.
46. den Hollander, M.-J.; Magis, J. G.; Fuchsenberger, P.; Aartsma, T. J.; Jones, M. R.; Frese, R. N. *Langmuir* **2011**, 27, (16), 10282–10294.
47. Yaghoubi, H.; Li, Z.; Jun, D.; Saer, R.; Slota, J. E.; Beerbom, M.; Schlaf, R.; Madden, J. D.; Beatty, J. T.; Takshi, A. *The Journal of Physical Chemistry C* **2012**, 116, (47), 24868–24877.
48. Magis, G. J.; den Hollander, M.-J.; Onderwaater, W. G.; Olsen, J. D.; Hunter, C. N.; Aartsma, T. J.; Frese, R. N. *Biochimica et Biophysica Acta (BBA) - Biomembranes* **2010**, 1798, (3), 637–645.

49. Popot, J.-L. *Annual Review of Biochemistry* **2010**, 79, (1), 737–775.
50. Swainsbury, D. J. K.; Scheidelaar, S.; van Grondelle, R.; Killian, J. A.; Jones, M. R. *Angewandte Chemie International Edition* **2014**, 53, (44), 11803–11807.
51. Badura, A.; Kothe, T.; Schuhmann, W.; Rogner, M. *Energy & Environmental Science* **2011**, 4, (9), 3263–3274.
52. Ravi, S. K.; Yu, Z.; Swainsbury, D. J.; Ouyang, J.; Jones, M. R.; Tan, S. C. *Advanced Energy Materials* **2017**, 7, (7), 1601821.
53. Ravi, S. K.; Udayagiri, V. S.; Suresh, L.; Tan, S. C. *Advanced Functional Materials* **2017**, 28, 1705305.
54. Ravi, S. K.; Sun, W.; Nandakumar, D. K.; Zhang, Y.; Tan, S. C. *Science Advances* **2018**, 4, (3), eaao6050.
55. Singh, V. K.; Ravi, S. K.; Ho, J. W.; Wong, J. K. C.; Jones, M. R.; Tan, S. C. *Advanced Functional Materials* **2017**, 28, 1703689.
56. Gunther, D.; LeBlanc, G.; Prasai, D.; Zhang, J. R.; Cliffel, D. E.; Bolotin, K. I.; Jennings, G. K. *Langmuir* **2013**, 29, (13), 4177–4180.
57. Medintz, I. L.; Mattoussi, H. *Physical Chemistry Chemical Physics* **2009**, 11, (1), 17–45.
58. van Grondelle, R.; Novoderezhkin, V. I. *Nature* **2010**, 463, (7281), 614–615.
59. Schmitt, F. J.; Maksimov, E. G.; Hätti, P.; Weißenborn, J.; Jeyasangar, V.; Razjivin, A. P.; Paschenko, V. Z.; Friedrich, T.; Renger, G. *Biochimica et Biophysica Acta (BBA) - Bioenergetics* **2012**, 1817, (8), 1461–1470.
60. Hardin, B. E.; Hoke, E. T.; Armstrong, P. B.; Yum, J.-H.; Comte, P.; Torres, T.; Frechet, J. M. J.; Nazeeruddin, M. K.; Gratzel, M.; McGehee, M. D. *Nature Photonics* **2009**, 3, (7), 406–411.
61. Czechowski, N.; Nyga, P.; Schmidt, M. K.; Brotosudarmo, T. H. P.; Scheer, H.; Piatkowski, D.; Mackowski, S. *Plasmonics* **2012**, 7, (1), 115–121.
62. Beyer, S. R.; Ullrich, S.; Kudera, S.; Gardiner, A. T.; Cogdell, R. J.; Köhler, J. *Nano Letters* **2011**, 11, (11), 4897–4901.
63. Krassen, H.; Ott, S.; Heberle, J. *Physical Chemistry Chemical Physics* **2011**, 13, (1), 47–57.
64. Ryu, W.; Bai, S.-J.; Park, J. S.; Huang, Z.; Moseley, J.; Fabian, T.; Fasching, R. J.; Grossman, A. R.; Prinz, F. B. *Nano Letters* **2010**, 10, (4), 1137–1143.
65. Gordon, J. M.; Polle, J. E. W. *Applied Microbiology and Biotechnology* **2007**, 76, (5), 969–975.
66. Strik, D. P. B. T. B.; Hamelers, H. V. M.; Snel, J. F. H.; Buisman, C. J. N. *International Journal of Energy Research* **2008**, 32, (9), 870–876.
67. Snaith, H. J. *Nature Photonics* **2012**, 6, (6), 337–340.
68. Lewis, N. S.; Nocera, D. G. *Proceedings of the National Academy of Sciences* **2006**, 103, (43), 15729–15735.
69. Darwin, C. *The Origin of Species.* Lulu. com: Morrisville, 1872.

Index

Note: Page numbers in italic and bold refer to figures and tables respectively.